Your *Clinics* subscription just got better!

You can now access the FULL TEXT of this publication online at no additional cost! Activate your online subscription today and receive...

- Full text of all issues from 2002 to the present
- Photographs, tables, illustrations, and references
- Comprehensive search capabilities
- Links to MEDLINE and Elsevier journals

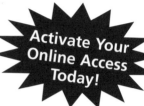

Plus, you can also sign up for E-alerts of upcoming issues or articles that interest you, and take advantage of exclusive access to bonus features!

To activate your individual online subscription:

1. Visit our website at **www.TheClinics.com**.

2. Click on "Register" at the top of the page, and follow the instructions.

3. To activate your account, you will need your subscriber account number, which you can find on your mailing label (note: the number of digits in your subscriber account number varies from six to ten digits). See the sample below where the subscriber account number has been circled.

This is your subscriber account number

```
*********************************************3-DIGIT
FEB00   J0167   C7   123456-89

J.H. DOE, MD
531 MAIN ST
CENTER CITY, NY  10001-001
```

D1593352

4. That's it! Your online access to the most trusted ... or clinical reviews is now available.

the**clinics**.com

ELSEVIER

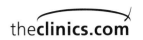

VETERINARY CLINICS

OF NORTH AMERICA

Small Animal Practice

Advances in Feline Medicine

GUEST EDITOR
James R. Richards, DVM

January 2005 • Volume 35 • Number 1

SAUNDERS

An Imprint of Elsevier, Inc.
PHILADELPHIA   LONDON   TORONTO   MONTREAL   SYDNEY   TOKYO

W.B. SAUNDERS COMPANY
A Division of Elsevier Inc.

The Curtis Center • Independence Square West • Philadelphia, Pennsylvania 19106

http://www.vetsmall.theclinics.com

THE VETERINARY CLINICS OF NORTH AMERICA: Volume 35, Number 1
SMALL ANIMAL PRACTICE   ISSN 0195-5616
January 2005   ISBN 1-4160-2843-9
Editor: John Vassallo

The ideas and opinions expressed in *The Veterinary Clinics of North America: Small Animal Practice* do not necessarily reflect those of the Publisher. The Publisher does not assume any responsibility for any injury and/or damage to persons or property arising out of or related to any use of the material contained in this periodical. The reader is advised to check the appropriate medical literature and the product information currently provided by the manufacturer of each drug to be administered to verify the dosage, the method and duration of administration, or contraindications. It is the responsibility of the treating physician or other health care professional, relying on independent experience and knowledge of the patient, to determine drug dosages and the best treatment for the patient. Mention of any product in this issue should not be construed as endorsement by the contributors, editors, or the Publisher of the product or manufacturers' claims.

The Veterinary Clinics of North America: Small Animal Practice (ISSN 0195-5616) is published bimonthly (For Post Office use only: volume 35 issue 1 of 6) by W.B. Saunders Company. Corporate and editorial offices: The Curtis Center, Independence Square West, Philadelphia, PA 19106-3399. Accounting and circulation offices: 6277 Sea Harbor Drive, Orlando, FL 32887-4800. Periodicals postage paid at Orlando, FL 32862, and additional mailing offices. Subscription prices are $170.00 per year for US individuals, $260.00 per year for US institutions, $85.00 per year for US students and residents, $215.00 per year for Canadian individuals, $325.00 per year for Canadian institutions, $225.00 per year for international individuals, $325.00 per year for international institutions and $113.00 per year for Canadian and foreign students/residents. To receive student/resident rate, orders must be accompanied by name of affiliated institution, date of term, and the *signature* of program/residency coordinator on institution letterhead. Orders will be billed at individual rate until proof of status is received. Foreign air speed delivery is included in all *Clinics* subscription prices. All prices are subject to change without notice. POSTMASTER: Send address changes to *The Veterinary Clinics of North America: Small Animal Practice*, Elsevier, Customer Service Department, 6277 Sea Harbor Drive, Orlando, FL 32887-4800, USA; phone: (+1)(877) 8397126 [toll free number for US customers], or (+1)(407) 3454020 [customers outside US]; fax: (+1)(407) 3631354; email: usjcs@elsevier.com

The Veterinary Clinics of North America: Small Animal Practice is also published in Japanese by Gakusosha Company Ltd., 2-16-28 Nishikata, Bunkyo-ku, Tokyo 113, Japan.

Reprints. For copies of 100 or more, of articles in this publication, please contact the Commercial Reprints Department, Elsevier Inc., 360 Park Avenue South, New York, New York 10010-1710. Tel. (212) 633-3813 Fax: (212) 462-1935, email: reprints@elsevier.com

The Veterinary Clinics of North America: Small Animal Practice is covered in *Current Contents/Agriculture, Biology and Environmental Sciences, Science Citation Index, ASCA, Index Medicus, Excerpta Medica, and BIOSIS.*

Printed in the United States of America.

GUEST EDITOR

JAMES R. RICHARDS, DVM, Director, Cornell Feline Health Center, Cornell University, College of Veterinary Medicine, Ithaca, New York; President, American Association of Feline Practitioners, Hillsborough, New Jersey

CONTRIBUTORS

SHARON A. CENTER, DVM, Diplomate, American College of Veterinary Internal Medicine; Professor, College of Veterinary Medicine, Cornell University, Ithaca, New York

DENNIS J. CHEW, DVM, Diplomate, American College of Veterinary Internal Medicine; Professor, Department of Clinical Sciences, The Ohio State University College of Veterinary Medicine, Columbus, Ohio

STEPHEN P. DIBARTOLA, DVM, Diplomate, American College of Veterinary Internal Medicine; Professor, Department of Clinical Sciences, The Ohio State University College of Veterinary Medicine, Columbus, Ohio

DANIÈLLE GUNN-MOORE, BVM&S, Phd, ILTM, MACVSc, MRCVS, RCVS Specialist in Feline Medicine, Nestlé Purina Senior Lecturer in Feline Medicine; Head of Feline Clinic, University of Edinburgh Hospital for Small Animals, Easter Bush Veterinary Clinics, Midlothian, Scotland

KATRIN HARTMANN, Dr med vet, Dr med vet habil, Diplomate, European College of Veterinary Internal Medicine-CA; Professor and Head, Small Animal Medicine Clinic, Ludwig-Maximilians-Universität München, Munich, Germany

ROGER A. HOSTUTLER, DVM, MS, Diplomate, American College of Veterinary Internal Medicine; Veterinary Specialty Hospital of the Carolinas, Cary, North Carolina; Clinical Instructor, Department of Clinical Sciences, The Ohio State University College of Veterinary Medicine, Columbus, Ohio

KATE F. HURLEY, DVM, MPVM, Assistant Clinical Professor of Shelter Medicine and Small Animal Population Health, Department of Medicine and Epidemiology; Shelter Medicine Program Director, Center for Companion Animal Health, University of California Davis School of Veterinary Medicine, Davis, California

A. ALAN KOCAN, PhD, Professor of Parasitology, Department of Veterinary Pathobiology, College of Veterinary Medicine, Oklahoma State University, Stillwater, Oklahoma

MICHAEL R. LAPPIN, DVM, PhD, Diplomate, American College of Veterinary Internal Medicine; Professor, Department of Clinical Sciences, College of Veterinary Medicine and Biomedical Sciences, Colorado State University, Fort Collins, Colorado

RHETT D. MARSHALL, BVSc, Centre for Companion Animal Health, School of Veterinary Science, The University of Queensland, Queensland, Australia; Creek Road Cat Clinic, Brisbane, Australia

JAMES H. MEINKOTH, DVM, PhD, Professor of Clinical Pathology, Department of Veterinary Pathobiology, College of Veterinary Medicine, Oklahoma State University, Stillwater, Oklahoma

JACQUIE S. RAND, BVSc, DVSc, Diplomate, American College of Veterinary Internal Medicine; Professor of Companion Animal Health, Centre for Companion Animal Health, School of Veterinary Science, The University of Queensland, Queensland, Australia

SHEILAH A. ROBERTSON, BVMS (Hons), PhD, MRCVS, Diplomate, American College of Veterinary Anesthesiologists; Diplomate, European College of Veterinary Anesthetists; Professor, Department of Large Animal Clinical Sciences, College of Veterinary Medicine, University of Florida, Gainesville, Florida

CONTENTS

systems remains an important goal. Management of chronic pain in cats is a challenge because of the potential problems with long-term NSAID use; however, reports of low doses given at extended intervals are encouraging. As we gain experience with less traditional analgesics, such as the tricyclic antidepressants, anticonvulsants, and N-methyl-D-aspartate antagonists, and critically evaluate complimentary therapies, our ability to provide comfort to this population of cats will improve.

recognizing the syndrome has improved case outcome by arresting this metabolic syndrome in its earliest stages. Simply ensuring adequate intake of a complete and balanced feline diet can rescue cats just developing clinical signs; however, full metabolic support as described herein provides the best chance for recovery of cats demonstrating the most severe clinicopathologic features. It remains possible that adjustments in recommended micronutrient and vitamin intake for healthy cats may pivotally change feline susceptibility to FHL over the coming years.

GOAL STATEMENT

The goal of the *Veterinary Clinics of North America: Small Animal Practice* is to keep practicing veterinarians up-to-date with current clinical practice in small animal medicine by providing timely articles reviewing the state of the art in small animal care.

ACCREDITATION

The *Veterinary Clinics of North America: Small Animal Practice* will be offering continuing education credits, to be awarded by a school of veterinary medicine, contract pending.

The aforementioned school of veterinary medicine is a designated provider of continuing veterinary education. Veterinarians participating in this learning activity may earn up to 6 credits per issue up to a maximum of 36 credits per year. Credits awarded may not apply toward license renewal in all states. It is the responsibility of each participant to verify the requirements of their state licensing board.

Credit can be earned by reading the text material, taking the examination online at *http://www.theclinics.com/home/cme*, and completing the program evaluation. Each test question must be answered correctly; you will have the opportunity to retake any questions answered incorrectly. Following successful completion of the test and the program evaluation, you may print your certificate.

TO ENROLL

To enroll in the *Veterinary Clinics of North America: Small Animal Practice* Continuing Education program, call customer service at 1-800-654-2452 or sign up online at http://www.theclinics.com/home/cme. The CME program is available to subscribers for an additional annual fee of $99.95.

FORTHCOMING ISSUES

RECENT ISSUES

VETERINARY
CLINICS
Small Animal Practice

ELSEVIER
SAUNDERS

Vet Clin Small Anim
35 (2005) xi–xii

Preface

Advances in Feline Medicine

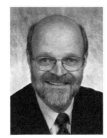

James R. Richards, DVM
Guest Editor

The *Veterinary Clinics of North America: Small Animal Practice* has a long history of presenting current and relevant information to veterinarians who are interested in cats. In fact, the second issue—Volume 1, Number 2, May 1971—was entitled "Symposium on Feline Medicine." Even the very first issue, "Physical Diagnosis in Small Animals," included an article on cats. Before that time, there were relatively few publications devoted to cats. The adage "cats are not small dogs" was popular at the time, perhaps to serve as a friendly reminder to veterinarians who too frequently were required to extrapolate what they knew about canine diseases and attempt to apply it to cats. But the *Veterinary Clinics of North America: Small Animal Practice* has done its part. By my count, 12 issues—including the one in your hand—have been devoted exclusively to cats, and articles relating to feline disorders abound, even in issues with a broader species focus.

The first task of a guest editor is to decide which topics to include. Rather than depending entirely on my own intuition, I asked e-mail–connected members of the American Association of Feline Practitioners (AAFP) to offer suggestions. Not surprisingly (I've found AAFP members to be *very* interested in cats), their response was enthusiastic. The phrase "by popular demand" perfectly characterizes this issue of the *Veterinary Clinics of North America: Small Animal Practice*, because every article was requested by practicing veterinarians.

The table of contents is interesting from a historical standpoint. With the exception of "Feline Infectious Disease Control in Shelters," each topic has

0195-5616/05/$ - see front matter © 2005 Elsevier Inc. All rights reserved.
doi:10.1016/j.cvsm.2004.10.014   *vetsmall.theclinics.com*

received coverage in previous issues. For example, feline infectious peritonitis first received attention in May 1971, then again in the August 1976, September 1984, and January 1993 issues. Articles on feline lower urinary tract disease were contained in the May 1971, August 1976, January 1993, and March and May 1996 issues. Various aspects of feline diabetes mellitus and other endocrinopathies, enteric protozoal diseases, feline zoonoses, hepatic lipidosis, and feline encephalopathies have all appeared in prior issues. At first blush, this might discourage some of us because we've still not eradicated these serious disorders. But the creativity and tenacity of veterinarians studying these conditions is being rewarded: the updates contained in this issue offer a wealth of insights into how to better understand and manage the frustrating diseases with which we've struggled for years.

I'm deeply indebted to the talented authors whose contributions enrich this issue. As with all people at the peak of their chosen field, none of them was looking for more to do, yet they believed in the merit of the project, met tight deadlines and graciously suffered through my naggings. Special thanks go to John Vassallo, editor of *The Veterinary Clinics of North America: Small Animal Practice*, for honoring me with the request to serve as guest editor, for his tireless dedication to the project, and for his sense of humor that lightened the burden. I'm especially grateful to my lovely wife, Anita, and my sons Jesse and Seth for bearing with yet another of my endless stream of projects. Lastly, I'm thankful to the Creator of heaven and earth who blesses us with good things, including cats. These fascinating little creatures have captivated me since childhood and made my life richer beyond measure.

James R. Richards, DVM
Cornell Feline Health Center
Cornell University
College of Veterinary Medicine
S3 111 Schurman Hall
Ithaca, NY 14853, USA

E-mail address: jrr1@cornell.edu

ELSEVIER
SAUNDERS

Vet Clin Small Anim
35 (2005) xiii

VETERINARY
CLINICS
Small Animal Practice

Dedication

This issue is dedicated to a lifelong devotee of cats and veterinarian of immeasurable importance to feline medicine: Jean Holzworth, DVM (Cornell, 1950) and staff member of the Angell Memorial Animal Hospital (1950–1986).

James R. Richards, DVM

ELSEVIER
SAUNDERS

Vet Clin Small Anim
35 (2005) 1–20

VETERINARY
CLINICS
Small Animal Practice

General Concepts in Zoonotic Disease Control

Michael R. Lappin, DVM, PhD

*Department of Clinical Sciences, College of Veterinary Medicine and Biomedical Sciences,
Colorado State University, Fort Collins CO 80523–1678, USA*

Zoonotic diseases are defined as being common to, shared by, or naturally transmitted between human beings and other vertebrate animals. Some agents might be transmitted to the person by direct contact with infected cats. Enteric zoonoses and those associated with bites and scratches are likely the most common feline zoonoses. Direct contact with respiratory secretions, urogenital secretions, or infected skin and exudates could also result in human infections. People could also be infected by a zoonotic agent via contaminated food or water, from shared vectors, or from the shared environment. Recommendations for cat ownership were recently made by a panel formed by the American Association of Feline Practitioners (AAFP) [1]. This article is adapted from those recommendations and a review written by the author [2]. General guidelines for cat owners and veterinarians from the AAFP are listed in Boxes 1 and 2.

Most of the agents discussed here can infect and cause disease in anyone who is exposed, but disease is sometimes more common or more severe in immunodeficient individuals. Zoonotic disease agents are generally not acquired from healthy cats; thus, the owner does not need to relinquish his or her pet in most cases. The US Centers for Disease Control and Prevention's on-line publication, *Preventing infections from pets; a guide for people with HIV infection*, states: "You do *not* have to give up your pet" (http://www.cdc.gov/hiv/pubs/brochure/oi_pets.htm). The AAFP's 2003 report on feline zoonoses states: "All human or animal care providers should provide accurate information to pet owners concerning the risks and benefits of pet ownership so that an informed decision about acquiring and keeping pets can be made" [1].

E-mail address: mlappin@colostate.edu

0195-5616/05/$ - see front matter © 2005 Elsevier Inc. All rights reserved.
doi:10.1016/j.cvsm.2004.08.005
vetsmall.theclinics.com

Box 1. Veterinarian guidelines for managing zoonotic diseases of cats

- Familiarize yourself and your staff with zoonotic issues.
- Take an active role in discussing the health risks and benefits of cat ownership with clients so that they can make logical decisions concerning cat ownership and management.
- Make it clear to your clients that you and your staff understand conditions associated with human immune deficiency, are discreet, and are willing to help.
- Provide information concerning veterinary or public health aspects of zoonoses to cat owners, but do not diagnose, treat, or make recommendations about diseases in human beings.
- Refer clinically ill cat owners to a physician for additional information and treatment.
- Veterinarians and physicians have different experiences concerning zoonoses; therefore, volunteer to speak to a cat owner's physician to clarify zoonotic issues when indicated.
- When public health–related advice is offered, document it in the medical record.
- When reportable zoonotic diseases are diagnosed, contact the appropriate public health officials.
- Vaccinate all cats for rabies.
- Routinely administer anthelmintics to kittens as early as 3, 5, 7, and 9 weeks of age to aid in controlling hookworms and roundworms.
- In *Dirofilaria immitis*–endemic areas, use monthly heartworm preventatives that control hookworms and roundworms.
- Test all cats for gastrointestinal parasites at least once yearly.
- Offer diagnostic plans to assess for presence of organisms with zoonotic potential, particularly if a cat is clinically ill.
- Consider the following minimal diagnostic plan for cats with diarrhea of a duration longer than 1 to 2 days and for all cats in homes with immunosuppressed human beings:
  — Zinc sulfate centrifugation and microscopic examination for oocysts, cysts, and eggs
  — Fecal wet mount to evaluate for trophozoites of *Giardia* and *Tritrichomonas*
  — Rectal cytology to look for white blood cells and spirochetes consistent with *Campylobacter* spp
  — *Cryptosporidium* spp screening by IFA, antigen enzyme-linked immunosorbent assay, or acid-fast stain
  — Fecal culture for *Salmonella* and *Campylobacter* spp

- Periodically (monthly in *Echinococcus multilocularis* endemic areas) administer taeniacides, particularly in cats allowed outdoors.
- Maintain flea and tick control at all times.
- Do not allow clients to restrain cats, and do not attempt to pull cats from their carriers.
- Train staff members how to avoid bites and scratches.
- Provide rabies vaccinations for all staff members who handle animals.
- Re-evaluate rabies antibody titers of staff members who handle animals every 2 years.
- Follow biosecurity measures for small animal hospitals.

From Brown RR, Elston TH, Evans L, Glaser C, Gulledge ML, Jarboe L, et al. American Association of Feline Practitioners 2003 report on feline zoonoses. Compend Contin Educ Pract Vet 2003;25:936–65; with permission.

Direct contact zoonoses

Enteric zoonoses

There are many infectious agents of the gastrointestinal tract that can be shared between cats and human beings (Table 1). Some enteric zoonotic agents like *Giardia* spp, *Cryptosporidium* spp, and the bacterial diseases are immediately infectious when passed with feces (see Table 1). Other infectious agents require time outside the host to become infectious, for example, *Toxoplasma gondii*, *Toxocara cati*, and *Ancylostoma tubaeforme*.

Prevalence rates for enteric zoonoses in cats were recently reported in two studies (Table 2) [3,4]. Most of the infectious agents were detected more frequently in cats with diarrhea than in healthy cats. These findings emphasize that diagnostic workups for enteric infections are indicated because of potential human health risks. The minimal diagnostic plan to assess for enteric zoonoses in cats with diarrhea that has been present for 1 to 2 days includes a fecal flotation, a *Cryptosporidium* spp screening procedure, a fecal wet mount, and rectal cytology [1]. Fecal culture should be considered if *Salmonella* spp or *Campylobacter* spp are on the list of differential diagnoses.

Parasitic enteric zoonoses

Visceral larva migrans and ocular larva migrans can be induced by infection of human beings with *T cati*. *A tubaeforme*, *Uncinaria stenocephala*, and *Strongyloides stercoralis* in infested cats have been associated with cutaneous larva migrans in people. Roundworm and hookworm eggs require an incubation period when passed into the environment in feces. Thus, these infectious are not direct contact zoonoses but occur from contact with the

Box 2. Cat owner guidelines for avoiding zoonotic transfer of disease

- If adopting a new cat, the cat least likely to be a zoonotic risk is a clinically normal, arthropod-free, adult animal from a private family.
- Once the cat to be adopted is identified, quarantine it from immunocompromised people until a thorough physical examination and zoonoses risk assessment are performed by a veterinarian.
- Seek immediate veterinary care for all unhealthy cats.
- Seek veterinary care at least once or twice yearly for a physical examination, fecal examination, deworming recommendations, and a vaccine needs assessment.
- Get cats vaccinated for rabies at appropriate intervals.
- Avoid handling unhealthy cats, particularly those with gastrointestinal, respiratory, skin, neurologic, or reproductive disease.
- Do not handle cats with which you are unfamiliar.
- Do not allow cats to drink from the toilet.
- Wash hands after handling cats.
- Remove fecal material from the home environment daily.
- If possible, do not have immunocompromised humans clean the litterbox. If immunocompromised humans must clean the litterbox, they should wear gloves and wash hands thoroughly when finished.
- Use litterbox liners and periodically clean the litterbox with scalding water and detergent.
- Wear gloves when gardening, and wash hands thoroughly when finished.
- Cover children's sandboxes to avoid fecal contamination by outdoor cats.
- Only feed cats cooked or commercially processed food.
- Control potential transport hosts, such as flies and cockroaches, that may bring zoonotic agents into the home.
- Filter or boil water from sources in the environment.
- Housing cats indoors may reduce their exposure to other animals that may carry zoonotic agents, to the excrement of other animals, and to fleas and ticks.
- Seek veterinary advice concerning flea and tick control.
- Do not share food utensils with cats.
- Avoid being licked on the face by cats.

- Have your cat's claws clipped frequently to reduce the risk of skin penetration; nail caps or declawing could be considered in some cases.
- Consider behavior modification for cats prone to biting or scratching.
- Do not tease cats or attempt to pull them from their carriers.
- If bitten or scratched by a cat, seek medical attention.
- Cook meat for human consumption to (176°F [80°C]) for a minimum of 15 minutes (medium-well).
- Wear gloves when handling meat, and wash hands thoroughly with soap and water when finished.

From Brown RR, Elston TH, Evans L, Glaser C, Gulledge ML, Jarboe L, et al. American Association of Feline Practitioners 2003 report on feline zoonoses. Compend Contin Educ Pract Vet 2003;25:936–65; with permission.

organisms in the contaminated environment. Diagnosis of hookworm and roundworm infections of cats is by fecal flotation. Prevention of hookworm and roundworm infection in people is achieved by control of animal excrement in human environments. All kittens should have a fecal flotation performed and should be routinely treated with an anthelmintic, such as pyrantel pamoate, at least three times (Table 3). In heavily infected kittens, deworming with pyrantel can begin at 3 weeks of age and can be repeated at 2-week intervals (http://www.cdc.gov/ncidod/dpd/parasites/ascaris/prevention.htm). The queen should be dewormed as well for any patent infections that may exist. If the kitten is presented for the first time for vaccination, anthelmintics should be administered 21 days apart at least three times. Roundworm and hookworm infections are occasionally occult; thus, all kittens should receive an anthelmintic whether or not eggs are detected on microscopic examination of feces. Feces of adult cats should be periodically

Table 1
Prevalence of enteric zoonoses in adult cats in north-central Colorado and kittens in New York

	Adult cats % (n = 206) [3]	Cats less than 1 year old % (n = 263) [4]
Ancylostoma spp	0.0	0.0
Campylobacter spp	1.0	0.8
Cryptosporidium spp	5.4	3.8
Giardia spp	2.4	7.2
Salmonella spp	1.0	0.8
Toxocara canis	0.0	0.0
Toxocara cati	3.9	32.7
Toxoplasma gondii	0.0	1.1
Any zoonotic agent	13.1	40.7

Table 2
Characteristics of common enteric zoonoses

Organism	Incubation
Bacterial	
Campylobacter spp	Immediately infectious
Eschericia coli	Immediately infectious
Helicobacter spp[a]	Immediately infectious
Salmonella spp	Immediately infectious
Yersinia enterocolitica	Immediately infectious
Parasitic-amoeba	
Entamoeba histolytica[a]	Cysts are immediately infectious
Parasitic-cestodes	
Echinococcus multilocularis	Ova are immediately infectious
Parasitic-coccidians	
Cryptosporidium spp	Oocysts are immediately infectious
Toxoplasma gondii	Oocysts are infectious after 1–5 days of incubation-exposure from environment
Parasitic-flagellates	
Giardia spp	Cysts are immediately infectious
Parasitic-helminths	
Ancylostoma tubaeforme	Larva are infectious after >3 days of incubation-skin penetration from larva in environment
Strongyloides stercoralis	Larva are immediately infectious
Toxocara cati	Larvated ova are infectious after 1–3 weeks of incubation-exposure from environment
Uncinaria stenocephala	As for *Ancylostoma*

[a] Zoonotic potential from cats undetermined.

screened for roundworms and hookworms, and anthelmintics should be administered periodically. Administration of monthly heartworm preventatives that also control or eliminate hookworms and roundworms is indicated in areas with a high prevalence.

Dipylidium caninum and *Echinococcus multilocularis* are cestodes that can infect human beings and cats. *E multilocularis* can be transmitted in feces of cats after ingestion of an infected vole. Transmission to people occurs after ingestion of the intermediate host (flea, *Dipylidium immitum*) or by the ingestion of eggs (*Echinococcus* spp). Thus, *D caninum* is a shared-vector zoonotic agent. *E multilocularis* is most common in the northern and central parts of North America but seems to be spreading with the fox population (most common definitive host). Prevention or control of cestodes is based on sanitation procedures and use of taeniacides. Praziquantel is effective for the treatment of *Echinococcus* spp and *D caninum* infection in cats (see Table 3). Cats in endemic areas for *E multilocularis* should not be allowed to hunt; if outdoors, they should be administered taeniacides up to monthly.

Cryptosporidium spp, *T gondii*, *Giardia* spp, and *Entamoeba histolytica* are the enteric protozoans of cats with zoonotic potential. Cats are only rarely infected by *E histolytica*, whereas the other protozoal infections are common.

Cryptosporidium spp are now known to cause gastrointestinal tract disease in a number of mammalian species, including rodents, dogs, cats, calves, and human beings. *Cryptosporidium* spp have an enteric life cycle similar to that of other coccidians; it culminates in the production of environmentally resistant oocysts that are passed in feces. Oocysts (4–6 μm in diameter) are passed sporulated and are immediately infectious to other hosts. It is now apparent that there are multiple strains of *Cryptosporidium* spp, including *C parvum*, *C hominis*, *C felis*, and *C canis* [5–7]. Although some isolates infect multiple species, others have a limited host range. Strains that infect pets and people cannot be differentiated from those that only infect pets by light microscopy; thus, all *Cryptosporidium* spp should be considered potentially zoonotic. The prevalence of *Cryptosporidium* spp oocysts or antigens in cat feces approximates that of *Giardia* (see Table 1), leading to the recommendation that all cats with diarrhea be assessed for this infection [1,2]. In the United States, the seroprevalence of IgG antibodies in serum is 8.6% in cats, suggesting that exposure is common [8]. Person-to-person contact with oocysts by fecal-oral contamination or by ingesting contaminated water is the most likely route of exposure. *Cryptosporidium* spp infection of people after exposure to infected calves has been recognized for years. Human infection associated with contact with infected dogs and cats has been reported but is thought to be unusual [1,2]. In one study, cat ownership was not statistically associated with cryptosporidiosis in HIV-infected people [9]. Most cats and people with *Cryptosporidium* spp infections are healthy; small bowel diarrhea is most common when disease occurs. The small size (approximately 4–6 μm in diameter) of *Cryptosporidium* spp oocysts leads to difficulty in diagnosis. Routine salt solution flotation and microscopic examination at a magnification ×100 commonly lead to false-negative results. The combination of concentration techniques with fluorescent antibody staining or acid-fast staining seems to be more sensitive. Enzyme-linked immunosorbent assays for the detection of *C parvum* antigen in feces and immunofluorescent assays for detection of *C parvum* oocysts in feces are commercially available, but it is unknown whether they consistently detect *C felis* or *C canis*. Polymerase chain reaction (PCR) is the most sensitive test to date, but assays are not routinely available and are not standardized between laboratories [10]. No drug has been shown to eliminate *Cryptosporidium* spp from the gastrointestinal tract; however, clinical signs often resolve after administration of paromomycin, tylosin, or azithromycin (see Table 3) [2]. Avoiding exposure is the most effective prevention measure. Routine disinfectants require extremely long contact with the organism to be effective. Drying, freeze-thawing, and steam-cleaning can inactivate the organism. Surface water collected in the field for drinking should be boiled or filtered.

Giardia spp infection of cats and people is common, and the organism can be detected in feces of normal cats (see Table 1). Clinical signs of disease are generally more severe in immunodeficient individuals. Because the organism is immediately infectious when passed as cysts in stool, there is potential for

Table 3
Select drugs used in managing feline zoonotic diseases

Drug	Dosage and route of administration	Organisms
Amoxicillin	10–22 mg/kg PO q12h	*Streptococcus* group A
Amoxicillin-clavulanate	15 mg/kg PO q12h	*Bartonella* spp
		Bordetella bronchiseptica
		Pasteurella multocida
Ampicillin	22 mg/kg IV q8h	*Leptospira* spp
Azithromycin	7.5–10 mg/kg PO q12–72h	*Cryptosporidium* spp?
		Bartonella spp
Clarithromycin	7.5 mg/kg PO q12–24h	*Helicobacter* spp
Clindamycin	10–12 mg/kg PO q12h	*Toxoplasma gondii*
Doxycycline	5–10 mg/kg PO q12–24h	*B bronchiseptica*
		Bartonella spp
		Chlamydophila felis
		Ehrlichia spp
		Mycoplasma felis
Enrofloxacin	5 mg/kg/d PO	*Bartonella* spp
		Campylobacter spp
		M felis
		Yersinia pestis
	5 mg/kg/d SC or IV	*Salmonella* spp bacteremia
Erythromycin	10 mg/kg PO q8h	*Bartonella* spp
		Campylobacter spp
Fenbendazole	50 mg/kg/d PO	*Ancylostoma* spp
		Giardia
		Strongyloides stercoralis
		Toxocara cati
Fipronil	7.5–15 mg/kg topical 0.25% spray and 10% spot-on	Ticks, fleas
Fipronil/methoprene	7.5–15 mg/kg topical spot-on	Ticks, fleas
Fluconazole	50 mg PO q12–24h	Dermatophytes
		Sporothrix schenkii
Griseofulvin (microsize)	25 mg/kg PO q12hr	Dermatophytes
Griseofulvin (ultramicrosize)	5–10 mg/kg/d PO	Dermatophytes
Imidacloprid	10–20 mg/kg topical spot-on	Fleas
Itraconazole	5 mg/kg PO q12hr for 4 days and then 5 mg/kg/d PO	Dermatophytes
		S schenkii
Ivermectin	24 μg/kg/mo PO	*Dirofilaria immitis*
		Hookworms
	200–300 μg/kg/wk PO	*Cheyletiella*
		Sarcoptes scabiei
Lufenuron	80–100 mg/kg PO every 2 wk	Dermatophytes
	30 mg/kg PO every 30 days	Fleas
	10 mg/kg SC every 180 days	Fleas
Lime-sulfur	Dip every 5–7 days	Dermatophytes
Metronidazole	25 mg/kg PO q12h	*Entamoeba histolytica*
		Giardia

Table 3 (*continued*)

Drug	Dosage and route of administration	Organisms
Miconazole and 2% chlorhexidine	Dip every 3–4 days	Dermatophytes
Milbemycin	0.5–0.99 mg/kg/mo PO	*D immitis* Hookworms Roundworms
Paromomycin	150 mg/kg PO q12h for 5 days	*Cryptosporidium* spp
Praziquantel	5 mg/kg PO, SC, or IM once	*Dipylidium caninum* *Echinococcus multilocularis*
Pyrantel	20 mg/kg PO once, repeat in 3 weeks	*Ancylostoma* spp *S stercoralis* *T cati*
Pyrantel plus praziquantel	72.6 mg pyrantel and 18.2 mg praziquantel, 1 table per cat PO	Hookworms, roundworms, and cestodes
Selamectin	6 mg/kg/mo topically	Hookworms, roundworms, and fleas
Terbinafine	20 mg/kg PO q24–48h	Dermatophytes
Tylosin	10–15 mg/kg PO q12h	*Cryptosporidium* spp

Abbreviations: IM, intramuscular; IV, intravenous; PO, per os; q, every; SC, subcutaneous.

From Brown RR, Elston TH, Evans L, Glaser C, Gulledge ML, Jarboe L, et al. American Association of Feline Practitioners 2003 report on feline zoonoses. Compend Contin Educ Pract Vet 2003;25:936–55; with permission.

direct zoonotic transfer. Although it is known that some *Giardia* spp can infect human beings and cats, not all isolates cross-infect. In one study, cats were relatively resistant to infection by a *Giardia* species isolated from human beings [11]. Based on genetic studies, it is now known that there are multiple *Giardia* spp [12,13]. Assemblage A has been found in infected people and many other mammals, including cats. Assemblage F seems to be a cat-specific genotype of *Giardia* [13]. Because it is impossible to determine zoonotic strains of *Giardia* spp by microscopic examination, it seems prudent to assume that feces from all cats infected with *Giardia* spp are a potential human health risk. Fecal examination should be performed on all cats at least yearly, and treatment with drugs with anti-*Giardia* activity like fenbendazole or metronidazole should be administered if indicated [1,2]. Zinc sulfate centrifugation is considered the optimal fecal flotation technique by most parasitologists to demonstrate cysts. If fresh stool is available from cats with diarrhea, examination of a wet mount to detect the motile trophozoites is also indicated. Monoclonal antibody–based immunofluorescent antibody tests and fecal antigen tests are available but have not been fully validated for detection of cat strains. Thus, these techniques should be used in addition to and not in lieu of fecal flotation, which can also reveal other parasites. Metronidazole and fenbendazole as well as a product that contains febantel, praziquantel, and pyrantel have had varying results in the treatment of feline giardiasis (see Table 3) [14–16]. *Giardia* vaccines for subcutaneous adminis-tration are now available for dogs and cats. The feline *Giardia* vaccine is considered optional by the AAFP [17]. Vaccination against *Giardia* could be considered in cats with recurrent infection and has been evaluated as a therapeutic agent in dogs and cats, with variable results [18,19]. It is unknown whether treated cats are cured, and it is likely that if a treated cat is exposed again, it will be reinfected. Cats with normal stools are unlikely a *Giardia* risk for people, because small numbers of cysts are generally shed. Prevention of zoonotic giardiasis includes boiling or filtering surface water for drinking and washing hands that have handled material contaminated by feces, even if gloves were worn.

   T gondii is a ubiquitous coccidian with worldwide distribution [20]. Most seroprevalence studies performed in the United States suggest that at least 30% of cats and people have previously been exposed. Cats are the only known definitive host of the organism and complete the enteroepithelial cycle (sexual phase) that results in the passage of environmentally resistant unsporulated oocysts in feces. Oocyst sporulation occurs in 1 to 5 days in the presence of oxygen; sporulated oocysts are infectious to most warm-blooded vertebrates. After infection by *T gondii*, an extraintestinal phase develops, which ultimately leads to the formation of tissue cysts containing the organism. Infection by *T gondii* occurs after ingesting sporulated oocysts, after ingesting tissue cysts, or transplacentally. Transplacental infection of human beings and cats usually only occurs if the mother is infected for the first time during gestation.

   Infected immunocompetent people are generally asymptomatic; self-limiting fever, lymphadenopathy, and malaise occur occasionally. Trans-placental infection of human beings results in clinical manifestations that include stillbirth, hydrocephalus, hepatosplenomegaly, and retinochoroiditis. Chronic tissue infection in people can be reactivated by immunosuppression, leading to dissemination and severe clinical illness; this has commonly been associated with drug-induced immunosuppression as well as with acquired immunodeficiency syndrome (AIDS). Approximately 10% of human beings with AIDS develop toxoplasmic encephalitis. Oocysts are most effectively demonstrated in cat feces after sugar solution centrifugation. Clinical toxoplasmosis is difficult to diagnose in people and cats but usually involves the combination of clinical signs, serologic test results, organism demonstra-tion techniques, and response to anti-*Toxoplasma* drugs [21]. *T gondii* is rec-ognized as one of the most common zoonoses; however, people are usually not infected by direct contact with cats. The oocyst shedding period usually lasts several days to several weeks (approximately 7–10 days if the cat was infected by tissue cyst ingestion). Because oocysts have to sporulate to be infectious, contact with fresh feces cannot cause infection. Cats are fastidious and usually do not allow feces to remain on their skin long enough to lead to oocyst sporulation; oocysts were not isolated from the fur of cats 7 days after completing the oocyst shedding period [20]. There was no association between cat ownership and *T gondii* seroprevalence in a group of human immunodeficiency virus (HIV)–infected human beings [22]. Veterinary health care providers do not have an increased incidence of toxoplasmosis when compared with the general population. Thus, removing cats from households with immunodeficient or pregnant persons does not necessarily decrease the risk of acquiring toxoplasmosis. Because *T gondii* infection is not acquired from direct contact with cats, serologic screening of healthy cats is not indicated (Centers for Disease Control and Prevention, 1999) [1,2]. There is no reason to treat healthy seropositive cats. *T gondii* infection can be avoided by preventing the ingestion of sporulated oocysts in old feline feces and the ingestion of tissue cysts in undercooked meats (Box 3).

Bacterial enteric zoonoses

Salmonella spp, *Campylobacter* spp, *Escherichia coli*, *Yersinia enterocolitica*, and *Helicobacter* spp each infect cats and can cause disease in human beings. Although *Helicobacter pylori* was isolated from a colony of cats, infection of people from contact with cats seems unlikely [23]. In two recent enteric zoonoses prevalence studies, *Salmonella* spp and *Campylobacter* spp infections were uncommon in pet cats (see Table 1). Prevalence of *Salmonella* and *Campylobacter* infections is greater in young animals housed

---

Box 3. Prevention of human toxoplasmosis

Prevention of oocyst ingestion
  Avoid feeding cats undercooked meats
  Do not allow cats to hunt
  Clean the litterbox daily and incinerate or flush the feces
  Clean the litterbox periodically with scalding water or use
    a litterbox liner
  Wear gloves when working with soil
  Wash hands thoroughly with soap and hot water after
    gardening
  Wash fresh vegetables well before ingestion
  Keep children's sandboxes covered
  Boil water for drinking that has been obtained from the general
    environment
  Control potential transport hosts
  Treat oocyst shedding cats with anti-*Toxoplasma* drugs
Prevention of tissue cyst ingestion
  Cook all meat products to medium well (80°C for 15 minutes)
  Wear gloves when handling meats
  Wash hands thoroughly with soap and hot water after handling
    meats
  Freeze all meat for a minimum of 3 days before cooking

in unsanitary or crowded environments. Gastroenteritis can occur in cats after infection by *Salmonella* spp, *Campylobacter* spp, or *E coli*; *Y enterocolitica* is probably a commensal agent in cats but causes fever, abdominal pain, polyarthritis, and bacteremia in human beings. Approximately 50% of cats with clinical salmonellosis have gastroenteritis; most are presented with signs of bacteremia. Salmonellosis of cats and people has been associated with songbirds (songbird fever). Diagnosis of *Salmonella* spp, *Campylobacter jejuni*, *E coli*, and *Y enterocolitica* is based on culture of feces. A single negative culture may not rule out infection. Rectal cytology should be performed on all cats with diarrhea [1,2]. If neutrophils are noted, culture for enteric bacteria should be considered, particularly if the animal is owned by an immunodeficient individual. Antibiotic therapy can control clinical signs of disease from infection by *Salmonella* spp or *Campylobacter* spp but should not be administered orally to cats that are subclinical carriers of *Salmonella* because of the risk of antibiotic resistance (see Table 3). Strains of *Salmonella* that were resistant to most antibiotics have been detected in several cats [24]. Prevention of enteric bacterial zoonoses is based on sanitation and control of exposure to feces. Immunodeficient human beings should avoid young animals and animals from crowded or unsanitary housing, particularly if clinical signs of gastrointestinal tract disease are occurring.

Bite, scratch, or exudate exposure zoonoses

Bacteria

Approximately 300,000 emergency room visits per year are made by people bitten by animals in the United States [24,25]. Most of the aerobic and anaerobic bacteria associated with bite or scratch wounds only cause local infection in immunocompetent individuals. Nevertheless, 28% to 80% of cat bites become infected, and severe sequelae, including meningitis, endocarditis, septic arthritis, osteoarthritis, and septic shock, can occur. Most of the aerobic and anaerobic bacteria associated with cat bite or scratch wounds lead only to local infection in immunocompetent individuals. Immunodeficient persons or persons exposed to *Pasteurella* spp, *Capnocytophaga canimorsus* (DF-2), or *Capnocytophaga cynodegmi* more consistently develop systemic clinical illness. Splenectomized human beings are at increased risk of developing bacteremia.

Cats are subclinical carriers of multiple bacteria in the oral cavity, including *Mycoplasma* spp and *C canimorsus* [26]. After a person is bitten or scratched, local cellulitis is noted initially, followed by evidence of deeper tissue infection. Bacteremia and the associated clinical signs of fever, malaise, and weakness are common, and death can occur in hours after infection with *Capnocytophaga* spp in immunodeficient people. Treatment of bite or scratch wounds in clinically affected human beings includes local wound management and parenteral antibiotic therapy when indicated. Penicillin derivatives are effective against most *Pasteurella* infections; penicillins and cephalosporins are effective against *Capnocytophaga* spp in vitro.

Bartonella henselae is the most common cause of cat scratch disease as well as bacillary angiomatosis and bacillary peliosis, which are common disorders in human beings with AIDS. Cats can also be infected with *B clarridgeiae*, *B koehlerae*, and *B weissii* [27–29]. *B henselae* has been isolated from the blood of subclinically ill seropositive cats and also from some cats with a variety of clinical manifestations like fever, lethargy, lymphadenopathy, uveitis, gingivitis, and neurologic diseases. Seroprevalence in cats varies by region but is commonly greater than 50% in some geographic areas of the United States [30–32]. The organism is transmitted between cats by fleas; thus, prevalence is greatest in cats from states where fleas are common [30–32]. Many people with cat scratch disease have recent exposure to kittens. *B henselae* survives for days in flea feces, which may be involved in the transmission of the organism to people [33,34]. Blood culture, blood PCR, and serologic testing can be used to determine the infection status of individual cats. Cats that are culture-negative or PCR-negative and antibody-negative and cats that are culture-negative or PCR-negative and antibody-positive are probably not actively bacteremic. Bacteremia can be intermittent, however, and false-negative culture or PCR results may occur. With PCR, false-positive results can occur and positive results do not necessarily indicate that the organism is alive. Although serologic testing can be used to determine whether an individual cat has been exposed, seropositive and seronegative cats can be bacteremic, limiting the diagnostic utility of serologic testing. Thus, testing healthy cats for *Bartonella* spp infection is not currently recommended [1,2]. Testing should be reserved for cats with suspected clinical bartonellosis. Because *B henselae* is associated with fleas, strict flea control should be maintained in all cats. Kittens of unknown health status should be avoided by immunodeficient people. Cat claws should be kept clipped, and cats should never be teased. Cat-induced wounds should immediately be cleansed and medical advice sought. Administration of doxycycline, tetracycline, erythromycin, amoxicillin-clavulanate, azithromycin, or enrofloxacin can limit bacteremia but does not cure infection in all cats and has not been shown to lessen the risk of cat scratch disease (see Table 3) [1,2,35]. Thus, antibacterial treatment of healthy bacteremic cats is controversial. Treatment should be reserved for cats with suspected clinical bartonellosis (see Table 3) [1,2].

Feline plague is caused by *Yersinia pestis*, a gram-negative coccobacillus found most commonly in the midwestern and far western states, particularly New Mexico and Colorado [36,37]. Rodents are the natural hosts for this bacterium; cats are most commonly infected by ingesting bacteremic rodents or lagomorphs or by being bitten by *Yersinia*-infected rodent fleas. Human beings are most commonly infected by rodent flea bites, but there have been many documented cases of transmission by exposure to wild animals and infected domestic cats. From 1977 to 1998, 23 cases of human plague (7.7% of the total cases) resulted from contact with infected cats [38]. Infection can be induced by inhalation of respiratory secretions of cats with pneumonic plague, bite wounds, or contaminating mucous membranes or abraded skin with secretions or exudates. Bubonic, septicemic, and pneumonic plague can develop in cats and human beings; each form has accompanying fever, headache, weakness, and malaise. Because cats are most commonly infected by ingestion of bacteremic rodents, suppurative lymphadenitis (buboes) of the cervical and submandibular lymph nodes is the most common clinical manifestation. Exudates from cats with lymphadenopathy should be examined cytologically for the presence of large numbers of the characteristic bipolar rods. The diagnosis is confirmed by fluorescent antibody staining of exudates; culture of exudates, tonsillar area, and saliva; and documentation of increasing antibody titers. People who are exposed to infected cats should be urgently referred to physicians for antimicrobial therapy, and public health officials should be alerted. Doxycycline, enrofloxacin, chloramphenicol, and aminoglycosides can be used successfully for the treatment of plague (see Table 3). Parenteral antibiotics should be used during the bacteremic phase. Drainage of lymph nodes may be required. Cats with suppurative lymphadenitis should be considered plague suspects, and extreme caution should be exercised when handling exudates or treating draining wounds. Suspect animals should be treated for fleas and housed in isolation. Cats are not infectious to human beings after 4 days of antibacterial treatment.

Francisella tularensis is the gram-negative bacillus found throughout the continental United States that causes tularemia. *Dermacentor variabilis* (American dog tick), *Dermacentor andersoni* (American wood tick), and *Amblyomma americanum* (Lone Star tick) are known vectors. Human tularemia occurs most commonly after exposure to ticks and, less commonly, from contact with infected animals. There have been at least 51 cases of human tularemia resulting from contact with infected cats [39]. Dogs are not considered a source of human tularemia but may facilitate human exposure by bringing infected ticks into the environment. Cats are infected most frequently by tick bites or by ingesting infected rabbits or rodents and generally present with clinical signs consistent with bacteremia. Unlike plague, the organism is not often recognized in exudates or lymph node aspirates from infected cats. Cultures and documentation of increasing antibody titers can be used to confirm the diagnosis in cats and people. Most cases of tularemia in cats have been diagnosed at necropsy; thus, the optimal treatment is unknown. Streptomycin and gentamicin are the drugs used most commonly to treat human beings. Tetracycline and chloramphenicol administered orally can be used in cases not requiring hospitalization but may be associated with relapses. The disease is prevented by avoiding exposure to lagomorphs, ticks, and infected cats. All cats dying with bacteremia should be handled carefully.

Fungi

Of the many fungal agents that infect human beings and animals, only *Sporothrix schenckii* and the dermatophytes have been shown to infect people on direct exposure [40,41]. The reader is referred to recent review articles for management of dermatophytes in cats [1,41]. *Sporothrix* is cosmopolitan in distribution, and soil is thought to be the natural reservoir. Infection of cats and people usually occurs after the organism contaminates broken skin. Cats are thought to be infected by scratches from contaminated claws of other cats; infection is most common in outdoor male cats. People can be infected by contaminating cutaneous wounds with exudates from infected cats [40]. Cats commonly produce large numbers of the organism in feces, tissues, and exudates; thus, veterinary care personnel are at high risk when treating infected cats. The organism can be demonstrated by cytologic examination of exudates or culture. Fluconazole, itraconazole, or ketoconazole is an effective treatment (see Table 3). Gloves should be worn when handling cats with draining tracts, and hands should be cleansed thoroughly.

Viral zoonoses

Rabies is still the only significant small animal viral zoonosis in the United States. Since 1980, more cases of rabies have been reported in cats than in dogs in the United States. In 2001, 270 cases of feline rabies were reported versus 89 cases of canine rabies [42]. Rabies is a major, potentially lethal, occupational health hazard for those commonly working with animals with unknown vaccination status, including veterinary staff as well as humane shelter and rescue group employees. Pre-exposure vaccination should be offered to veterinarians and others who work with dogs and cats in areas that are enzootic for rabies [43]. In a recent survey, however, 85.1% of veterinary medical association members and managers of animal shelters or wildlife rehabilitation centers had been vaccinated versus only 17.5% of staff members [44]. The reader is referred to recently published reviews for further discussion of clinical rabies and vaccination recommendations [1,45].

To date, human beings have not been shown to be infected by feline leukemia virus (FeLV), FIV, or feline foamy virus (FeFV). In the most recent study, 204 veterinarians and others potentially exposed to feline retroviruses were assessed for antibodies against FIV and FeFV, FeLV p27 antigen, and FeLV provirus; all were negative [46]. Because FeLV and FIV can induce immunodeficiency, infected cats should be considered more likely than retrovirus-naive cats to be carrying other potential zoonotic agents, particularly if gastrointestinal tract signs are occurring.

Respiratory zoonoses

Bordetella bronchiseptica, *Chlamydophila felis* (formerly *Chlamydia psittaci*), *Y pestis* (see section on bites and scratches), and *Fransicella tularensis* (section on bites and scratches) are the most important respiratory zoonoses of cats [47–49]. Human beings rarely develop clinical disease caused by *B bronchiseptica* unless they are immune compromised. Only 39 cases of

B bronchiseptica infection in people had been reported by 1998; most infected individuals were immunodeficient [47]. In Japan, the prevalence rates of antibodies against an isolate of *C felis* were 51.1% in stray cats, 15.0% in pet cats, 3.1% in the general human population, and 5.0% in small animal clinic veterinarians, suggesting that transfer between cats and people may occur [49]. Illness is rare, however, and is usually just a mild conjunctivitis. Cats with upper or lower respiratory tract inflammatory disease should be kept away from immunodeficient people until clinically normal. Treated cats can still shed *B bronchiseptica* and *C felis* for varying times, however. Care should be taken to avoid direct conjunctival contact with discharges from the respiratory or ocular secretions of cats. Employees should be directed to wear gloves or wash their hands carefully when handling cats with conjunctivitis.

Human beings are the principal natural hosts for *Streptococcus* group A bacteria, *Streptococcus pyogenes* and *Streptococcus pneumoniae*, which cause "strep throat" in people. Cats in close contact with infected people can develop transient subclinical colonization of pharyngeal tissues and can transmit the infection to other people [50]. This is poorly documented, however, and thought to be unusual. The organism can be cultured from the tonsillar crypts. Culture-positive cats should be treated with penicillin derivatives. If cats are to be treated in a household with chronic recurrent strep throat, all people should also be treated because they also could be chronic subclinical carriers.

Genital zoonosis

Coxiella burnetii is a rickettsial agent found throughout the world, including North America. Many ticks, including *Rhipicephalus sanguineus*, are naturally infected with *C burnetii*. Cattle, sheep, and goats are commonly subclinically infected and pass the organism into the environment in urine, feces, milk, and parturient discharges. Infection of cats most commonly occurs after tick exposure, ingestion of contaminated carcasses, or aerosolization from a contaminated environment [1,2]. Fever, anorexia, and lethargy develop in some experimentally infected cats. Infection has been associated with abortion in cats, but the organism can also be isolated from normal parturient cats. Infection of cats seems to be common; 20% of cats from a humane society in southern California and in maritime Canada were seropositive, and the organism was grown from the vagina of healthy cats in Japan [51]. Human illness (Q fever) associated with direct contact with infected cats occurs after aerosol exposure to the organism passed by parturient or aborting cats; clinical signs develop 4 to 30 days later [52,53]. Human beings commonly develop acute clinical signs similar to those associated with other rickettsial diseases, including fever, malaise, headache, pneumonitis, myalgia, and arthralgia. After primary infection, chronic Q fever develops in approximately 1% and can manifest as hepatic inflammation or valvular endocarditis. Gloves and masks should be worn when handling parturient or aborting cats. People who develop fever or respiratory tract disease after exposure to parturient or aborting cats should seek medical attention.

Shared vector zoonoses

Some zoonotic agents are transmitted between animals and human beings by shared vectors like fleas, ticks, or mosquitoes. *Rickettsia felis* (fleas), *B henselae* (fleas), *D caninum* (fleas), *Ehrlichia* spp (ticks), *Anaplasma phagocytophilum* (ticks), *D immitis* (mosquitoes), and West Nile virus (mosquitoes) are examples of vector-borne zoonoses. In some instances, the cat brings the vector of the organism into the environment, resulting in exposure of the human being. There could be a slight increased risk of exposure to veterinary health care providers because they handle cats infested with fleas and ticks. Nevertheless, it is the vector rather than direct contact with the infected animal that results in infection of the human being. Flea and tick control should always be maintained as indicated, and infested cats that are seen in the clinic should be treated immediately.

Shared environment zoonoses

Some zoonotic agents, including *Histoplasma capsulatum*, *Coccidioides immitis*, *Blastomyces dermatitidis*, *Cryptococcus neoformans*, and *Aspergillus* spp, do not usually infect human beings from direct contact with an infected cat but are acquired from the same environmental source.

Summary

It is unlikely that human beings acquire a zoonotic infection from healthy cats without ectoparasites [1,2]. The benefits of cat ownership to human mental health are well established [1,54–57]. Veterinarians and physicians should work together closely to provide accurate information to cat owners so that logical decisions concerning cat ownership can be made by the owner [1,58].

References

[1] Brown RR, Elston TH, Evans L, Glaser C, Gulledge ML, Jarboe L, et al. American Association of Feline Practitioners 2003 report on feline zoonoses. Compend Contin Educ Pract Vet 2003;25:936–65.
[2] Lappin MR. Zoonoses. In: Nelson RW, Couto CG, editors. Small animal internal medicine. 3rd edition. Philadelphia: Elsevier; 2003. p. 1229–321.
[3] Hill S, Lappin MR, Cheney J, et al. Prevalence of enteric zoonotic agents in cats. J Am Vet Med Assoc 2000;216:687–92.

[4] Spain CV, Scarlett JM, Wade SE, McDonough P. Prevalence of enteric zoonotic agents in cats less than 1 year old in central New York State. J Vet Intern Med 2001;15:33–8.

[5] Morgan UM, Constantine CC, Forbes DA, et al. Differentiation between human and animal isolates of *Cryptosporidium parvum* using rDNA sequencing and direct PCR analysis. J Parasitol 1997;83:825–30.

[6] Morgan U, Weber R, Xiao L, et al. Molecular characterization of *Cryptosporidium* isolates obtained from human immunodeficiency virus-infected individuals living in Switzerland, Kenya, and the United States. J Clin Microbiol 2000;38:1180–3.

[7] Morgan U, Xiao L, Sulaiman I, et al. Which genotypes/species of *Cryptosporidium* are humans susceptible to? J Eukaryot Microbiol 1999;46(Suppl):42–3.

[8] McReynolds C, Lappin MR, McReynolds L, et al. Regional seroprevalence of *Cryptosporidium parvum* IgG specific antibodies of cats in the United States. Vet Parasitol 1998;80:187–95.

[9] Glaser CA, Angulo FJ, Rooney JA. Animal associated opportunistic infections among persons infected with the human immunodeficiency virus. Clin Infect Dis 1994;18: 14–24.

[10] Scorza AV, Brewer MM, Lappin MR. Polymerase chain reaction for the detection of *Cryptosporidium* spp. in cat feces. J Parasitol 2003;89:423–6.

[11] Kirkpatrick CE, Green GA. Susceptibility of domestic cats to infections with *Giardia lamblia* cysts and trophozoites from human sources. J Clin Microbiol 1985;21:678–80.

[12] Thompson RCA, Hopkins RM, Homan WL. Nomenclature and genetic groupings of *Giardia* infecting mammals. Parasitol Today 2000;16:210–3.

[13] Monis PT, Andrews RH, Mayrhofer G, et al. Genetic diversity within the morphological species *Giardia intestinalis* and its relationship to host origin. Infect Genet Evol 2003;3:29–38.

[14] Keith CL, Radecki SV, Lappin MR. Evaluation of fenbendazole for treatment of *Giardia* infection in cats concurrently infected with *Cryptosporidium parvum*. Am J Vet Res 2003; 64:1027–9.

[15] Scorza V, Lappin MR. Metronidazole for treatment of giardiasis in cats. J Feline Med Surg 2004;6:157–60.

[16] Scorza V, Radecki SV, Lappin MR. Efficacy of febantel, praziquantel, and pyrantel for the treatment of giardiasis in cats. Presented at the American College of Veterinary Internal Medicine Forum, June, 2004.

[17] Richards J, Rodan I, Elston T, et al. Feline vaccine selection and administration. Compend Contin Educ Pract Vet 2001;23:71–80.

[18] Olson ME, Hannigan C, Gaviller R, et al. The use of a *Giardia* vaccine as an immunotherapeutic agent in dogs. Can Vet J 2001;42:865–8.

[19] Stein JE, Radecki SV, Lappin MR. Efficacy of *Giardia* vaccination for treatment of giardiasis in cats. J Am Vet Med Assoc 2003;222:1548–51.

[20] Dubey JP, Lappin MR. Toxoplasmosis and neosporosis. In: Greene CE, editor. Infectious diseases of the dog and cat. 2nd edition. Philadelphia: WB Saunders; 1998. p. 493–503.

[21] Lappin MR. Feline toxoplasmosis: interpretation of diagnostic test results. Semin Vet Med Surg 1996;11:154–60.

[22] Wallace MR, Rossetti RJ, Olson PE. Cats and toxoplasmosis risk in HIV-infected adults. JAMA 1993;269:76–7.

[23] Simpson K, Neiger R, DeNovo R, et al. The relationship of *Helicobacter* spp. infection to gastric disease in dogs and cats. J Vet Intern Med 2000;14:223–7.

[24] Wall PG, Threlfall EJ, Ward LR, et al. Multiresistant *Salmonella typhimurium* DT104 in cats: a public health risk. Lancet 1996;348:471–2.

[25] Talan DA, Citron DM, Abrahamian FM, et al. Bacteriologic analysis of infected dog and cat bites. N Engl J Med 1999;340:84–92.

[26] Valtonen M, Lauhio A, Carlson P, et al. *Capnocytophaga canimorsus* septicemia: fifth report of a cat-associated infection and five other cases. Eur J Clin Microbiol Infect Dis 1995; 14:520–3.

[27] Regnery RL, Anderson BE, Clarridge JE III, et al. Characterization of a novel *Rochalimaea* species, *R. henselae* sp. nov., isolated from blood of a febrile, human immunodeficiency virus-positive patient. J Clin Microbiol 1992;30:265–74.

[28] Breitschwerdt EB, Kordick DL. *Bartonella* infection in animals: carriership, reservoir potential, pathogenicity, and zoonotic potential for human infection. Clin Microbiol Rev 2000;13:428–38.

[29] Pretorius AM, Kelly PJ. An update on human bartonelloses. Cent Afr J Med 2000;46: 194–200.

[30] Jameson PH, Greene CE, Regnery RL, et al. Prevalence of *Bartonella henselae* antibodies in pet cats throughout regions of North America. J Infect Dis 1995;172:1145–9.

[31] Chomel BB, Kasten RW, Floyd-Hawkins K, et al. Experimental transmission of *Bartonella henselae* by the cat flea. J Clin Microbiol 1996;34:1952–6.

[32] Foley JE, Chomel B, Kikuchi Y, et al. Seroprevalence of *Bartonella henselae* in cattery cats: association with cattery hygiene and flea infestation. Vet Q 1998;20:1–5.

[33] Finkelstein JL, Brown TP, O'Reilly KL, et al. Studies on the growth of *Bartonella henselae* in the cat flea (*Siphonaptera: Pulicidae*). J Med Entomol 2002;39:915–9.

[34] Higgins JA, Radulovic S, Jaworsk DC, et al. Acquisition of the cat scratch disease agent *Bartonella henselae* by cat fleas (*Siphonaptera:Pulicidae*). J Med Entomol 1996;33:490–5.

[35] Kordick DL, Papich MG, Breitschwerdt EB. Efficacy of enrofloxacin or doxycycline for treatment of *Bartonella henselae* or *Bartonella clarridgeiae* infection in cats. Antimicrob Agents Chemo 1997;41:2448–55.

[36] Eidson M, Thilsted JP, Rollag OJ. Clinical, clinicopathologic and pathologic features of plague in cats: 119 cases (1977–1988). J Am Vet Med Assoc 1991;199:1191–7.

[37] Macy DW. Plague. In: Greene CE, editor. Infectious diseases of the dog and cat. 2nd edition. Philadelphia: WB Saunders; 1998. p. 295–300.

[38] Gage KL, Dennis DT, Orloski KA, et al. Cases of cat-associated human plague in the Western US, 1977–1998. Clin Infect Dis 2000;30:893–900.

[39] Capellan J, Fong IW. Tularemia from a cat bite: case report and review of feline-associated tularemia. Clin Infect Dis 1993;16:472–5.

[40] Dunston RW, Langham RF, Reimann DA, et al. Feline sporotrichosis: a report of five cases with transmission to humans. J Am Acad Dermatol 1986;15:37.

[41] Morriello KA, DeBoer DJ. Feline dermatophytosis: recent advances and recommendations for therapy. Vet Clin N Am Small Animal Pract 1995;25:901–21.

[42] Krebs JW, Noll HR, Rupprecht CE. Rabies surveillance in the United States during 2001. J Am Vet Med Assoc 2002;221:1690–701.

[43] Centers for Disease Control Prevention (CDC). Human rabies prevention—United States, 1999. Recommendations of the Advisory Committee on Immunization Practices (ACIP). MMWR Morb Mortal Wkly Rep 1999;48(RR-1):1–21.

[44] Trevejo RT. Rabies preexposure vaccination among veterinarians and at-risk staff. J Am Vet Med Assoc 2000;217:1647–50.

[45] Jenkins SR, Auslander M, Conti L, et al. Compendium of animal rabies prevention and control. J Am Vet Med Assoc 2003;222:156–61.

[46] Butera ST, Brown J, Callahan ME, et al. Survey of veterinary conference attendees for evidence of zoonotic infection by feline retroviruses. J Am Vet Med Assoc 2000;217:1475–9.

[47] Dworkin MS, Sullivan PS, Buskin SE, et al. *Bordetella bronchiseptica* infection in human immunodeficiency virus-infected patients. Clin Infect Dis 1999;28:1095–9.

[48] Sykes JE. Feline upper respiratory tract pathogens: *Chlamydophila felis*. Compend Contin Educ Pract Vet 2001;23:231–41.

[49] Yan C, Fukushi H, Matsudate H, et al. Seroepidemiological investigation of feline chlamydiosis in cats and humans in Japan. Microbiol Immunol 2000;44:155–60.

[50] Greene CE, Prescott JF. Streptococcal and other gram-positive bacterial infections. In: Greene CE, editor. Infectious diseases of the dog and cat. 2nd edition. Philadelphia: WB Saunders; 1998. p. 205–14.

[51] Nagaoka H, Sugieda M, Akiyama M, et al. Isolation of *Coxiella burnetii* from the vagina of feline clients at veterinary clinics. J Vet Med Sci 1998;60:251–2.

[52] Pinsky RL, Fishbein DB, Greene CR, et al. An outbreak of cat-associated Q fever in the United States. J Infect Dis 1991;164:202–4.

[53] Marrie TJ. *Coxiella burnetii* (Q fever) pneumonia. Clin Infect Dis 1995;21(Suppl):S253–64.

[54] Angulo FJ, Glaser CA, Juranek DD, et al. Caring for pets of immunocompromised persons. J Am Vet Med Assoc 1994;205:1711–8.

[55] Burton B. Pets and PWAs: claims of health risk exaggerated. AIDS Patient Care 1989;34–7.

[56] Carmack B. The role of companion animals for persons with AIDS/HIV. Hol Nurs Pract 1991;5:24–31.

[57] Spencer L. Study explores health risks and the human animal bond. J Am Vet Med Assoc 1992;201:1669.

[58] Grant S, Olsen CW. Preventing zoonotic diseases in immunocompromised persons: the role of physicians and veterinarians. Emerg Infect Dis 1999;5:159–63.

ELSEVIER
SAUNDERS

Vet Clin Small Anim
35 (2005) 21–37

VETERINARY
CLINICS
Small Animal Practice

Feline Infectious Disease Control in Shelters

Kate F. Hurley, DVM, MPVM

*Center for Companion Animal Health, University of California
Davis School of Veterinary Medicine, Davis, CA 95616, USA*

Managing feline infectious disease in animal shelters is an immensely challenging task. Financial resources are limited, facilities are often less than ideal, and cats are highly susceptible to the effects of a stressful and crowded environment. Carrier states are common for feline infectious conditions, which means a constant influx of potentially contagious animals. High turnover of caretakers necessitates clearly written systems of communication and constant training to maintain consistency. Adding to the challenge, the medical program must contribute to the overall goals of the shelter, including adoption of cats into permanent homes. Moving cats promptly through the shelter for placement sometimes conflicts with ideal infectious disease control. A clearly thought out and systematic approach is required to develop an effective program in the face of all these challenges.

Disease in feline shelter populations

Infectious diseases of greatest concern in shelters include respiratory disease (feline viral rhinotracheitis, feline calicivirus [FCV], and others), skin disease (particularly dermatophytosis), gastrointestinal disease (eg, panleukopenia, protozoal and parasitic infestation), and systemic disease, such as feline infectious peritonitis [1,2]. In addition, shelter cats may present with infections that are virtually unheard of in private veterinary practice or may develop relatively severe signs of common infectious conditions [3,4]. Specific strategies for management of shelter infections are beyond the scope of this article and are detailed elsewhere [1,2,5]. Visible disease is often only the tip of the iceberg, however. High levels of upper respiratory infection (URI), for example, often reflect an overall breakdown in husbandry and

E-mail address: kfhurley@ucdavis.edu

infectious disease control. All too commonly, veterinary services in shelters are used only in reaction to occurrences of a particular disease. Although admittedly difficult to implement in the hectic environment typical of many shelters, a proactive preventive approach to disease control is more effective, more humane, and less costly in the long run.

Principles of prevention

Contact with a pathogen does not guarantee that infection and disease are going to result. It is common to find evidence of exposure to various pathogens in healthy cats raised in a low-density and low-stress environment [6–8]. These same pathogens can cause significant morbidity and mortality in a shelter or cattery. The outcome of disease is determined by an interaction of environmental, host, and agent factors. This provides three general targets for a preventive medicine program:

1. Environment: prevent disease from building up or spreading in the environment.
2. Host: support the host's immune response.
3. Agent: develop written procedures for control of specific pathogens of importance, based on an understanding of pathogen life cycle.

Box 1 lists some of the factors that should be considered when developing a comprehensive prevention program.

Environmental management

Reducing environmental contamination provides a powerful tool for prevention. Environmental control offers broad protection for the entire population. The list in Box 1 should be systematically reviewed with shelter management, and each factor should be optimized to the extent possible. Management of population density, effective cleaning and disinfection, and accurate disease recognition and segregation are particularly critical.

Population density

Population density is a key determinant of health, well-being, and productivity in many species, ranging from livestock to human hospital settings [9–13]. Crowding increases the overall environmental pathogen load and contact rate and intensifies the effects of many other negative factors, such as poor air quality, excessive noise, and stress. Controlling density is particularly critical in cats. Although cats may choose to live in loose-knit groups in the wild, they are poorly adapted to close confinement [14]. Managing population density in a shelter can be an emotional as well as logistic challenge, however. The constant excess of homeless cats often leads well-meaning shelter managers to house more cats than the facility can

---

Box 1. Environmental, host, and agent determinants of disease

Environment factors
    Population density
    Sanitation/disinfection
    Disease recognition
    Segregation/animal flow
    Air quality/ventilation
    Temperature/humidity
    Noise control
    Light cycles
    Pest control
Host factors
    Stress
    Age
    Immunity
      Natural exposure
      Vaccination
      Maternal antibodies
    Genetics
    Nutritional status
    Physiologic state (eg, pregnancy)
    Concurrent disease
    Internal or external parasites
    Drug treatment
Agent factors
    Virulence
    Strain differences
    Dose
    Method of spread
    Route of infection
    Incubation and shedding
    Carrier state

---

readily accommodate. It is important to recognize that crowding is likely to cost rather than save lives in the long run, through increased infectious disease, a damaged shelter reputation, and reduced adoptions.

Some guidelines are available regarding recommended cat-housing density. For individually housed cats, a minimum cage space of 2.55 m^2 (8.4 ft^2) has been recommended [15]. For group-housed cats, the recommended minimum is 1.67 m^2 per cat (5.5 ft^2), with a maximum group size of 10 cats [15–17]. The number of cats available for adoption should be driven by the expected number of adoptions rather than by the maximum physical capacity of the shelter [18]. Overflow space for busy seasons or large-scale emergencies should be planned in advance (eg, development of a foster home network or temporary caging). Although minimum space guidelines are helpful, the number of cats that can be kept without overcrowding is not simply a matter of cage space; rather, maximum capacity depends on many factors, including facility design, ventilation, and staff availability. If the population outstrips the staff's ability to provide adequate care, overcrowding is present, regardless of the number of cats. Indications of serious overcrowding are provided in Box 2.

For a given facility size and staffing level, crowding can be controlled through limiting admissions, euthanasia, or decreasing the amount of time each cat is in the shelter (turnover time). Clearly, the latter would be the preferred choice whenever possible. Turnover time is reduced by daily assessment of every cat in the shelter to make decisions and take any needed action at the earliest possible point. This includes medical and behavioral assessment, surgical sterilization or other preadoption procedures, resolution of legal issues, and placement for public viewing. The less time a cat spends in the shelter, the less likely it is to become ill, further reducing the population burden on the facility [19]. The impact on turnover should be kept in mind when developing policies that delay placement for adoption.

Box 2. Indications of overcrowding in a shelter

Animals are routinely housed in inappropriate areas of the facility or in inappropriate cages (eg, cats remain in short-term intake areas rather than being moved to stray-holding or adoption areas; cats are housed in carriers, wire cages, or other housing not intended for long-term use).

Animals with infectious disease remain in the general population rather than being moved to isolation.

More animals are placed in a kennel or cage than it was designed for, or frequent aggressive incidents are observed in group housing.

There is a noticeable smell of animal waste in the facility.

Cleaning and disinfection are compromised because of crowding (eg, cats are placed in a transport carrier or cage without thorough cleaning between occupants).

Vaccines are not given promptly at intake because of overwhelming animal numbers or lack of staff time.

Sick animals often do not receive needed treatment.

Serious disease spreads repeatedly within the shelter or common infections, such as URI, are noticeably more severe or persistent than expected.

Such polices are not necessarily wrong, but the effect on population density must be considered. Even a few days make a big difference when multiplied by many cats. The average turnover time per cat to avoid overcrowding can be estimated as follows:

$$\text{Average Turnover Time in Days} = (\text{Total Cage/Cat Holding Spaces} \div$$
$$\text{Total Yearly Cat Intake}) \times 365 \text{ Days}$$

Sanitation and disinfection

Substantial time and energy are spent cleaning and disinfecting shelters, and this is relied on as a major barrier against disease. A clean shelter encourages adoptions and public support as well as protecting animal health. Because of its importance, cleaning should be approached systematically. A well-conceived plan needs to be developed, implemented, and periodically revisited to make sure it is still functional. Incorrectly performed disinfection can be ineffective or actually serve to spread disease [20].

Choice of cleaning and disinfectant products should reflect the pathogens most likely to be present and the type of surface to be cleaned. Other considerations include cost, ease of application, and staff tolerance. No single product is ideal under all circumstances; advantages and disadvantages of various products are presented in Table 1. Unenveloped viruses, such as panleukopenia and FCV, are resistant to many commonly used disinfectants but are susceptible to sodium hypochlorite and potassium peroxymonosulfate [21–24]. Dermatophytes are inactivated by sodium hypochlorite at higher concentrations with repeated applications (5% bleach diluted at a ratio of 1:10) [25]. Disinfectants must be applied to a clean surface free of organic matter, with the correct concentration and adequate contact time to be effective. This requires careful ongoing staff training.

No disinfectant can be relied on to inactivate all pathogens. Careful handwashing can reduce the effects of residual environmental contamination [26]. Mechanical cleaning, desiccation, and exposure to ultraviolet light are important adjuncts to chemical disinfection, and cat-housing areas should be designed to take advantage of these factors. Scratching posts, soft furniture, and home-like environments can become heavily contaminated over time. Ideally, bedding and toys should be washable, and larger items, such as scratching posts, if used, should be periodically replaced (particularly after a known contamination with a durable agent, such as ringworm or parvovirus). Some pathogens, such as ascarid eggs and coccidial cysts, are virtually impossible to inactivate or remove from porous surfaces [27]. Kittens and cats should be tested or treated for these infections before being placed in environments that are hard to clean. It is particularly important that kitten-housing areas be readily cleanable because of the frequency of infectious disease in this population.

Table 1
Characteristics of commonly used disinfectants

Disinfectant	Advantages	Disadvantages
Quaternary ammonium compounds	Some detergent activity Moderate inactivation by organic matter (less so than with bleach) Low tissue toxicity Inexpensive	Unreliable efficacy against unenveloped viruses (eg, feline panleukopenia, calicivirus) or dermatophytes Inactivated by soaps and detergents
Sodium hypochlorite (bleach)	Completely inactivates unenveloped viruses when used correctly Inactivates dermatophytes at higher concentration Low tissue toxicity Inexpensive Can be combined with quaternary ammonium compounds	Significantly inactivated by organic matter, exposure to light, or extended storage No detergent activity Fumes can be irritating at high concentration Corrosive to metal Hard water reduces effectiveness
Potassium peroxymonosulfate (Virkon or Trifectant)	Completely inactivates unenveloped viruses when used correctly. Some detergent activity Low tissue toxicity Less corrosive to metal than bleach Relatively good activity in the face of organic matter	Comes in powdered form, cannot be applied through hose-end applicator systems Leaves visible residue on some surfaces More costly than bleach
Chlorhexidine (Nolvasan)	Extremely low tissue toxicity	Relatively expensive Ineffective against unenveloped viruses, ringworm
Alcohol (usually in hand sanitizer)	Less irritating to tissue than quaternary ammonium or bleach Ethanol (70% concentration) moderately effective against calicivirus	Ineffective against unenveloped viruses, dermatophytes Adequate contact time required (15–30 seconds recommended by manufacturer) May encourage false sense of security

The logistics of cat cage cleaning can be problematic. Many shelters house cats in single cages, necessitating removal and extensive handling to clean. Moving cats from cage to cage can cause sufficient stress to activate latent feline herpesvirus (FHV) infection [28]. Extensive fomite spread is almost inevitable in this circumstance. Ideally, individually housed cats should be provided with double-sided cages or switched between the same two cages throughout their shelter stay. An alternative is to assign each cat its own carrier or "feral cat" box for use during cleaning. If the cage size is sufficient, the carrier can remain in the cage to provide a hiding place, providing the added benefit of stress reduction [29]. Less frequent cage cleaning (within reason) has been correlated with improved health in laboratory rodents [30]. In shelters that house healthy cats for extended periods, intensive daily cleaning may not be required, although frequent litter box cleaning and removal of any visible debris are necessary under all circumstances. It may be beneficial to leave bedding with the animal if it is not heavily soiled [31].

Fomite transmission on human hands and clothing is, of course, a significant means of disease spread. This poses a particularly vexing problem in the shelter population, where human interaction must be encouraged to some extent to promote socialization and adoption of the shelter's charges. Friendly signs can be posted to remind the public not to touch cats, but unless given a reasonable alternative, the desire to interact with the animals often outweighs caution. Alcohol hand sanitizers are commonly used and better than nothing in most cases, although they do not reliably inactivate some important feline pathogens, such as panleukopenia virus, FCV, and dermatophytes [24,25,32,33]. When possible, thorough handwashing or a change of gloves is greatly preferred. This is important for prevention of zoonotic disease transmission as well as for shelter cat health. Handwashing stations for the public and staff should be planned in new facilities. Lightweight plastic gloves used in food service can be obtained inexpensively; some shelters require that the public as well as staff wear gloves and change gloves between cats. Other shelters house cats in solid-fronted cages with an attached toy that can be used for interaction. If solid-fronted cages are used, careful attention must be paid to ensure adequate ventilation.

Segregation and animal flow

Segregation of subpopulations is an essential principle of population health management. In addition to health, categories for segregation include age, intake date, and intake type (stray/recent intakes from adoptable/longer term cats). Increasing the number of separate subpopulations facilitates infectious disease control. At a minimum, separate housing areas must be provided for cats with active signs of infectious disease. Ideally, isolation areas should be further subdivided to separate cats with respiratory infections from those with skin or gastrointestinal infections. If space permits, it is preferable to separate mildly ill cats or cats recently recovering from URIs from more severely ill cats. Even separating healthy cats into smaller populations is useful. This should be kept in mind when designing new facilities.

Handling, cleaning, and foot traffic should proceed from the most vulnerable or healthiest populations to those that are relatively less vulnerable to disease or more likely to be shedding infectious pathogens. For example, handling could proceed from kittens to adult adoptable cats, to stray/recent intakes, and, finally, to sick cats housed in isolation. If the design of the shelter prohibits an ideal handling/traffic pattern, careful handwashing and use of protective clothing should be particularly encouraged to prevent cross-contamination of areas.

Disease recognition

To segregate animals appropriately, a system for disease recognition and reporting must be in place. All staff and volunteers should be trained to look for general signs of disease, and a clear reporting system should be developed. In addition to noting signs on the animal's cage card or other record, concerns should be recorded in a central location so that medical staff can follow up efficiently. Medical problem reports should include the signs; signalment, including animal identification number and name if available; the animal's location in the shelter; the date and time the problem was observed; and the initials of the person making the report. This is especially important in a high-turnover shelter, where the animal may have been moved from its original cage by the time the veterinarian is able to check up on medical concerns.

The next level of disease recognition is an individual examination of each animal. Ideally, this is performed by a veterinarian. An initial examination by a trained technician can be a valuable screening tool to identify animals requiring additional veterinary attention, however. This examination is ideally performed at intake, particularly at shelters that place virtually every animal they admit. At shelters where a higher percentage of cats are euthanized, it may be more practical to perform the screening examination after completion of a stray-holding period but before placement for adoption. An additional brief examination at the time of adoption can catch problems, such as URI, that develop during the shelter stay and allow adopters to be counseled accordingly.

Identification of specific diseases also has an important place in a preventive medicine program. Diagnostic testing allows segregation or removal of potentially infectious individuals, protects adopters from taking home an unexpected veterinary bill or heartache, and allows the shelter to invest resources in animals most likely to benefit. For treatable conditions (which vary greatly according to a shelter's resources), diagnostic testing also allows the animal to receive appropriate care promptly. Diagnostic testing is not without cost, however, in terms of scarce resources of money and time as well as in the consequences of inaccurate results. It is critical that diagnostic tests be used, interpreted, and documented carefully.

Accuracy of diagnostic testing is always a concern, and in a shelter, the stakes are particularly high. A false-negative result can lead to exposure of the entire population to a devastating disease, whereas a false-positive result may cause an individual animal to be needlessly isolated or euthanized. Choice and interpretation of test results should reflect the relative risk of each of these scenarios. For diseases like ringworm or panleukopenia, which pose a high population risk, testing strategies should be chosen to minimize the risk of false-negative results. For diseases like feline immunodeficiency virus (FIV), which are not readily spread but may prove devastating to the individual, a testing strategy should be selected to decrease the risk of false-positive results. Staff performing these tests should be carefully trained and should understand the reliability and possible causes of inaccurate results for all tests commonly used in the shelter [34].

Air quality

Poor ventilation and high humidity contribute to disease by promoting buildup of pathogens in the environment and by direct irritation of the respiratory tract from airborne debris and fumes from urine and cleaning products. Air quality is of particular importance in shelters, given the frequency of respiratory syndromes. Although true aerosol transmission is not thought to be a significant method of spread for feline URI, droplet spread can transmit respiratory infections for distances up to 4 ft (1.2 m) [35,36].

Three general strategies exist for maintaining indoor air quality [37]. In order of decreasing effectiveness, these strategies are:

1. Source control: reducing the amount of contaminants in the air
2. Ventilation: bringing outside air indoors
3. Air cleaning: processing indoor air through a filter (ie, HEPA filter)

Indoor air contamination is reduced by decreasing population density, cleaning litter boxes frequently, using low-dust litter, and applying cleaning products at the correct dilution. Cleaning products themselves can be respiratory irritants and should not be sprayed around cats. A fresh air exchange rate of 10 to 12 air exchanges per hour is commonly recommended [38]. The relevant air exchange rate is at the level of the cat's nose, however, which may be quite a bit lower than the overall air exchange rate in the room, especially if cats are housed in cages that are enclosed on three sides [39]. High air exchange rates are costly in terms of heating and cooling; thus, design of caging to take full advantage of ventilation systems is crucial. In shelters with poor air exchange systems, air filters are sometimes used as an adjunct to improve air quality. The efficacy of this approach in reducing feline disease has not been documented. Frequent filter changes are required, which may lead to substantial costs. Investment in fresh air sources, such as adding a window or skylight with a fan, may provide a better return in the long run, especially in mild climates. The importance of source control should never be overlooked.

Other environmental factors

Noise, temperature, humidity, and light cycles affect feline health and well-being [14,40]. Exposure to noise from dogs should be minimized, and temperature should be maintained between 10°C and 29°C (50°F–85°F), with humidity between 10% and 50%. Lights should be turned off at night. Overall environmental comfort for cats and visiting adopters is an important contributor to population health and the ultimate outcome of successful adoptions. Environmental enrichment is discussed in greater detail elsewhere in this article.

Selected host factors

Given that some level of exposure to pathogens is inevitable, support of the host's immune response is a crucial part of disease prevention. As with environmental control, no single factor is adequate in itself. Stress reduction, vaccination, nutrition, and other factors listed in Box 1 all contribute to the cat's ability to resist disease.

Stress reduction/environmental enrichment

Mental wellness is key to maintaining feline health, particularly given the frequency of stress-activated herpesvirus infection in cats [28]. Stress in cats also results in decreased play and exploration, increased hiding, and stereotypic behaviors, all of which may lead to a lower likelihood of adoption [15,41]. Stress results from aversive stimuli, such as noise; odors; uncomfortable temperatures; unfamiliar people, animals, and environments; and unpredictable handling. Even minor changes, such as moving from one cage to another or being placed in a carrier, can be significantly stressful for cats [29,35]. Stressful effects of aversive stimuli are amplified when events are unpredictable or the animal lacks the opportunity to modulate their effects through behavioral responses [29,40]. A feline stress-scoring system has been proposed, which may help to monitor the success of interventions [42]. Efforts at enrichment must take each cat's individuality into account. What is relaxing to one cat may be highly stressful to another, depending on past experience, genetics, and individual temperament [43,44].

Recommendations for environmental enrichment include provision of adequate quantity of space as described in the section on population density. Quality of space is also important, and an optimal cage should include a place to hide, an elevated resting area, feeding and litter areas separated as widely as possible, comfortable bedding, and a scratching surface [40,45–48]. Solitary cats in double-sided housing have more control over their environment and are more interactive with strange people than solitary cats in traditional single cages [41]. Space limitations make some of these provisions impractical in some shelters, but even simple interventions, such as toys and a paper bag or box to hide in, can reduce stress and improve adoptability [49]. Additional recommendations for group-housed cats include provision of multiple litter boxes of various types (including at least one or two uncovered litter boxes) and multiple feeding stations to avoid competition around resources. Regardless of housing type, cats benefit from reduction of noise, exposure to natural light and fresh air, a variety of toys, and consistent friendly interaction with known caretakers. Feeding, cleaning, and socialization should follow set schedules as much as possible.

Group cat housing is increasingly popular in shelters and affords an opportunity to provide more of the features of an enriched environment while conserving the amount of space required to house each cat [17]. The effect of group versus single housing on feline stress levels is variable, however, and depends on the density and quality of housing, the temperament and prior experience of the cats, and the rate of turnover. Boarding cats observed for their first 14 days in a cattery did not show significant differences in stress levels between cats housed singly, in pairs, or in small low-density groups (<10 cats per group with 2–3 m^2 of space per cat) in a boarding cattery [42]. In animal shelters, cats housed at high density or in large groups displayed more signs of stress than cats housed singly [16,50]. Cats that had not been socialized to other cats also experienced more stress in group housing [51]. Stable groups are preferred to the extent possible, because the introduction and departure of new animals inevitably create some stress as well as disease control challenges [41,50]. Group housing should not be viewed as a way to inexpensively house large numbers of cats, regardless of individual needs, but may be valuable as an alternative to single caging as long as it is used appropriately, particularly in shelters that often house cats for more than a few weeks [52].

Many shelters have programs that allow volunteers to pet, groom, and play with cats. Such programs can foster goodwill in the community and provide cats with extra attention. Poorly controlled volunteer interactions may actually increase stress for some cats, however. Interaction with strangers and being moved from a familiar cage are potentially stressful events, especially if the cat is taken to a room filled with the smells of many unfamiliar animals [44,47]. Cats' willingness to approach unfamiliar people is highly variable and often follows a slower schedule than if the interaction is initiated by the person [53]. Cat socialization programs should be responsive to the individual cat's needs. Some cats may do better if allowed to initiate interaction at their own pace, and it may be preferable to groom or play with cats in their own cage rather than moving them to another room, especially in shelters where cats stay short term. Limiting indirect exposure to other cats is also preferable from a disease control perspective. An advantage of group housing (or spacious single cat housing) is that it allows interaction with cats on their own turf and offers cats the opportunity to withdraw at will.

Incorporating infectious disease control with enrichment is critical, especially in areas where new intake cats are housed and in shelters with high population turnover. Illness and the attendant isolation and medication are highly stressful—there is no benefit to an enrichment program that fosters spread of infectious disease. Toys and bedding should be washable, disposable, or go home with the cat at the time of adoption. Volunteers should be trained to scan carefully for signs of illness, and careful precautions should be taken before and after handling cats. A well-designed enrichment program fosters overall mental and physical health of sheltered cats.

Vaccination

The best vaccination strategy depends somewhat on characteristics of the shelter population, facility, staff resources, and prevalent diseases in the region. Factors to consider include which pathogens to vaccinate against, whether to use modified live versus killed vaccines, route of administration, timing, and revaccination schedule. Some general recommendations can be made, but, ultimately, the vaccine program must be tailored to the particular population.

Core vaccines generally recommended for all shelter cats are: FHV type 1 (feline viral rhinotracheitis), FCV, and feline panleukopenia (FPV). FPV has been reported with increasing frequency in many areas of the United States. For communities in which FPV is an active threat, prevention of this deadly disease is a priority. The best protection is afforded by a modified live parenteral vaccine given immediately on shelter entry to all cats (including injured and mildly ill cats), with the exception of pregnant cats and kittens less than 5 weeks old. Modified live FPV vaccine is currently only available as part of three-way combination products also containing FHV and FCV vaccines.

If FPV is not a concern, parenteral or intranasal products may be chosen. Intranasal products have several theoretic advantages, including relatively rapid onset of protection, generation of local immunity, and efficacy in the face of maternal antibodies [54,55]. A disadvantage of intranasal vaccines (and, to a lesser extent, modified live vaccines in general) is the possibility of mild signs induced by the vaccine. For shelters that euthanize all symptomatic cats, this is a tremendous drawback. Anecdotally, shelters report varying results from use of an intranasal rather than parenteral vaccine to control URI; some have reported an increase, some have reported a decrease, and some have appreciated little change in overall URI levels. One study suggested that use of an intranasal respiratory virus vaccine in addition to a parenteral three-way feline viral rhinotracheitis-calicivirus-panleukopenia (FVRCP) vaccine resulted in decreased severity of URI in shelter cats [56].

Noncore vaccines include *Chlamydia* and *Bordetella bronchiseptica* vaccines. Use of these vaccines should be reserved for shelters in which infection has been confirmed by laboratory diagnostics as an ongoing problem. Other vaccines, such as feline leukemia virus (FeLV), FIV, and rabies, are best given after adoption, when the cat's individual circumstances can be better evaluated (although shelters that hold cats long term may consider vaccinating for rabies according to local regulations). Feline coronavirus and *Giardia* vaccines are not recommended because of a lack of demonstrated efficacy.

All staff members responsible for vaccination must be carefully trained in correct vaccine handling and administration. Staff should be aware of possible adverse consequences of vaccination, including recognition of anaphylactic shock. If parenteral modified live FVRCP is used, staff should be aware of the potential to cause severe URI if given inadvertently by the oronasal route [55]. Vaccines should be drawn up away from the cat's face. Vaccine spilled on cats' fur should be cleaned promptly with alcohol, and the environment should be wiped down with bleach solution.

Nutrition

Adequate nutrition is important to an animal's ability to mount an effective immune response [57]. Maintaining adequate nutritional intake for sheltered cats can be challenging for several reasons. Cats in a shelter may not eat enough because of stress, illness, competition for food in group housing, an unpalatable or novel diet, or simple underfeeding. Cats tend to be neophobic and may take some time to acclimate to an unfamiliar food [58]. Because of this, it is particularly important to feed cats a consistent diet rather than a variety of donated foods, as is sometimes practiced in shelters. Poor-quality or spoiled donated food also may lead to vomiting and diarrhea, which obscures recognition of infectious conditions and creates a poor public image. A high-quality readily absorbed diet can help to compensate for slightly decreased intake, although the benefits of a premium diet must balance the increased cost. The diet should be appropriate to the life stage of the cat. If donated food is used, a consistent brand or gift certificates to a local feed store are preferable to a random mix. If a consistent brand absolutely cannot be obtained, donations should be carefully inspected to make sure they are not damaged or spoiled and food should be thoroughly mixed to provide as consistent a blend as possible rather than switching from one brand to another [59].

Cats generally prefer taking multiple small meals and should have food freely available throughout the day [60]. Because cats have marked individual dietary preferences, wet and dry food should be offered, at least initially [61]. Food should be fed in consistent measured quantities to allow determination of how much is eaten daily. Cats in short-term shelter care should be offered the high end of the amount recommended by the manufacturer. This may need to be modified for cats in long-term care to prevent obesity. Monitoring and documentation of intake are important, especially when multiple caretakers are involved. Daily written notation should be made as to whether a cat seems to be eating (food should be measured if in doubt), and cats should be weighed at least every 2 weeks. Cats that do not eat for more than 1 or 2 days should be carefully evaluated for a medical condition and offered a variety of foods. Correction of B-vitamin deficiency through parenteral supplementation may be helpful in the treatment of anorexia, especially in sick cats. An appetite stimulant, such as cyproheptadine, may be helpful in the short term [62].

Cats, especially kittens, often enter shelters in a precarious nutritional state and may thus be more susceptible to dietary deficiencies. For this reason, homemade diets should be used with great care, under the supervision of a veterinarian, and only as indicated for treatment of diet-responsive disorders. In general, additional nutritional supplementation is not needed for healthy shelter cats fed a balanced commercial diet. The addition of L-lysine at a dose of 500 mg twice daily in adult cats has been recommended to reduce recrudescence and shedding of FHV, although the efficacy of this in a shelter population is unknown [63]. L-lysine is generally palatable to cats and may be added as a powder sprinkled on wet or dry food.

Other host factors

Concurrent infections and parasitic infestation reduce the animal's ability to respond to infectious challenge. External parasites, such as fleas, reduce adoptability as well as compromising health and causing discomfort and can facilitate transmission of zoonotic agents, such as *Bartonella spp* [64]. A variety of safe and effective flea and tick control products are available and should be used as needed. All kittens should be treated with a product effective against ascarids, and cats should be treated for other internal parasites based on results of diagnostic testing [7]. Antibiotic use should be reserved for cases in which a bacterial infection is confirmed or strongly suspected based on clinical signs. Overuse of antibiotics may select for antibiotic-resistant bacteria and compromise the cat's normal flora, increasing the cat's vulnerability to disease.

Planning for agent factors

Agent risk factors for disease are generally inherent to the specific pathogen and cannot be manipulated in the same way as environmental or host risk factors. Nevertheless, it is helpful to develop specific strategies for control of the most common diseases seen in a given population. Written infectious disease control protocols should include a description of the disease (including case definition, mode of transmission, and whether or not the disease is zoonotic) and considerations for protection of the population as well as care of the individual animal. Population considerations include requirements for environmental decontamination, length of quarantine for exposed animals, and level of infectious risk while symptomatic and after apparent recovery. Policies with respect to treatment and adoption of cats affected with various conditions should be developed in consultation with shelter management, based on the risk posed by the disease and the shelter's philosophy and resources.

Summary

No single factor determines whether a population remains healthy or disease rages out of control. All host and environmental factors taken together provide a number of tools to protect the vulnerable feline shelter population, however. A well-conceived infectious disease control program contributes to improved public perception, increased adoptions, and a healthier feline population within the shelter and in the community in general.

References

[1] Pedersen NC. Common infectious diseases of multiple-cat environments. In: Feline husbandry: diseases and management in the multiple cat environment. 1st edition. St. Louis: Mosby; 1991. p. 163–289.

[2] Foley JE. Infectious diseases of dogs and cats. In: Miller L, Zawistowski S, editors. Shelter medicine for veterinarians and staff. Ames (IA): Blackwell; 2004. p. 235–84.

[3] Binns SH, Dawson S, Speakman AJ. Prevalence and risk factors for Bordetella bronchiseptica infection. Vet Rec 1999(144):575–80.

[4] Hurley KF, Pesavento PA, Pedersen NC, Poland AM, Wilson E, Foley JE. An outbreak of virulent systemic feline calicivirus disease. J Am Vet Med Assoc 2004;224(2):241–9.

[5] Lawler DF. Prevention and management of infection in catteries. In: Greene CE, editor. Infectious diseases of the dog and cat. 2nd edition. Philadelphia: WB Saunders; 1990. p. 701–6.

[6] Binns SH, Dawson S, Speakman AJ, et al. A study of feline upper respiratory tract disease with reference to prevalence and risk factors for infection with feline calicivirus and feline herpesvirus. J Feline Med Surg 2000;2(3):123–33.

[7] Spain CV, Scarlett JM, Wade SE, McDonough P. Prevalence of enteric zoonotic agents in cats less than 1 year old in central New York State. J Vet Intern Med 2001;15(1):33–8.

[8] Wardley RC, Gaskell RM, Povey RC. Feline respiratory viruses—their prevalence in clinically healthy cats. J Small Anim Pract 1974;15(9):579–86.

[9] Flint M, Murray P. Lot-fed goats: the advantages of using an enriched environment. Aust J Exp Agric 2001;41(4):473–6.

[10] Sevi A, Massa S, Annicchiarico G, Dell'Aquila S, Muscio A. Effect of stocking density on ewes' milk yield, udder health and microenvironment. J Dairy Res 1999;66(4):489–99.

[11] Maes D, Deluyker H, Verdonck M, et al. Herd factors associated with the seroprevalences of four major respiratory pathogens in slaughter pigs from farrow-to-finish pig herds. Vet Res (Paris) 2000;31(3):313–27.

[12] Borg MA. Bed occupancy and overcrowding as determinant factors in the incidence of MRSA infections within general ward settings. J Hosp Infect 2003(54):316–8.

[13] Bugajski J, Borycz J, Glod R, Bugajski AJ. Crowding stress impairs the pituitary-adrenocortical responsiveness to the vasopressin but not corticotropin-releasing hormone stimulation. Brain Res 1995;681(1–2):223–8.

[14] Pedersen NC. Feline husbandry: diseases and management in a multiple cat environment. 1st edition. St. Louis (MO): Mosby; 1991.

[15] Rochlitz I. Recommendations for the housing of cats in the home, in catteries and animal shelters, in laboratories and in veterinary surgeries. J Feline Med Surg 1999;1(3):181–91.

[16] Kessler MR, Turner DC. Effects of density and cage size on stress in domestic cats (Felis silvestris catus) housed in animal shelters and boarding catteries. Anim Welf 1999;8(3): 259–67.

[17] Dowling J. All together now: group housing for cats. Anim Sheltering 2003;26:13–26.

[18] Seif D, Freed J. Operational guide for animal care and control agencies: sanitation and disease control. Denver (CO): American Humane Association; 1999.

[19] Dinnage J, Scarlett JM, Richards J. Epidemiology of upper respiratory tract infections in animal shelter cats. Presented at the American Humane Conference. Garden Grove, CA, September 7–10, 2003.

[20] Dharan S, Mourouga P, Copin P, Bessmer G, Tschanz B, Pittet D. Routine disinfection of patients' environmental surfaces. Myth or reality? J Hosp Infect 1999;42(2):113–7.

[21] Doultree JC, Druce JD, Birch CJ, Bowden DS, Marshall JA. Inactivation of feline calicivirus, a Norwalk virus surrogate. J Hosp Infect 1999;41(1):51–7.

[22] Eleraky NZ, Potgieter LN, Kennedy MA. Virucidal efficacy of four new disinfectants. J Am Anim Hosp Assoc 2002;38(3):231–4.

[23] Kennedy MA, Mellon VS, Caldwell G, Potgieter LN. Virucidal efficacy of the newer quaternary ammonium compounds. J Am Anim Hosp Assoc 1995;31(3):254–8.

[24] Scott FW. Virucidal disinfectants and feline viruses. Am J Vet Res 1980;41(3):410–4.

[25] Moriello KA. Management of dermatophyte infections in catteries and multiple-cat households. Vet Clin North Am Small Anim Pract 1990;20(6):1457–74.

[26] Wilcox MH, Fawley WN, Wigglesworth N, Parnell P, Verity P, Freeman J. Comparison of the effect of detergent versus hypochlorite cleaning on environmental contamination and incidence of Clostridium difficile infection. J Hosp Infect 2003;54(2):109–14.

[27] Bowman D. Georgi's parasitology for veterinarians. 7th edition. Philadelphia: WB Saunders; 1999.

[28] Gaskell RM, Povey RC. Experimental induction of feline viral rhinotracheitis virus re-excretion in FVR-recovered cats. Vet Rec 1977;100(7):128–33.

[29] Carlstead K, Brown JL, Strawn W. Behavioral and physiologic correlates of stress in laboratory cats. Appl Anim Behav Sci 1993;38:143–58.

[30] Reeb-Whitaker CK, Paigen B, Beamer WG, et al. The impact of reduced frequency of cage changes on the health of mice housed in ventilated cages. Lab Anim 2001;35(1):58–73.

[31] Van Loo PL, Van Der Meer E, Kruitwagen CL, Koolhaas JM, Van Zutphen LF, Baumans V. Long-term effects of husbandry procedures on stress-related parameters in male mice of two strains. Lab Anim 2004;38(2):169–77.

[32] Kramer A, Rudolph P, Kampf G, Pittet D. Limited efficacy of alcohol-based hand gels. Lancet 2002;359(9316):1489–90.

[33] Gehrke C, Steinmann J, Goroncy-Bermes P. Inactivation of feline calicivirus, a surrogate of norovirus (formerly Norwalk-like viruses), by different types of alcohol in vitro and in vivo. J Hosp Infect 2004;56(1):49–55.

[34] Hurley KF. Diagnostic testing in the shelter environment. Presented at the American Humane Conference, Anaheim, CA, September 7–10, 2003.

[35] Gaskell RM, Povey RC. Transmission of feline viral rhinotracheitis. Vet Rec 1982;111(16):359–62.

[36] Wardley RC, Povey RC. Aerosol transmission of feline caliciviruses. An assessment of its epidemiological importance. Br Vet J 1977;133(5):504–8.

[37] Environmental Protection Agency. Residential air cleaning devices: a summary of available information. Washington, DC: EPA Office of Air and Radiation; 1990.

[38] American Humane Society. Operational guide for animal care and control agencies. Planning and building an animal shelter. Denver: American Humane Society; 2000.

[39] Keller LS, White WJ, Snider MT, Lang CM. An evaluation of intra-cage ventilation in three animal caging systems. Lab Anim Sci 1989;39(3):237–42.

[40] Carlstead K. Stress, stereotypic pacing and environmental enrichment in leopard cats (Felis bengalensis). Presented at the American Association of Zoological Parks and Aquariums/Canadian Association of Zoological Parks and Aquariums Annual Conference, Wheeling, WV, 1992.

[41] Overall KL. Recognizing and managing problem behavior in breeding catteries. In: August JR, editor. Consultations in feline internal medicine, vol. 3. Philadelphia: WB Saunders; 1997. p. 634–46.

[42] Kessler MR, Turner DC. Stress and adaptation of cats (Felis silvestris catus) housed singly, in pairs and in groups in boarding catteries. Anim Welf 1997;6(3):243–54.

[43] Mendl M, Harcourt R. Individuality in the domestic cat: origins, development and stability. In: Turner DC, Bateson P, editors. The domestic cat: the biology of its behavior. Cambridge: Cambridge University Press; 2000. p. 47–64.

[44] Podberscek AL, Blackshaw JK, Beattie AW. The behaviour of laboratory colony cats and their reactions to a familiar and unfamiliar person. Appl Anim Behav Sci 1991;31(1–2): 119–30.

[45] Rochlitz I, Podberscek AL, Broom DM. Welfare of cats in a quarantine cattery. Vet Rec 1998;143(2):35–9.

[46] Monte MD, Pape GL, De Monte M, Le Pape G. Behavioural effects of cage enrichment in single-caged adult cats. Anim Welf 1997;6(1):53–66.

[47] Buffington T. External and internal influences on disease risk in cats. J Am Vet Med Assoc 2002;220(7):994–1002.

[48] Loveridge GG, Horrocks LJ, Hawthorne AJ. Environmentally enriched housing for cats when housed singly. Anim Welf 1995;4(2):135–41.

[49] Wells DL, Hepper PG. The influence of environmental change on the behaviour of sheltered dogs. Appl Anim Behav Sci 2000;68(2):151–62.

[50] Ottway DS, Hawkins DM. Cat housing in rescue shelters: a welfare comparison between communal and discrete-unit housing. Anim Welf 2003(12):173–89.

[51] Kessler MR, Turner DC. Socialization and stress in cats (Felis silvestris catus) housed singly and in groups in animal shelters. Anim Welf 1999;8(1):15–26.

[52] Smith D, Durman K, Roy D, Bradshaw JWS. Behavioral aspects of the welfare of rescued cats. J Feline Advisory Bur 1994;31:25–8.

[53] Mertens C, Turner DC. Experimental analysis of human-cat interactions during first encounters. Anthrozoos 1989;2(2):83–97.

[54] Cocker FM, Newby TJ, Gaskell RM, et al. Responses of cats to nasal vaccination with a live, modified feline herpesvirus type 1. Res Vet Sci 1986;41(3):323–30.

[55] Greene C. Immunoprophylaxis and immunotherapy. In: Infectious diseases of the dog and cat. 2nd edition. Philadelphia: WB Saunders Company; 1998. p. 717–50.

[56] Edinboro CH, Janowitz LK, Guptill-Yoran L, Glickman LT. A clinical trial of intranasal and subcutaneous vaccines to prevent upper respiratory infection in cats at an animal shelter. Feline Pract 1999;27(6):7–13.

[57] Ford RB, Greene RT. The influence of host factors on the outcome of a viral infection. Vet Clin North Am Small Anim Pract 1986;16(6):1041–8.

[58] Bradshaw JW. Mere exposure reduces cats' neophobia to unfamiliar food. Anim Behav 1986;34(2):613–4.

[59] Shelter Speak. Feeding protocols for shelter animals. Anim Sheltering 2001;25:29.

[60] Kane E, Burger IH, Rivers JP. Feeding behaviour of the cat. In: Nutrition of the dog and cat. Waltham Symposium 7. Cambridge, UK: Cambridge University Press; 1989. p. 147–58.

[61] Bradshaw JWS, Healey LM, Thorne CJ, Macdonald DW, Arden-Clark C. Differences in food preferences between individuals and populations of domestic cats Felis silvestris catus. Appl Anim Behav Sci 2000;68(3):257–68.

[62] Michel K. Management of anorexia. Presented at the Atlantic Coast Veterinary Conference. Atlantic City, NJ, October 2002.

[63] Maggs DJ. Ocular feline herpes virus. Presented at the Western Veterinary Conference. Las Vegas, February 11–14, 2002.

[64] Foley JE, Chomel B, Kikuchi Y, Yamamoto K, Pedersen NC. Seroprevalence of Bartonella henselae in cattery cats: association with cattery hygiene and flea infestation. Vet Q 1998; 20(1):1–5.

ELSEVIER
SAUNDERS

Vet Clin Small Anim
35 (2005) 39–79

VETERINARY
CLINICS
Small Animal Practice

Feline Infectious Peritonitis

Katrin Hartmann, Dr med vet, Dr med vet habil

*Clinic of Small Animal Medicine, Ludwig-Maximilians-Universität München,
Veterinaerstrasse 13, 80539 Munich, Germany*

Feline infectious peritonitis (FIP) is a common disease and a frequent reason for referral; approximately 1 of every 200 new feline cases presented to American veterinary teaching hospitals represents a cat with FIP [1]. It is also a major factor in kitten mortality [2]. FIP is a fatal immune-mediated disease triggered by infection with a feline coronavirus (FCoV) [3]. FCoV belongs to the family Coronaviridae, a group of enveloped positive-stranded RNA viruses that are frequently found in cats [4]. Coronavirus-specific antibodies are present in up to 90% of cats in catteries and in up to 50% of those in single-cat households [5–8]. Only approximately 5% of FCoV-infected cats develop FIP in a cattery situation, however [5,9–11]. Because FIP is not only common but deadly and has no effective long-term man-agement, a rapid and reliable diagnosis is critical for prognostic reasons. A reliable diagnostic test would lessen the suffering of affected patients while avoiding euthanasia of unaffected cats; however, unfortunately, such a test is not currently available. Difficulties in definitively diagnosing FIP arise from nonspecific clinical signs; lack of pathognomonic, hematologic, and biochemical abnormalities; and low sensitivity and specificity of tests routinely used in practice.

It was initially hypothesized that FCoV strains causing FIP are different from avirulent enteric FCoV strains [12]. Those former strains, however, are serologically and genetically indistinguishable [13–18] and represent virulent variants of the same virus rather than separate virus species [19]. It is now known that cats are infected with the primarily avirulent FCoV that replicates in enterocytes. In some instances, however, a mutation occurs in a certain region of the FCoV genome [20–22], leading to the ability of the virus to replicate within macrophages, which seems to be a key pathogenic event in the development of FIP [9,23]. Although intensive research has continuously led to new knowledge and understanding about FIP, it has

E-mail address: hartmann@uni-muenchen.de

produced even more questions that still have to be answered. The objective of this article is to review recent knowledge and to increase understanding of the complex pathogenesis of FIP.

Etiology

The disease FIP was first described in 1963 as a syndrome in cats characterized by immune-mediated vasculitis and pyogranulomatous inflammatory reactions [24]. In 1978, a virus was identified as the etiologic agent, and in 1979, it was classified as a coronavirus labeled "feline infectious peritonitis virus" (FIPV) [25]. FIP has become an increasingly important disease for veterinarians and must now be considered to account for most infectious disease-related deaths in pet cats, thus taking over this title in recent years from feline leukemia virus (FeLV) infection, which is decreasing in prevalence and importance. A possible explanation for an increase in the prevalence of FIP is that management of domestic cats has changed [20]. With the introduction of litter boxes, more cats are kept permanently indoors, exposing them to large doses of FCoV in the feces that would previously have been buried outdoors. More and more cats are spending part of their life in crowded environments, such as at cat breeders or shelters, which increases their stress and exposure to FCoV while in such an environment [26].

Coronaviruses can cause harmless and mostly clinically inapparent enteral infections in cats, but they can also cause FIP. In earlier days, it was the common hypothesis that two different coronaviruses existed in cats, the "feline enteric coronavirus" (FECV) and the FIPV. Since then, it has become known that FIPV develops out of FECV spontaneously within the infected cat. Both viruses are identical with regard to their antigenetic properties and, with the exception of a single mutation, their genetic properties, but they are different with regard to their pathogenicity. This is why only the term *feline coronavirus* FCoV should be used to describe all coronaviruses in cats.

FCoV is an RNA virus and belongs to the genus *Coronavirus* of the family Coronaviridae. Coronaviruses are pleomorphic enveloped particles that average 100 nm in diameter (range: 60–120 nm) and contain single-stranded RNA. Characteristic petal-shaped projections called peplomers (range: 12–24 nm) protrude from the viral surface [29]. These peplomers are responsible for the crown-like ("corona") appearance of the virus when visualized under the electron microscope, which led to the term *coronavirus*. The peplomer proteins are used for virus attachment to cellular surface proteins, which act as receptors for the virus. They are shaped so that they can bind specifically to topical enterocytes. Replication of nonmutated FCoV is thus primarily restricted to enterocytes. The mutated FIP-causing FCoV has a broader cell spectrum, including macrophages.

FCoV belongs to the same taxonomic cluster of coronaviruses as transmissible gastroenteritis virus (TGEV), porcine respiratory coronavirus, canine coronavirus (CCV) [16,30–32], and some human coronaviruses [33]. In many species of animals, coronaviruses have a relatively restricted organ tropism, mainly infecting respiratory or gastrointestinal cells [34]. In cats and mice, however, coronavirus infections can, under certain circumstances, involve several organs. Coronaviruses have a relatively low species specificity. CCV that can cause diarrhea in dogs is closely related to FCoV and can also infect cats. After contact with CCV-containing dog feces, cats develop antibodies that cross-react with FCoV. One CCV strain induced diarrhea in laboratory cats after experimental infection. In a cat infected with another CCV strain, histologic changes identical to changes typically seen in enteral FCoV infection were detected. In one study, CCV even caused FIP [35].

Depending on their antigenetic relation to CCV, FCoV strains can be classified into the subtypes serotype I and serotype II. Antibodies against CCV neutralize FCoV serotype II but not FCoV serotype I. FCoV serotype II strains are genetically more closely related to CCV than are FCoV serotype I strains, and FCoV serotype II strains seem to have arisen by recombination between FCoV serotype I strains and CCV [19,21,32]. Aside from the different degree of neutralization by antisera to CCV, serotypes I and II are different in their growth characteristics in cell culture and in their cytopathogenicity in vitro. FCoV serotype I strains are difficult to grow in cell culture and cause a slowly developing cytopathogenic effect. FCoV serotype II strains, however, grow more rapidly and produce a pronounced cytopathogenic effect [36]. Serotype I is the more prevalent serotype in field infections; between 70% and 95% of isolated FCoV strains in the field in the United States and Europe belong to serotype I. In Japan, however, serotype II predominates [19,37]. Most cats with FIP are infected with FCoV serotype I. Both serotypes can cause FIP, however, and both can cause clinically inapparent FCoV infections [38].

Epidemiology

FCoV and FIP are major problems in multiple-cat households and, to a much lesser extent, in free-roaming cats.

Prevalence

FCoV is distributed worldwide in household and wild cats [27,28]. The virus is endemic especially in environments in which many cats are kept together in a small space (eg, catteries, shelters, pet stores). There is virtually no multiple-cat household without endemic FCoV. At least 50% of cats in the United States and Europe have antibodies against coronaviruses. In Switzerland, 80% of breeding cats and 50% of free-roaming cats tested positive for antibodies. In Great Britain, 82% of show cats, 53% of cats in breeding institutions, and 15% of cats in single-cat households had antibodies [8,27]. FCoV is relatively rare in free-roaming ownerless cats because stray cats are usually loners without close contact with each other. Most importantly, they do not use the same locations for dumping their feces, which is the major route of transmission in multiple-cat households. In a study in Gainesville, Florida, 250 adult feral cats in a trap-neuter-return program were tested for antibodies to coronavirus; 88% of the sera were negative, confirming that most of these cats were not infected [39]. In another study, feral cats were tested at the time they were brought into local shelters (in which multiple cats were kept together) and at 1-to 2-week intervals thereafter. At the time of entering, only a small number of cats had antibodies (approximately 15%); the percentage, however, increased rapidly until virtually all cats in the shelters were infected with FCoV [40].

Although the prevalence of FCoV infection is high, only approximately 5% of cats in multiple-cat household situations develop FIP; the number is even lower in a single-cat environment [5,9,10]. The risk of developing FIP is higher for young and immune-compromised cats, because the replication of FCoV in these animals is less controlled, and the critical mutation is thus more likely to occur. More than half of the cats with FIP are younger than 12 months of age [41].

FCoV is also an important pathogen in nondomestic felids [42]. Kennedy et al [43] found evidence of FCoV infection in 195 of 342 investigated nondomestic felids in southern Africa, which included animals from wild populations and animals in captivity. There is also a high incidence of FIP in wild felids in captivity in the United States and Europe (eg, in zoos). Cheetahs are highly susceptible to development of FIP, and a genetic deficiency in their cellular immunity is thought to predispose them to the disease [44].

Transmission

Infection usually takes place oronasally.

Infection

Cats are usually infected with nonpathogenic FCoV through FCoV-containing feces shed by a cat with a harmless FCoV enteric infection or by a cat with FIP. Mutated FIP-causing FCoV has not been found in secretions or excretions of cats with FIP. Thus, transmission of the mutated FIP-causing FCoV is considered unlikely under natural circumstances. FIP-causing FCoV can, however, be transmitted iatrogenically or under experimental conditions if, for example, effusion from a cat with FIP containing infected macrophages is injected into a naive cat [45].

FCoV is a relatively fragile virus (inactivated at room temperature within 24 to 48 hours), but in dry conditions (eg, in carpet), it has been shown to survive for up to 7 weeks outside the cat [46]. Indirect fomite transmission is thus possible, and the virus can be transmitted through clothes, toys, and grooming tools. In organ homogenates, it is even resistant to repeated freezing at -70°C for many months. The virus is destroyed by most household disinfectants and detergents, however.

The most common mode of infection is through virus-containing feces. Thus, the major source of FCoV for uninfected cats is litter boxes shared with infected cats [47]. If multiple cats are using the same litter box, they readily infect each other. Continuous reinfection through the contaminated litter box of a cat already infected also seems to play an important role in the endemic survival of the virus. Rarely, virus can be transmitted through saliva, by mutual grooming, by sharing the same food bowl, or through close contact. Sneezed droplet transmission is also possible. Whether or not FCoV transmission occurs to a significant degree at cat shows is still a point of discussion. In one survey, attending cat shows seemed to be a factor of minor significance affecting the incidence of FIP [48], but in another survey, more than 80% of cats at shows in the United Kingdom were found to have antibodies [8]. Transmission by lice or fleas is considered unlikely [33]. Transplacental transmission can occur, because FIP was found in a 4-day-old kitten and in stillborn and weak newborn kittens born to a queen that had FIP during the later stages of pregnancy [26]. This mode of transmission is uncommon under natural circumstances, however. Most kittens that are removed from contact with adult virus-shedding cats at 5 to 6 weeks of age do not become infected [7]. Most commonly, kittens are infected at the age of 6 to 8 weeks, at a time when their maternal antibodies wane, mostly through contact with feces from their mothers or other FCoV-excreting cats.

Virus shedding

FCoV is shed mainly in the feces. In early infection, it may be found in saliva when the virus replicates in tonsils and, possibly, in respiratory secretions and urine [49,50]. It is likely that when naive cats in a multiple-cat household first encounter FCoV all become infected (and develop antibodies) and most probably shed virus for a period of weeks or months. With extremely sensitive reverse transcriptase (RT)–polymerase chain reaction (PCR) techniques, it has been shown that many naturally infected healthy carrier cats shed FCoV for at least up to 10 months [50]. Most cats shed virus intermittently, but some become chronic FCoV shedders for years to lifelong, providing a continuous source for reinfection of other cats [51]. Cats that are antibody-negative are unlikely to shed [51,52], whereas approximately one third of FCoV antibody–positive cats shed virus [10]. It has been shown that cats with high antibody titers are more likely to shed FCoV and to shed more consistently and higher amounts of the virus [51]. Thus, the height of the titer is directly correlated with virus replication and the amount of virus in the intestines. Most cats with FIP also shed (nonmutated) FCoV [53]; however, the virus load in feces seems to decrease after a cat has developed FIP [51].

Pathogenesis

Nonmutated FCoV replicates in enterocytes, causing asymptomatic infection or diarrhea, whereas mutated FCoV replicates in macrophages, leading to FIP. It was once believed that avirulent FCoV remained confined to the digestive tract, could not cross the gut mucosa, and was not spread beyond the intestinal epithelium and regional lymph nodes [12], whereas FIP-causing FCoV disseminated to other organs, most likely via bloodborne monocytes [54–56]. FCoV can be detected in the blood using RT-PCR, however, not only in cats with FIP but in healthy cats from households with endemic FCoV that never develop FIP [50,57–59], indicating that non-mutated FCoV may also cause viremia. It is likely that this viremia in cats that do not develop FIP may be only short term and low grade.

Pathogenesis of enteric feline coronavirus infection

After a cat becomes infected with FCoV by ingestion (or, rarely, by inhalation), the main site of viral replication is the intestinal epithelium. The specific receptor for FCoV (at least FCoV serotype I) is an enzyme, aminopeptidase-N, found in the intestinal brush border [60–62]. Replication of FCoV in the cytoplasm can cause destruction of intestinal epithelium cells. Cats may sometimes develop diarrhea, depending on the degree of virus replication. In many cats, infection persists over a long period without causing any clinical signs. These cats shed FCoV intermittently or continuously and act as a source of infection for other cats.

Pathogenesis of feline infectious peritonitis

FIP itself is not an infectious but a sporadic disease caused by a virus variant that has developed within a specific cat.

Occurrence of the mutation

FIP develops when there is a spontaneous mutation in a certain region of the FCoV genome (the genes 3C and 7B are being discussed as most important) [19]. Whenever FCoV infection exists, so does the potential for the development of FIP [11,63]. The critical mutation always occurs in those same genes, but the exact location varies. Comparison of the genome of the mutated virus with the parent virus revealed 99.5% homology [21,64,65]. The mutation leads to changes in the surface structures of the virus that allow the virus phagocytized by macrophages to bind to the ribosomes in these macrophages. Thus, this mutated virus, in contrast to its harmless relative, is all of a sudden able to replicate within macrophages; this is considered the key event in the pathogenesis of FIP.

Decreased suppression of the virus in the intestines by the immune system may allow for increased virus replication; this, in turn, predisposes the cat to FIP development through increased virus load, because increased virus replication makes the occurrence of a "virulent mutation" more likely [20,66]. Any factors that increase FCoV replication in the intestines increase the probability of the mutation to occur. These factors include physical characteristics (eg, young age and breed predisposition); immune status of the cat, which may be compromised by infections (eg, feline immunodeficiency virus [FIV] or FeLV infection); stress; glucocorticoid treatment; surgery as well as dosage and virulence of the virus; and the reinfection rate in multiple-cat households [66]. It is likely that kittens developing FIP do so because they are subjected to a large virus dose at a time of life when their still undeveloped immune systems are also coping with other infections and the stresses of vaccination, relocation, and neutering [11,66]. The question as to why one cat develops FIP and many others do not is a subject of intensive research. A recent study failed to detect a correlation between genetic differences in the feline leukocyte antigen complex (class II polymorphisms) and susceptibility to FIP [67].

Development of the disease

FIP is an immune complex disease involving virus or viral antigen, antiviral antibodies, and complement. It is not the virus itself that causes major damage but the cat's own immune reaction that leads to the fatal consequences. Within approximately 14 days after the mutation has occurred, mutated viruses that have been distributed by macrophages in the whole body, are found in the cecum, colon, intestinal lymph nodes, spleen, liver, and central nervous system (CNS). There are two possible explanations for the events occurring after viral dissemination from the intestines. The first proposed mechanism is that FCoV-infected macrophages leave the bloodstream and enable virus to enter the tissues. The virus attracts antibodies, complement is fixed, and more macrophages and neutrophils are attracted to the lesion [20]; as a consequence, typical granulomatous changes develop. The alternative explanation is that FIP occurs as a result of circulating immune complexes exiting from the circulation into blood vessel walls, fixing complement [68] and leading to the development of the granulomatous changes. It is assumed that these antigen antibody complexes are recognized by macrophages but are not, as they should be, presented to killer cells and thus are not destroyed. The consequences of the formation of immune complexes in cats depend on their size, antibody concentration, and antigen content. Immune complex deposition most likely occurs at sites of high blood pressure and turbulence, and such conditions occur at blood vessel bifurcations. FIP lesions are common in the peritoneum, kidney, and uvea, all of which are sites of high blood pressure and turbulence [26].

Not only virus but chemotactic substances, including complement and inflammatory mediators, are released from infected and dying macrophages. Complement fixation leads to the release of vasoactive amines, which causes endothelial cell retraction and thus increased vascular permeability. Retraction of capillary endothelial cells allows exudation of plasma proteins, hence the development of characteristic protein-rich exudates [36]. Inflammatory mediators activate proteolytic enzymes that cause tissue damage. The immune-mediated vasculitis leads to activation of the coagulatory system and to disseminated intravascular coagulation (DIC).

An imbalance in certain cytokines (eg, increase in tumor necrosis factor-α [TNFα], decrease in interferon-γ) can be found early in experimentally induced FIP [69–71]. Acute-phase proteins are altered in cats with FIP [72]. It has been suggested that increase of the acute-phase protein $α_1$-acid glycoprotein and changes in its glycosylation play a role in the pathogenesis of FIP [73]. The tissue distribution of the $α_1$-acid glycoprotein–related protein is, however, not dependent on the presence of FCoV, suggesting that this protein is not directly involved in the pathogenesis of FIP [74].

Antibody-dependent enhancement

In many infectious diseases, preexisting antibodies protect against subsequent challenge. In experimentally induced FIP, however, an enhanced form of disease may occur in cats that already have preexisting antibodies [75–79]. The proposed mechanism of this so-called "antibody-dependent enhancement" (ADE) is that antibodies facilitate the uptake of FCoV into macrophages [18,80–83]. Because of ADE, a higher proportion of antibody-positive cats died compared with antibody-negative controls, and the antibody-positive cats developed disease earlier (12 days compared with 28 days or more for controls) [78]. These findings have complicated the search for an effective and safe vaccine, because ADE occurred after vaccination in many vaccine experiments. ADE does not seem to play a major role in the field, however. Antibody-positive pet cats that were naturally reinfected by FCoV showed no evidence of ADE [26].

Clinical findings

The clinical signs totally depend on whether the "virulent mutation" occurs or not.

Feline coronavirus infection

After initial FCoV infection, there may be a short episode of upper respiratory tract signs, although these signs are usually not severe enough to warrant veterinary attention [26]. FCoV infection can cause a transient and clinically mild diarrhea or vomiting [20] as a result of replication of FCoV in enterocytes. Kittens infected with FCoV generally more commonly develop diarrhea, sometimes have a history of stunted growth, and occasionally have upper respiratory tract signs [7]. Rarely, the virus can be responsible for severe acute or chronic vomiting or diarrhea with weight loss, which may be unresponsive to treatment and continue for months. Most FCoV-infected cats, however, are asymptomatic.

Feline infectious peritonitis

Clinical signs of FIP can be variable, because many organs, including the liver, kidneys, pancreas, and eyes, as well as the CNS can be involved. The clinical signs and pathologic findings that occur in FIP are a direct consequence of the vasculitis and organ failure resulting from damage to the blood vessels that supply them. In all cats with nonspecific clinical signs, such as chronic weight loss or fever of unknown origin resistant to antibiotic treatment or recurrent in nature, FIP should be on the list of differential diagnoses.

In the case of natural infection, the exact duration of time between mutation and development of clinical signs is unknown and almost certainly depends on the immune system of the individual cat. Most likely, the disease becomes apparent a few weeks to 2 years after the mutation has occurred. The time between infection with "harmless" FCoV and the development of FIP is even more unpredictable and depends on the event of spontaneous mutation. It has been shown that cats are at greatest risk of developing FIP in the first 6 to 18 months after infection with FCoV and that the risk falls to approximately 4% at 36 months after infection [11].

Three different forms of FIP have been identified: (1) an effusive, exudative, wet form; (2) a noneffusive, nonexudative, dry, granulomatous, parenchymatous form; and (3) a mixed form. The first form is characterized by a fibrinous peritonitis, pleuritis, or pericarditis with effusions in the abdomen, thorax, and/or pericardium, respectively. The second form without obvious effusions is characterized by granulomatous changes in different organs, including the eyes, as well as the CNS. In the meantime, it has been shown that differentiation between these forms is not useful (and is only of value for the diagnostic approach), because there is always effusion to a greater or lesser degree in combination with more or less granulomatous organ changes present in each cat with FIP. In addition, the forms can transform into each other. FIP can thus simply be more or less exudative or productive in a certain cat at a given time point.

Effusions

Many cats with FIP develop effusions. Cats with effusions have ascites (Fig. 1), thoracic effusions, and/or pericardial effusion. In a survey of 390 cats with FIP with effusions, 62% had ascites, 17% had thoracic effusions, and 21% had effusions in both body cavities [41]. Nevertheless, it is important to consider that of all cats with effusions, less than 50% actually have FIP. In a study including 197 cats with effusions caused by various reasons, approximately 30% of cats with thoracic effusions and 30% of cats with both abdominal and thoracic effusions had FIP. Of the cats with ascites, approximately 60% had FIP [84].

In cats with ascites, an abdominal swelling is commonly noticed by the owner and sometimes may be confused with pregnancy. Fluctuation and a fluid wave may be present; in less severe cases, fluid can be palpated between the intestinal loops. Abdominal masses may sometimes be palpated, reflecting omental and visceral adhesion or enlarged mesenteric

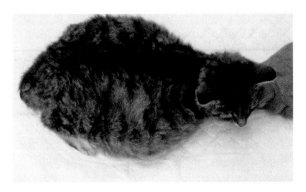

Fig. 1. Cat with ascites caused by FIP.

lymph nodes. Thoracic effusions usually manifest in dyspnea and tachypnea, and sometimes in open-mouth breathing and cyanotic mucous membranes. Auscultation reveals muffled heart sounds [84]. Pericardial effusions may be present in addition to or without other effusions. In these cats, heart sounds are muffled and typical changes can be seen on EKG and echocardiography. In one survey, FIP accounted for 14% of cats with pericardial effusion, second to congestive heart failure (28%) [85].

Some cats with effusions may be bright and alert, whereas others are depressed. Some of these cats eat with a normal or even increased appetite, whereas others are anorectic. Some cats have a fever, and some show weight loss. Signs of organ failure can be present in addition to the effusion (eg, icterus). Effusions can be visualized by diagnostic imaging (eg, radiographs, ultrasound). Their presence is verified by tapping the fluid.

Changes in abdominal and thoracic organs

In cats without effusion, signs are often vague and include fever, weight loss, lethargy, and decreased appetite. Cats may be icteric. If the lungs are involved, cats may be dyspneic and thoracic radiographs may reveal patchy densities in the lungs [86]. Abdominal palpation may reveal enlarged mesenteric lymph nodes and irregular kidneys or nodular irregularities in other viscera. Presenting clinical signs can be unusual. In some cats, abdominal tumors are suspected, but FIP is finally diagnosed at necropsy [87]. Other cats are presented with only gastrointestinal obstruction [88]. In one case report, a cat suffered from necrotizing orchitis because of FIP but had no other signs [89]. Although believed to be so in the 1970s, reproductive disorders, neonatal deaths, and fading of kittens are not usually associated with FIP [26].

Sometimes, the main or only organ affected by granulomatous changes is the intestine. Lesions are commonly found only in the ileocecocolic junction but may also be present in other areas (eg, colon or small intestine). Cats may have a variety of clinical signs as a result of these lesions, most commonly chronic diarrhea but sometimes vomiting. Obstipation can also occur [26,90,91]. Palpation of the abdomen often reveals a thickened intestinal area. Hematology sometimes shows increased numbers of Heinz bodies, which is a result of decreased absorption of vitamin B_{12}.

Ocular changes

Cats with FIP frequently have ocular lesions. The most common but not obvious ocular lesions are retinal changes. Therefore, a retinal examination should be performed in all cats in which FIP is suspected. FIP can cause cuffing of the retinal vasculature, which appears as fuzzy grayish lines on either side of the blood vessels. Occasionally, granulomatous changes are seen on the retina [26]. Retinal hemorrhage or detachment may also occur. The changes, however, are not pathognomonic. Similar changes can be seen in other systemic infectious diseases, including toxoplasmosis, systemic fungus infections and FIV and FeLV infection.

Another common manifestation is uveitis (Fig. 2) [92]. Uveitis is an inflammation of the uveal coat of the eye, which consists of the iris, ciliary body, and choroidal vessels. The uveal coat can be seeded by immunologically competent cells that migrate into the eye. The eye can thus undergo all types of immunologically mediated inflammation [93]. Mild uveitis can manifest as color change of the iris. Usually, part of or all the iris becomes brown, although blue eyes occasionally appear to be green. Uveitis may also manifest as aqueous flare, with cloudiness of the anterior chamber, which can sometimes be detected only in a darkened room using focal illumination. Large numbers of inflammatory cells in the anterior chamber settle out on the back of the cornea and cause keratic precipitates, which may be hidden by the nictitating membrane. In some cats, there is hemorrhage into the anterior chamber. If aqueous humor is tapped, it may reveal elevated protein and pleocytosis [26].

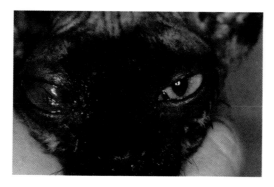

Fig. 2. Cat with uveitis caused by FIP.

Neurologic signs

FIP is a common reason for neurologic disorders in cats. In a retrospective study of 286 cats with neurologic signs, more than half of the cats (47) in the largest disease category (inflammatory diseases) had FIP [94]. Of all cats with FIP, approximately 13% have neurologic signs [95]. These are variable and reflect the area of CNS involvement. Usually, the lesions are multifocal [96]. The most common clinical sign is ataxia, followed by nystagmus and seizures [97]. In addition, incoordination, intention tremors, hyperesthesia, behavioral changes, and cranial nerve defects can be seen [98,99]. If cranial nerves are involved, neurologic signs like visual deficits and loss of menace reflex may be present, depending on which cranial nerve is damaged. When the FIP lesion is located on a peripheral nerve or the spinal column, lameness, progressive ataxia, tetraparesis, hemiparesis, or paraparesis may be observed [26]. In a study of 24 cats with FIP with neurologic involvement, 75% were found to have hydrocephalus on postmortem examination. Finding hydrocephalus on a CT scan is suggestive of neurologic FIP, because other diseases, such as cryptococcosis, toxoplasmosis, and lymphoma, have not been reported to cause these findings [97].

Diagnosis

Diagnosing enteral FCoV can be performed by RT-PCR in feces [51,100] or by electron microscopy of fecal samples. Intestinal biopsies are of limited value, because the histopathologic features of villus tip ulceration, stunting, and fusion are nonspecific [26]. FCoV infection as the cause of diarrhea can only be confirmed if immunohistochemical or immunofluorescent staining of intestinal biopsies is positive.

Definitively diagnosing FIP antemortem can be extremely challenging in many clinical cases. FIP is often misdiagnosed [29]. Many times, its general clinical signs (eg, chronic fever, weight loss, anorexia, malaise) are nonspecific. A fast and reliable diagnosis would be critical for prognostic reasons and to avoid suffering of the patient. Difficulties in definitively diagnosing FIP, however, arise from unspecific clinical signs; lack of pathognomonic, hematologic, and biochemical abnormalities; and low sensitivity and specificity of tests routinely used in practice. The diagnostic value of frequently used parameters is only known in experimental settings, and some tests have not been widely used in clinical patients. A weighted score system for FIP diagnosis that takes several parameters into account, including background of the cat, history, presence of clinical signs, laboratory changes, and height of antibody titers, has been suggested [95]. This, however, only leads to a certain score or percentage of likelihood of FIP, and thus does not help to confirm the diagnosis definitively. There are, however, certain tests available in the meantime (eg, staining of antigen in macrophages in effusion or tissue) that, at least in the case of a positive result, confirm the diagnosis of FIP 100% [101].

Laboratory changes

There are a number of laboratory changes that are common in cats with FIP; they are not pathognomonic, however, and FIP cannot be diagnosed based on these findings.

Complete blood cell counts and coagulation parameters

Blood cell counts are often changed in cats with FIP [102,103]; however, changes are not pathognomonic. White blood cells can be decreased or increased. Although it is often stated that lymphopenia and neutrophilia are typical for FIP, this change can be interpreted as a typical "stress leukogram" that occurs in many severe systemic diseases in cats [101]. In up to 65% of cats with FIP, anemia is present, usually with only a mild decrease in hematocrit. The anemia can be regenerative; in these cases, it is caused mainly by a secondary autoimmune hemolytic anemia (AIHA) in which autoantibodies to erythrocytes can be found and Coomb's test results are positive. In cats with severe intestinal changes, Heinz bodies can be found in large numbers in erythrocytes [26], and this can also lead to hemolysis. Alternatively, anemia can be nonregenerative and is then mainly caused by anemia associated with chronic inflammation [41]. Approximately 50% of cats with FIP have nonspecific reactive changes of the bone marrow at necropsy [104]. Thrombocytopenia can commonly be found in cats with FIP as a result of DIC. In experimental infection, thrombocytopenia was detected as early as 4 days after infection [105]. Other parameters indicating DIC, including fibrinogen degradation products (FDPs) and D-dimers, are also commonly increased.

Serum chemistry

The most consistent laboratory finding in cats with FIP is an increase in total serum protein concentration [41,101,106]. This is found in approximately 50% of cats with effusion and 70% of cats without effusion [107]. This increase in total protein is caused by increased globulins, mainly γ-globulins, also leading to a decrease in the albumin-to-globulin ratio [101,108,109]. In experimental infections, an early increase of α_2-globulins was reported [49], whereas γ-globulins and antibody titers increase just before the appearance of clinical signs [5,49,69,77]. The characteristically high levels of γ-globulins [110,111] and the increased antibody titers [5,112] invite the conclusion that hypergammaglobulinemia is caused by a specific anti-FCoV immune response. Antibody titers and hypergammaglobulinemia show a linear correlation, but the wide variation in anti-FCoV titers at a given concentration of γ-globulins indicates that additional (autoimmune) reactions occur during the pathogenesis of FIP [113,114]. It has been discussed that stimulation of B cells by interleukin-6, which is produced as part of the disease process, additionally contributes to the increase in γ-globulins [115]. Total protein in cats with FIP can reach high concentrations of up to 12 g/dL (120 g/L) and more. This, however, only reflects the chronic antigenic stimulation that generally can be caused by any chronic infection the cat is not able to clear through its immune response. Even if the serum total protein concentration is 120 g/L or greater, the likelihood of FIP is only 90%. Cats with these high serum protein concentrations that do not have FIP may suffer from severe chronic stomatitis, chronic upper respiratory disease, dirofilariasis, or multiple myeloma [101].

In a recent study of cats with FIP, comparison of total serum protein concentration, γ-globulins, and the albumin-to-globulin ratio revealed that the albumin-to-globulin ratio has a statistically significantly better diagnostic value than the other two parameters [101]. Thus, not only the increase in globulins but the decrease in albumin concentrations seems to be characteristic of FIP. A decrease in serum albumin occurs through decreased production because of liver failure or through protein loss. Protein loss can be attributed to glomerulopathy caused by immune complex deposition, loss of protein caused by exudative enteropathy in case of granulomatous changes in the intestines, or loss of protein-rich fluid in vasculitis. It can also be explained by decreased production in the liver (without compromised liver function), because not only albumin but globulins contribute (although not as importantly) to the plasma oncotic pressure. Thus, an increase in globulins may cause a negative feedback on albumin production in the liver. An optimum cutoff value (maximum efficiency) of 0.8 was determined for the albumin-to-globulin ratio. If the serum albumin-to-globulin ratio is less than 0.8, the probability that the cat has FIP is high (92% positive predictive value); if the albumin-to-globulin ratio is higher than 0.8, the cat likely does not have FIP (61% negative predictive value) [101].

Electrophoresis is often performed, and the rational behind it is to quantify γ-globulins and to distinguish a polyclonal from a monoclonal hypergammaglobulinemia so as to differentiate FIP (and other chronic infections) from tumors like multiple myelomas or other plasma cell tumors. Quantification of γ-globulins is not more useful than measurement of total proteins [101], however. In addition, polyclonal and monoclonal hypergammaglobulinemia can occur in cats with FIP, and the same is true in multiple myeloma. Thus, the value of electrophoresis is limited.

Other laboratory parameters (eg, liver enzymes, bilirubin, urea, creatinine) can be variably increased depending on the degree and localization of organ damage [116,117], but they are not helpful in making an etiologic diagnosis. Hyperbilirubinemia and icterus are often observed and are frequently a reflection of hepatic necrosis, despite the fact that alkaline phosphatase (ALP) and alanine aminotransferase (ALT) activities are often not increased as dramatically as they are with other liver diseases, such as cholangiohepatitis and hepatic lipidosis [26]. Hyperbilirubinemia is caused rarely by hemolysis as a result of secondary AIHA; however, the hemolysis has to be severe to cause icterus. Bilirubin is sometimes increased in cats with FIP without evidence of hemolysis, liver disease, or cholestasis. It has been speculated that the bilirubin metabolism and excretion into the biliary system are compromised in cats with FIP, similar to the findings in sepsis.

Measurement of α_1-acid glycoprotein may be helpful in the diagnosis of FIP [118]. This acute-phase protein is increased in several infectious diseases of cats, and thus is not specific for FIP. Nevertheless, α_1-acid glycoprotein levels in plasma (or effusion) are usually greater than 1500 µg/mL in cats with FIP, which may help to distinguish FIP from other clinically similar conditions [26].

Tests on effusion fluid

If there is effusion, the most important diagnostic step is to sample the fluid, because tests of effusion have a much higher diagnostic value than tests performed using blood. Thus, fluid should be collected before blood is taken to avoid a waste of money with expensive blood tests. Only approximately half of the cats with effusions suffer from FIP [84]. Thus, although effusions of a clear yellow color and sticky consistency are often called "typical," the presence of this type of fluid in body cavities alone is not diagnostic (Fig. 3). The effusion in FIP may be clear, straw-colored, or viscous and may froth on shaking because of the high protein content. The effusion may clot when stored refrigerated [26]. If the sample is bloody, pus filled, or foul smelling or is chylus, FIP is less likely [95], although effusions in FIP can be different and sometimes red, pink, or almost colorless in appearance. Some cases of cats with FIP with pure chylus effusion have even been reported [119].

The effusion in FIP is usually classified as a modified transudate or exudate typically combining characteristics of both transudates and exudates. The protein content is usually high (>35 g/L), reflecting the composition of the serum, whereas the cellular content is low and approaches that of a pure transudate (<1000 nucleated cells per milliliter). The protein content of effusion is high because of the high concentration of γ-globulins. Other diseases causing similar effusions include lymphoma, heart failure, cholangiohepatitis, and bacterial peritonitis or pleuritis.

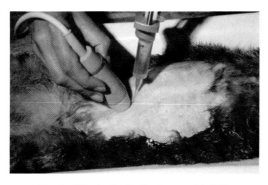

Fig. 3. "Typical" effusion in cat with FIP.

Measurement of enzyme activity in effusion also is an indication that FIP might be the underlying disease. Lactate dehydrogenase (LDH) is typically high (>300 IU/L) in effusions caused by FIP because it is released from inflammatory cells. Activity of α-amylase also is often high, likely as a result of common pancreatic involvement. The enzyme adenosine deaminase (AD) has been used to distinguish different causes of effusions, and its activity was significantly high in cats with FIP [120].

Cytologic evaluation of effusion in cats with FIP typically shows a pyogranulomatous character, predominantly with macrophages and neutrophils (Fig. 4). Cytologic findings may appear similar in cats with bacterial serositis or, sometimes, with lymphoma; these effusions often can be differentiated, however, by the presence of malignant cells or bacteria, respectively. Bacterial cultures should be performed in unclear cases.

A simple test, the so-called "Rivalta's test," (Fig. 5) has been used to differentiate transudates from exudates. This test was originally developed by an Italian researcher named Rivalta around 1900 and was used to differentiate transudates and exudates in human patients [121]. Other methods have replaced this test in human medicine because of its limited diagnostic value in people. It has not been shown to be diagnostically helpful in dogs with effusion [122]. Nevertheless, this test seems to be useful in cats to differentiate between effusions caused by FIP and effusions caused by other diseases [101]. It is not only the high protein content but the high concentrations of fibrin and inflammatory mediators that induce a positive reaction. To perform this test, three quarters of a reagent tube is filled with distilled water, to which one drop of acetic acid (98%) is added and is mixed thoroughly. On the surface of this solution, one drop of the effusion fluid is carefully layered. If the drop disappears and the solution remains clear, the Rivalta's test result is defined as negative. If the drop retains its shape, stays attached to the surface, or slowly floats down to the bottom of the tube (drop-like or jellyfish-like), the Rivalta's test result is defined as positive. In

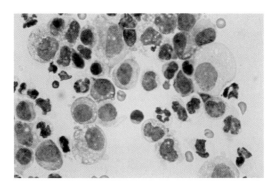

Fig. 4. Typical cytology of the effusion in a cat with FIP.

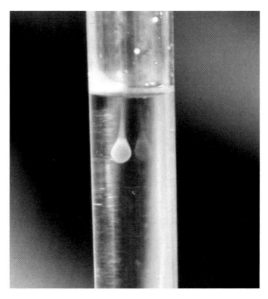

Fig. 5. Positive Rivalta's test in a cat with FIP.

a recent study, the Rivalta's test had a positive predictive value of 86% and a negative predictive value of 97% [101]. There are some false-positive results in cats with bacterial peritonitis. Those effusions, however, are usually easy to differentiate (through macroscopic examination, cytology, and bacterial culture). Some cats with lymphoma also have a positive Rivalta's test result, but many of these cases can be differentiated cytologically [101]. Overall, the Rivalta's test is an easy and inexpensive method that does not require special laboratory equipment and can be easily performed in private practice. It provides good predictive values, and thus is a helpful diagnostic test.

Tests on cerebrospinal fluid

Analysis of cerebrospinal fluid (CSF) from cats with neurologic signs caused by FIP lesions may reveal elevated protein (50–350 mg/dL, with a normal value of less than 25 mg/dL) and pleocytosis (100–10,000 nucleated cells per milliliter) containing mainly neutrophils, lymphocytes, and macrophages [97,123,124], which is a relatively nonspecific finding, however. Many cats with FIP and neurologic signs have normal CSF taps.

Measurement of antibodies

Antibody titers measured in serum are an extensively used diagnostic tool [6,125]. In view of the facts that a large percentage of the healthy cat population is FCoV antibody–positive, that high and rising titers are frequently found in asymptomatic cats, and that most of those cats never develop FIP [126], antibody titers must be interpreted extremely cautiously [7,10,127,128]. From the time when the first "FIP test" was described more than two decades ago [9] to the present, the inadequacies and pitfalls of the test have been the topic of continuous discussion and controversy. Meanwhile, the so-called "FIP test" is referred to as the "feline coronavirus antibody test," emphasizing that the latter more correctly describes the antibodies that are detected and react with a large group of closely related coronaviruses. At times, clinicians have mistakenly taken a positive titer to equate with a diagnosis of FIP, and it has been assumed that more cats have died of FCoV antibody tests than of FIP [77]. FCoV tests are often performed for inappropriate reasons. There are five major indications to test for FCoV antibodies: (1) for the diagnosis of FCoV-induced enteritis or to narrow the diagnosis of FIP, (2) for a healthy cat that has had contact with a suspected or known excretor of FCoV, (3) for a cat-breeding facility with the aim of obtaining an FCoV-free environment, (4) to screen a cattery for the presence of FCoV, and (5) to screen a cat for introduction into a FCoV-free cattery [26].

Antibodies in blood

Although frequently criticized, antibody testing has a certain role in the diagnosis and, more importantly, in the management of FCoV infection when it is performed by appropriate methodologies and results are properly interpreted. Antibody testing can only be useful if the laboratory is reliable and consistent. Methodologies and antibody titer results may vary significantly. A single serum sample divided and sent to five different laboratories in the United States yielded five different results [26]. The antigen used in a test, for example, can play an important role in test sensitivity and specificity (eg, if the antigen used for the test is derived from nonfeline viruses, which is practiced by many commercial laboratories). Thus, it is essential that antibody results that are interpreted and compared by the clinician are always obtained with the same method performed by the same laboratory, and it is essential to use antibody tests validated by the scientific community. Evaluating titers of antibodies gives an idea of the amount of antibodies present. In contrast, tests (eg, in-house tests) that only indicate the presence of antibodies without quantification are not useful. They also produce a high number of false-positive and false-negative results [129]. The choice of the laboratory to be used is critical, and only those that perform quantitative titer evaluations should be used. The laboratory should have established two levels: one is its least significant level of reactivity (or lowest positive titer), and the other is its highest antibody titer value. In searching for a reliable laboratory, repeat samples from the same animal should be sent without warning to the same laboratory and to an FCoV-referenced laboratory for comparison to enable useful interpretation. Serum or plasma samples store well at $-20°C$ without loss of antibody concentration [26].

The presence of antibodies does not indicate FIP, and the absence of antibodies does not exclude FIP. Many authors agree that low or medium titers do not have any diagnostic value [101,130,131]. Approximately 10% of the cats with clinically manifest FIP have negative results. It has been shown that in cats with fulminant FIP, titers decrease terminally [77]. Cats with effusions sometimes have low titers or even no antibodies. This is because large amounts of virus in the cat's body bind to antibodies and render them unavailable to bind antigen in the antibody test or because the antibodies are lost in effusion when protein is translocated in vasculitis. Extremely high titers are of a certain diagnostic value. If the highest measurable titer is present in a cat (thus, it is important to know what the highest titer in a specific laboratory is), it increases the likelihood of FIP. In a recent study, the probability of FIP was 94% in cats with the highest titer when investigating a cat population in which FIP was suspected [101]. The diagnostic value of a high titer is also dependent on the background of the cat. The highest titer in a cat coming out of a multiple-cat household situation is not extremely predictive, because in those households, FCoV is endemic and many cats have high titers, whereas the highest titer in a cat from a single-cat environment is unusual and a stronger indicator of FIP.

Although antibody testing in sick cats that are suspected to have FIP is of limited value, there are a number of other situations in which antibody testing is a useful tool. A healthy cat that has no antibodies is considered likely to be free of FCoV, and thus is not infectious to others, does not shed FCoV, and does not develop FIP [10]. It has been shown that the height of the antibody titer directly correlates with the amount of virus that is shed with feces; cats with high antibody titers are more likely to shed FCoV and to shed more consistently with higher amounts of the virus [51]. Thus, height of the titer is directly correlated with the virus replication rate and the amount of virus in the intestines. Antibody measurement is important for the common situation in practice in which a cat is presented because it has been in contact with a cat with FIP or a suspected or known virus excretor. The owner wants to know the prognosis for an exposed cat or wishes to obtain another cat and needs to know whether the exposed cat is shedding FCoV. Also, cat breeders may request testing, with the goal of creating an FCoV-free cattery. Screening a cattery for the presence of FCoV and screening a cat before introduction into an FCoV-free cattery are also important indications.

Antibodies in effusion

Some studies have evaluated the diagnostic value of antibody detection in fluids other than serum, such as in effusions [132]. The presence of antibodies in effusion is correlated with the presence of antibodies in blood [133]. In a study by Kennedy et al [132], antibody titers in effusions were not helpful, because all cats in their study had medium antibody titers irrespective of whether they had FIP or not. In a study by Hartmann et al [101], however, the presence of anti-FCoV antibodies in effusion had a high positive predictive value (90%) and a high negative predictive value (79%), although height of titers was not correlated with the presence of FIP. The measurement of antibodies in effusions is at least more useful than the measurement of antibodies in blood.

Antibodies in cerebrospinal fluid

Foley et al [134] determined the diagnostic value of antibody detection in CSF and found a good correlation to the presence of FIP when compared with histopathologic findings, whereas in a study by Boettcher et al [135], there was no significant difference in antibody titers in CSF from cats with neurologic signs caused by FIP compared with cats with other neurologic diseases confirmed by histopathologic findings.

Polymerase chain reaction

Compared with serology, RT-PCR provides the obvious advantage of directly detecting the ongoing infection rather than documenting a previous immune system encounter with a coronavirus.

Polymerase chain reaction in blood

RT-PCR can be performed to reverse-transcribe coronavirus RNA to cDNA and then to make large quantities of DNA visually detectable. Although FIP-causing viruses are genetic mutants of harmless enteric FCoV, numerous sites exist in the 3C and 7B genes that can be mutated or deleted and confer on the virus the capability to infect and replicate within macrophages. Sometimes, the change can be a single RNA base. As a result, PCR primers to discriminate between FIP-causing viruses and harmless enteric FCoV cannot be designed, and it is not possible to distinguish between a mutated and nonmutated virus by PCR [136]. There are a number of reasons why RT-PCR results are not always easy to interpret. There are several plausible explanations for false-negative PCR results. The assay requires reverse transcription of viral RNA to DNA before amplification of DNA, and degradation of RNA could be a potential problem, because RNases are virtually ubiquitous. There may be sufficient strain and nucleotide sequence variation such that the target sequence chosen for the assay may not detect all strains of FIPV [19]. There are also a number of explanations for false-positive results. First, the assay does not distinguish between "virulent" and "avirulent" FCoV strains, nor does it differentiate FCoV from CCV or TGEV. Although the role of these viruses in the field is unknown, cats can be experimentally infected with CCV and TGEV [35,137,138]; these infections could result in a positive PCR result. Second, recent studies support the hypothesis that viremia occurs not only in cats with FIP but in healthy carriers. FCoV RNA could be detected in the blood of cats with FIP as well as in the blood of healthy cats that did not develop FIP for a period of up to 70 months [50,57,58,136,139]. In a study by Gunn-

Moore et al [59], it was shown that in households in which FCoV is endemic, up to 80% of the cats can be viremic, irrespective of their health status, and that the presence of viremia does not seem to predispose the cats to the development of FIP. Therefore, the results of PCR tests must be interpreted in conjunction with other clinical findings and cannot be used as the sole criterion for diagnosing FIP.

Polymerase chain reaction in effusion

RT-PCR in effusion has been discussed as an interesting diagnostic tool. Data on the usefulness of this approach are limited, however. So far, only one study including information about RT-PCR on ascites fluid of a limited number of cats has been reported. In this study, six of six cats with confirmed FIP had positive RT-PCR results, and one of one cat with ascites caused by another disease had a negative RT-PCR result [101]. These numbers are, however, not sufficient to judge that approach sufficiently.

Polymerase chain reaction in cerebrospinal fluid

CSF has not been recommended for RT-PCR because it may contain low numbers of virus also in cats that do not have FIP if the blood-brain barrier is compromised. Accurate studies are needed, however.

Polymerase chain reaction in feces

RT-PCR has been used to detect FCoV in fecal samples and is sensitive and useful for documenting that a cat is shedding FCoV in feces [100]. Because cats vary in how much FCoV is shed in feces, repeated PCR should be performed daily over 4 to 5 days to detect accurately whether a given cat is shedding FCoV. Samples for RT-PCR must be carefully handled, kept frozen, and protected from RNA-degrading enzymes (which are ubiquitous in most environments). PCR should be performed as quickly as possible after collection, even if samples are frozen; delays in testing may result in false-negative results. Positive RT-PCR results in fecal samples document FCoV infection. The strength of the PCR signal in feces correlates with the amount of virus present in the intestines [51].

Antibody antigen complex detection

Because FIP is an immune-mediated disease and antibody antigen complexes play an important role, it has been suggested to look for circulating complexes in serum and effusions [113,140]. Antibody antigen complex detection can be performed using a competitive ELISA. Usefulness, however, is limited; the positive predictive value of the test was not high (67%) in one study, because there were many false-positive results [101].

Antigen detection

Other methods to detect the virus include searching for the presence of FCoV antigen (Fig. 6).

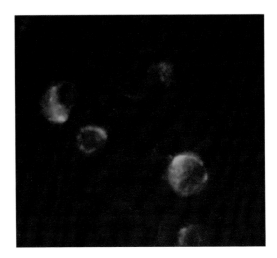

Fig. 6. Immunofluorescent staining of macrophages.

Immunofluorescence staining of feline coronavirus antigen in effusion

In a study by Parodi et al [141], an immunofluorescence assay detecting intracellular FCoV antigen in cells within effusion was used; however, the number of cats enrolled in that study was limited. Hirschberger et al [84] detected FCoV antigen in 34 of 34 samples from cats with FIP-induced effusions. In a recent study involving a large number of cats, immunofluorescence staining of intracellular FCoV antigen in macrophages of effusion had a positive predictive value of 100%. There were no false-positive results. This means that if this staining test is positive, it predicts 100% that the cat has FIP. Unfortunately, the negative predictive value was not high (57%). Cases that stained negative (although the cats did have FIP) can be explained by the fact that the number of macrophages on the effusion smear is sometimes insufficient. Another explanation is a potential masking of the antigen by competitive binding of FCoV antibodies in effusion that displace binding of fluorescence antibodies [101].

Antigen in tissue

Immunohistochemistry can also be used to detect the expression of FCoV antigen in tissue [142]. Tammer et al [143] used immunohistochemistry to detect intracellular FCoV antigen in paraffin-embedded tissues of euthanized cats and found FCoV antigen only in macrophages of cats that had FIP and not in control cats. Hök [144] was able to demonstrate FCoV antigen in the membrana nictitans of cats with FIP. It was shown that positive staining of macrophages in effusion predicts FIP 100% [101]; the same seems to be true for immunohistochemical staining of tissue macrophages. Immunostaining cannot differentiate between the "harmless" nonmutated FCoV and the mutated FIP-causing FCoV. Obviously, only FIP-causing virus is able to replicate in sufficiently large amounts in macrophages, which results in positive staining. Therefore, in addition to histopathology (if pathognomonic lesions are present), detection of intracellular FCoV antigen by immunofluorescence or immunohistochemistry is the only way to diagnose FIP definitively. This tool should be used whenever possible.

Histology

Diagnosis of FIP can be established in many cases with just histopathologic testing of biopsy or necropsy samples. Hematoxylin and eosin–stained samples typically contain localized perivascular mixed inflammation with macrophages, neutrophils, lymphocytes, and plasma cells. Pyogranulomas may be large and consolidated, sometimes with focal tissue necrosis, or numerous and small. Lymphoid tissues in cats with FIP often show lymphoid depletion caused by apoptosis [26,145,146]. If histologic testing is not diagnostic, staining of antigen in macrophages [146] or detection of nucleic acids in tissue [147] can be used to confirm FIP (Fig. 7).

Therapy

Virtually every cat with confirmed FIP dies. Fast and reliable diagnosis of FIP and differentiating it from harmless enteric FCoV infection are crucial for prognostic reasons.

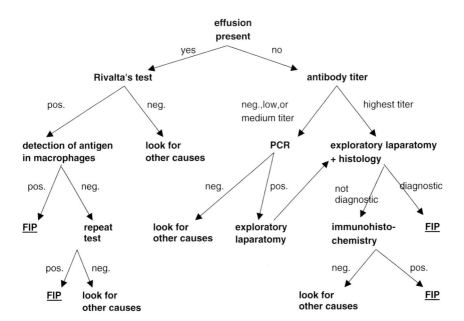

Fig. 7. Algorithm for the diagnosis of FIP.

Treatment of healthy feline coronavirus antibody–positive cats

There is no indication that any treatment of a healthy antibody-positive cat would prevent development of FIP [26]. Treatment with corticosteroids can conceivably prevent clinical signs from occurring (once the mutation has occurred) for a certain period of time, but immune suppression might have the opposite effect and precipitate clinical FIP because it can increase the risk of mutation (if the mutation has not occurred yet). Thus, immune suppression is contraindicated as long as the cat is only infected with harmless FCoV. Because stress is an important factor in the development of FIP [95], avoidance of unnecessary stress, such as rehoming, elective surgery, or placement in a boarding cattery, may be beneficial. IFNs (eg, feline IFN-ω, which is available commercially in Europe and Japan) have been discussed in this situation, but controlled studies are missing to date.

Treatment of cats with feline coronavirus–induced enteritis

Most cases of diarrhea caused by nonmutated FCoV are self-limiting. Cats with chronic diarrhea that have antibodies against FCoV, in which other possible causes have been eliminated or in which FCoV has been detected in the feces by electron microscopy, can only be treated supportively with fluid and electrolyte replacement and dietary intervention [20]. Treatment with lactulose or living natural yogurt may be beneficial because it regulates the intestinal bacterial flora and increases passage time. No specific antiviral treatment has yet been demonstrated to cure this condition. These cases can be a challenge because they are sometimes difficult to distinguish from cats with FIP, which can manifest solely as granulomatous changes in the intestines leading to diarrhea. FIP diarrhea can only be treated with immune suppression if it is identified, which, conversely, is contraindicated in harmless FCoV infection. In both cases, cats usually have antibodies and sometimes high titers but can only be differentiated by exploratory surgery, which should be avoided in cats with harmless intestinal FCoV infection.

Symptomatic treatment of cats with feline infectious peritonitis

Treatment for FIP is almost invariably doomed to failure, because cats with clinical FIP eventually die. Some cats with milder clinical signs may survive for several months and enjoy some quality of life with treatment, however. Once clinical signs become debilitating and weight and appetite decline, the owner must be prepared for the reality that the cat is dying.

Because FIP is an immune-mediated disease, treatment is aimed at controlling the immune response to FCoV, and the most successful treatments consist of relatively high doses of immunosuppressive and anti-inflammatory drugs. Immunosuppressive drugs, such as prednisone (4 mg/kg administered orally every 24 hours) or cyclophosphamide (2.5 mg/kg administered orally for four consecutive days every week), may slow disease progression but do not produce a cure. Some cats with effusion benefit from tapping and removal of the fluid and injection of dexamethasone (1 mg/kg) into the abdominal or thoracic cavity (every 24 hours until no effusion is produced anymore). Cats with FIP should also be treated with broad-spectrum antibiotics and supportive therapy (eg, subcutaneous fluids) for as long as they are comfortable. A thromboxane synthetase inhibitor (ozagrel hydrochloride), which inhibits platelet aggregation, has been used in a few cats and has led to some improvement of clinical signs [148].

Some veterinarians prescribe immune modulators (eg, *Propionibacterium acnes*, acemannan) to treat cats with FIP, with no documented controlled evidence of efficacy. Immune modulators and IFN inducers are widely used and induce synthesis of IFNs and other cytokines. It has been suggested that these agents may benefit infected animals by restoring compromised immune function, thereby allowing the patient to control viral burden and recover from the disease. Nonspecific stimulation of the immune system is contra-indicated however in cats with FIP, because clinical signs develop and progress as a result of an immune-mediated response to the mutated FCoV.

Antiviral chemotherapy in cats with feline infectious peritonitis

The search for an effective antiviral treatment for cats with FIP, unfortunately, has not been successful, although several studies have been performed.

Ribavirin

Ribavirin, 1-β-D-ribofuranosyl-1H-1,2,4-triazole-3-carboxamide (RTCA), is a broad-spectrum triazole nucleoside that has marked in vitro antiviral activity against a variety of DNA and RNA viruses, including FCoV. Ribavirin is a nucleoside analogue, but in contrast to the most common antiviral compounds, which act primarily to inhibit polymerases, ribavirin allows DNA and RNA synthesis to occur but prevents the formation of viral proteins, most likely by interfering with capping of viral mRNA. In vivo, therapeutic concentrations are difficult to achieve because of toxicity, and cats are extremely sensitive to the side effects.

Although active against FCoV in vitro [149,150], ribavirin was not effective in the treatment of cats with FIP. In one study, ribavirin was administered (16.5 mg/kg orally, intramuscularly, or intravenously every 24 hours for 10 to 14 days) to specific pathogen-free kittens 18 hours after experimental challenge exposure with an FIP-causing virus. All kittens, including ribavirin-treated and untreated kittens, succumbed to FIP. Clinical signs of disease were even more severe in the ribavirin-treated kittens, and their mean survival times were shortened [151]. The most common side effect in cats reported in several studies (already using a low dose of 11 mg/kg) is hemolysis. This develops as a result of sequestration of the drug in red blood cells. In addition, a dose-related toxic effect on bone marrow occurs, primarily on megakaryocytes (resulting in thrombocytopenia and hemorrhage), and erythroid precursors. Later on or at higher dosages, neutrophil numbers are suppressed. Liver toxicity has also been reported [152,153]. Weiss et al [151] tried to decrease the toxicity of ribavirin by incorporating it into lecithin-containing liposomes and giving it intravenously at a lower dose (5 mg/kg) to cats challenged with an FIP-causing virus. They were, however, not able to reach a therapeutic concentration with this regimen.

Human interferon-α

Human IFNα has immunomodulatory and antiviral activity. IFNα is active against many DNA and RNA viruses, including FCoV. IFNα has a direct antiviral effect by inducing a general "antiviral state" of INFα-containing cells that protects against virus replication. It is not virucidal but merely inhibits viral nucleic acid and protein synthesis. It binds to specific cell receptors that activate enzymes, inhibiting synthesis, assembly, and release of viruses. Human IFNα is marketed as a recombinant product (rHuIFNα) produced by a cloned human IFNα gene expressed in *Escherichia coli*. There are two common treatment regimens for use of human IFNα in cats: subcutaneous injection of high-dose IFNα (10^4 to 10^6 IU/kg every 24 hours) or oral application of low-dose IFNα (1–50 IU/kg every 24 hours). When given parenterally in high doses, application leads to detectable serum levels. When given parenterally to cats, it becomes ineffective after 3 to 7 weeks because of the development of neutralizing antibodies against the human IFNα, which limits its activity. In a study in which cats were treated with human IFNα subcutaneously, cats became refractory to therapy after 3 or 7 weeks, respectively, depending on whether a high (1.6×10^6 IU/kg) or a lower (1.6×10^4 IU/kg) dose was used [154].

In vitro, antiviral activity of human IFNα against FIP-causing FCoV strains was demonstrated. Combination of IFNα with ribavirin in vitro resulted in antiviral effects significantly greater than the sum of the observed effects from ribavirin or IFNα alone, indicating synergistic interactions [149]. Human IFNα treatment was used in 74 cats (52 treated cats, 22 controls) with experimentally induced FIP that received IFNα, *P acnes*, a combination, or placebo. The prophylactic and therapeutic administration of high doses (10^4 or 10^6 IU/kg) of IFNα did not significantly reduce the mortality in treated versus untreated cats; only in cats treated with IFNα and *P acnes* at a dose of 10^6 IU/kg, the mean survival time was significantly prolonged by a few days [155].

Orally, human IFNα can be given for a longer period, because no antibodies develop. Given orally, however, IFNα is inactivated by gastric acid and, like other proteins, destroyed by trypsin and other proteolytic enzymes in the duodenum; therefore, it is not absorbed and cannot be detected in the blood after oral administration [156]. Thus, direct antiviral effects are unlikely after oral administration; instead, it only seems to have immunomodulatory activity. IFNα may bind to mucosal receptors in the oral cavity, stimulating the local lymphoid tissue and leading to cytokine release on lymphatic cells in the oral or pharyngeal area, which triggers a cascade of immunologic responses that finally act systemically [157]. Tomkins [158] showed that orally administered IFNα induced cytokine responses in buccal mucosal lymph nodes, including upregulation of IFNγ expression and downregulation of interleukin-4. In studies in mice, it was shown that subcutaneous administration of murine IFNα had an antiviral effect, whereas oral administration caused an immunomodulatory effect. Infection of mice with encephalomyocarditis virus resulted in death in 100% of mice if not treated, in 40% survival of mice when treated with murine IFNα orally at a dose of 2×10^5 IU per mouse, and in 90% survival of mice when given the same dose intraperitoneally [159] confirming the immune modulatory effect after oral application. Therefore, low-dose oral IFNα treatment should not be used in cats with FIP because of its immunomodulatory activity, which may lead to progression of disease.

Feline interferon-ω

Recently, the corresponding feline IFN, feline IFNω, was licensed for use in veterinary medicine in some European countries and Japan. IFNs are species specific, and the human IFN clearly differs from the feline one not only regarding its antigenicity (thus causing antibody development in animals) but with respect to its antiviral efficacy in feline cells. Even if feline IFNω is used long term, cats do not develop antibodies. In addition, because it is the homologous species of IFN in cats, it is expected to be more effective than human IFNα. Feline IFNω is a recombinant product, which is produced by baculoviruses containing the feline sequence for this IFN that replicate in silkworms after infection; subsequently, feline IFNω is purified out of homogenized silkworm preparations [160]. Data on the efficacy of feline IFNω in cats with FIP are limited. FCoV replication is inhibited by feline IFNω in vitro [161]. In one study (not controlled and only including a small number of cats), 12 cats that were suspected of having FIP were treated with IFNω in combination with glucocorticoids and supportive care [162]. IFNω was given at a rate of 10^6 IU/kg subcutaneously every 48 hours initially until clinical improvement and, subsequently, once every 7 days. Glucocorticoids were given in the form of dexamethasone in case of effusion (1 mg/kg intrathoracic or intraperitoneal injection every 24 hours) or prednisolone (initially, 2 mg/kg administered orally every 24 hours until clinical improvement, then gradually tapered to 0.5 mg/kg administered every 48 hours). Although most cats died, 4 cats survived over a period of 2 years; all had initially presented with effusions. Even though there was no control group in this study and FIP was not even confirmed in the 4 surviving cats, these results are somewhat interesting (because cats with other effusion-associated diseases would not be expected to survive for 2 years without proper treatment), and further studies would certainly be interesting.

Prevention

Unfortunately, preventing FIP is extremely difficult. The only way to prevent the development of FIP is to prevent infection with FCoV. Vaccination prevents neither FIP nor FCoV infection effectively. Testing and removing strategies are ineffective. Management of FIP should be directed at minimizing the population impact and accurately diagnosing and supporting individual affected cats. Thus, veterinarians need to be knowledgeable regarding successful and unsuccessful strategies so as to provide useful counsel to their clients.

Management

Different situations have to be considered depending on the environment.

Management of a cat after contact

If a cat with FIP is euthanized and there are no remaining cats, the owner should wait approximately 3 months before obtaining another cat, because FCoV can stay infectious for at least 7 weeks in the environment. If there are other cats in the household, they are most likely infected with and shedding FCoV. In natural circumstances, cats go outside to defecate and bury their feces, in which case the virus remains infectious hours to days (slightly longer in freezing conditions). Domesticated cats have been introduced to litter boxes, however, in which FCoV may survive for several days, and possibly up to 7 weeks in dried-up feces. Thus, FCoV-shedding cats most likely have a better chance to eliminate the virus if allowed to go outside (optimum situation is in a fenced yard).

It is a common practice for clients to present a cat to the veterinarian that has been in contact with a cat with FIP or a suspected or known virus excretor. The owner may want to know the prognosis for the exposed cat or may want to obtain another cat and needs to know whether the exposed cat is shedding FCoV. It is likely that the cat is antibody-positive, because 95% to 100% of cats exposed to FCoV become infected and develop antibodies approximately 2 to 3 weeks after FCoV exposure. There are a few cats, however, that may be resistant to FCoV infection. It has been shown that a low number of cats in FCoV endemic multiple-cat households continuously remain antibody-negative [163]. The mechanism of action for this resistance is still unknown. The owner should be advised that the cat in contact is likely to have antibodies and reassured that this is not necessarily associated with a poor prognosis. Most cats infected with FCoV do not develop FIP, and many cats in single- or 2-cat households eventually clear the infection and become antibody-negative in a few months to years. Cats can be retested (using the same laboratory) every 6 to 12 months until the results of the antibody test are negative. Cats exposed only once often have a quicker reduction in antibodies. To exclude any risk at all, the owner should be advised to wait until antibody titers of all cats are negative before obtaining a new cat. Some cats, however, remain antibody-positive for years. A rise in antibody titer or maintenance at a high level does not necessarily indicate a poor prognosis for the cat. In a study following cats with high titers, the titers of 50 of these cats remained at a high level on at least three occasions, yet only 4 cats died of FIP [26]. In contrast, in a situation of endemic infection, a constantly low titer is highly indicative that a cat is not going to develop FIP.

Management of multiple-cat households with endemic feline coronavirus

Households of less than 5 cats can spontaneously and naturally become FCoV-free, but in households of more than 10 cats, this is almost impossible, because the virus passes from one individual cat to another, maintaining the infection. This holds true for virtually all multiple-cat households, such as breeding catteries, shelters, foster homes, and other homes with more than 5 cats.

When a cat in a household develops FIP, all other cats in contact with that cat have already been exposed to the same FCoV. There is virtually nothing to prevent FIP in other cats that are in contact with the cat with FIP. Although the risk is only 5% to 10%, full-sibling litter mates of kittens with FIP have a higher likelihood of developing FIP than other cats in the same environment [164] indicating a certain genetic component.

Various tactics have been used to eliminate FCoV from a household. Reducing the number of cats (especially kittens less than 12 months old) and keeping possibly FCoV-contaminated surfaces clean can minimize population loads of FCoV. Antibody testing and segregating cats are aimed at stopping exposure. Approximately one third of antibody-positive cats excrete virus [10,11,130,165,166]; thus, every antibody-positive cat has to be considered infectious. After 3 to 6 months, antibody titers can be retested to determine whether cats have become negative. Alternatively, RT-PCR testing of (several) fecal samples can be performed to detect shedders. It is important to detect chronic FCoV carriers so that they can be removed. In large multiple-cat environments, 40% to 60% of cats shed virus in their feces at any given time. Approximately 20% shed virus persistently. Approximately 20% are immune and do not shed virus. Repeated PCR testing of feces should be performed at weekly intervals for 2 months or more to document carriers. If the cats remain persistently PCR-positive for more than 6 weeks, they should be eliminated from the cattery and placed in single-cat environments [164].

Early weaning and isolation

More than any other factor, management of kittens determines whether or not they become infected with FCoV. Kittens of FCoV-shedding queens should be protected from infection by maternally derived antibody until they are 5 to 6 weeks old. An early weaning protocol for the prevention of FCoV infection in kittens has been proposed by Addie and Jarrett [26], which consists of isolation of queens 2 to 3 weeks before parturition, strict quarantine of queens and kittens, and early weaning at 4 to 6 weeks of age. This procedure is based on the findings that some queens do not shed the virus and some queens stop shedding after several weeks if not re-exposed. Even if queens do shed, young kittens have maternal resistance to the virus [7]. Early removal of kittens from the queen and prevention of infection from other cats may succeed in preventing infection in these kittens. Although straightforward in concept, isolation of queens and early weaning is not as simple as it may seem. The procedure requires quarantine rooms and procedures that absolutely ensure a new virus does not enter. It is an advantage when the isolated queens are not shedding FCoV, when they are shedding low levels, or when they can clear the infection early after being isolated. The single most important factor is the number of animals. The success of early weaning and isolation in FCoV control depends on effective quarantine and low numbers of cats (<5 cats) in the household. Also, human abodes do not easily allow adequate quarantine space for large numbers of queens and kittens, and the time and money required to maintain quarantine increase in proportion to the number of queens and litters under quarantine. In a study in large catteries in Switzerland in which the same protocol was followed, early weaning failed and viral infection of kittens as young as 2 weeks old was demonstrated [167]. It is clear that low FCoV exposure can delay infection, whereas high exposure can overcome maternally derived immunity at an early age.

There are two essential downsides of isolation and early weaning. It is not easy to do, and it fails if appropriate conditions are not maintained. Additionally, some breeders believe that early weaning exacts a social price on the kittens. In recognition of both concerns, it is recommended that early weaning not be undertaken without careful consideration. FCoV-free households do not require routine isolation and early weaning. When kittens are isolated with their queen, special care must be taken during the period from 2 to 7 weeks of age to socialize the kittens. The success of early weaning should also be monitored, and it should not be continued if it is not successful. Kittens that have been successfully reared free of FCoV should be antibody-negative at 12 weeks of age. Even if kittens can be raised free of FCoV, they may become infected sooner or later. Therefore, the objective of isolation and early weaning should not be to prevent infection but to delay it [164]. For early weaning to be effective, it is best for kittens to be taken to a new home (with no other cats) at 5 weeks of age. Even then, however, early weaning is not always successful.

Recommendations for breeding catteries

It has been suggested to maximize heritable resistance to FIP in breeding catteries. Genetic predisposition is not completely understood, however. It is known that susceptible cats are approximately twice as likely to develop FIP as other cats [168]. If a cat has two or more litters in which kittens develop

FIP, that cat should not be bred again. Particular attention should be paid to pedigrees of males, in which FIP is overrepresented. Because line breeding often uses valuable tomcats extensively, eliminating such animals may have a small but important effect on improving overall resistance [164].

Screening of a cattery for the presence of FCoV is important. If there are many cats housed in a group, a random sampling of 3 to 4 cats should indicate whether FCoV is endemic. If cats are housed individually, it may be necessary to test them all. Cats in households with fewer than 10 cats and no new acquisitions and cats that are isolated from each other in groups of 3 or less often eventually lose their FCoV infection [169]. Once they have been established, antibody-negative catteries can be maintained free of FCoV by monitoring new cats before they are introduced. Thus, cats should be screened before introduction, and antibody-positive cats should never be taken into the household. Cat breeders often also request that their cats be screened for FCoV antibodies before mating. If the cat is healthy and antibody-negative, it can be safely mated with another antibody-negative cat. If the cat is antibody-positive, it should not be mated with a cat from an FCoV-free environment [164].

Recommendations for shelters

Prevention of FIP in a shelter situation is virtually impossible unless cats are strictly kept in separate cages and handled only by means of sterile handling devices (comparable to isolation units). Isolation is often not effective because of the ease with which FCoV is transported on clothes, shoes, dust, and cats. Comparison of shelters with different types of handling revealed a significant correlation between an increase in the number of handling events outside the cages and an increase in the percentage of antibody-positive cats. In a study in which feral cats were tested at the time they were brought into local shelters (in which multiple cats were kept together) and at 1-to 2-week intervals thereafter, only a low number of cats had antibodies at the time point of entering, but the percentage increased rapidly until virtually all cats in the shelters were infected with FCoV [40].

Shelter managers should use education and communication to minimize adverse effects of FIP in cat populations. Shelter managers should have written information sheets or contracts informing adopters about FCoV and FIP. They should understand that FCoV is unavoidable in multiple-cat environments and that FIP is an unavoidable consequence of endemic FCoV. Shelters need to optimize facilities and husbandry so that the facilities can be cleaned easily and virus spread is minimized. It is essential to decrease viral load and stress levels [164].

Vaccination

There have been many attempts to develop effective vaccines, but, unfortunately, most have failed, mainly because of ADE [75,78,170,171].

Nevertheless, a vaccine was licensed (Primucell, Pfizer Animal Health) incorporating a temperature-sensitive mutant of the FCoV strain DF2-FIPV, which can replicate in the cool lining of the upper respiratory tract but not at higher internal body temperatures [172–175]. This vaccine, administered intranasally, produces local immunity (IgA antibodies) at the site where FCoV first enters the body (the oropharynx) and also induces cell-mediated immunity. The vaccine has been available in the United States since 1991 and has been introduced in many European countries. The concerns of such a vaccine are safety and efficacy. Safety concerns focus on whether the vaccine could cause FIP or produce ADE. Although some experimental vaccine trials with vaccines that never appeared on the market have recorded ADE on challenge [176,177], field studies have demonstrated that this intranasal vaccine is safe. In two extensive placebo-controlled double-blind field trials there was no development of FIP or ADE [178–180]. There were a few immediate side effects after application, such as sneezing, vomiting, or diarrhea, which were not statistically different in the vaccinated group and the placebo group [178].

The efficacy of this vaccine is questioned constantly, however. Experimental studies have reported preventable fractions between 0% [176,177] and 50% to 75% [175,181], depending on the investigator. In a survey of 138 cats belonging to 15 cat breeders in which virtually all the cats had antibodies, no difference was found in the development of FIP between the vaccinated group and the placebo group [178]. Thus, vaccination in an FCoV endemic environment or in a household with known cases of FIP is not effective. In one of the placebo-controlled double-blind trials that was performed in Switzerland in a group of cats that did not have contact with FCoV before vaccination, a small but statistically significant reduction in the number of cats that developed FIP was noted [178,182]. Because the vaccine is ineffective when cats have already had contact with FCoV, antibody testing may be beneficial before vaccination. One disadvantage is that most cats develop antibodies after vaccination, thus making the establishment and control of an FCoV-free household difficult. In conclusion, study results do not clearly identify whether vaccination has no effect versus a small effect. Although only marginally if at all efficacious, the vaccine is at least safe and does not induce ADE.

Public health considerations

Concerns have arisen about a possible danger of FCoV to people because there is a close antigenetic relation between coronaviruses of different domestic animal species (eg, CCV, TGEV) and a coronavirus deriving from animals in close contact with humans recently caused the so-called "severe acute respiratory syndrome" (SARS) that seemed to be a threat to thousands of people. There is, however, no indication that people can be infected with FCoV.

References

[1] Rohrbach BW, Legendre AM, Baldwin CA, et al. Epidemiology of feline infectious peritonitis among cats examined at veterinary medical teaching hospitals. J Am Vet Med Assoc 2001;218:1111–5.

[2] Cave TA, Thompson H, Reid SW, et al. Kitten mortality in the United Kingdom: a retrospective analysis of 274 histopathological examinations (1986 to 2000). Vet Rec 2002; 151:497–501.

[3] Pedersen NC. Coronavirus diseases (coronavirus enteritis, feline infectious peritonitis). In: Holzworth J, editor. Diseases of the cat. Medicine and surgery, vol. 1. Philadelphia: WB Saunders; 1987. p. 193–214.

[4] Pedersen NC. Morphologic and physical characteristics of feline infectious peritonitis virus and its growth in autochthonous peritoneal cell cultures. Am J Vet Res 1976;37: 567–72.

[5] Pedersen NC. Serologic studies of naturally occurring feline infectious peritonitis. Am J Vet Res 1976;37:1449–53.

[6] Loeffler DG, Ott RL, Evermann JF, et al. The incidence of naturally occurring antibodies against feline infectious peritonitis in selected cat populations. Feline Pract 1978;8:43–7.

[7] Addie DD, Jarrett O. A study of naturally occurring feline coronavirus infections in kittens. Vet Rec 1992;130:133–7.

[8] Sparkes AH, Gruffydd-Jones TJ, Harbour DA. Feline coronavirus antibodies in UK cats. Vet Rec 1992;131:223–4.

[9] Pedersen NC. Feline infectious peritonitis: something old, something new. Feline Pract 1976;6:42–51.

[10] Addie DD, Jarrett O. Feline coronavirus antibodies in cats. Vet Rec 1992;131:202–3.

[11] Addie DD, Toth S, Murray GD, et al. Risk of feline infectious peritonitis in cats naturally infected with feline coronavirus. Am J Vet Res 1995;56:429–34.

[12] Pedersen NC, Boyle JF, Floyd K, et al. An enteric coronavirus infection of cats and its relationship to feline infectious peritonitis. Am J Vet Res 1981;42:368–77.

[13] Pedersen NC, Black JW, Boyle JF, et al. Pathogenetic differences between various feline coronavirus isolates. Adv Exp Med Biol 1983;173:365–80.

[14] Boyle JF, Pedersen NC, Evermann JF, et al. Plaque assay, polypeptide composition and immunochemistry of feline infectious peritonitis virus and feline enteric coronavirus isolates. Adv Exp Med Biol 1984;173:133–47.

[15] Fiscus SA, Teramoto YA. Antigenic comparison of feline coronavirus isolates: evidence for markedly different peplomer glycoproteins. J Virol 1987;61:2607–13.

[16] Hohdatsu T, Okada S, Koyama H. Characterization of monoclonal antibodies against feline infectious peritonitis virus type II and antigenic relationship between feline, porcine, and canine coronaviruses. Arch Virol 1991;117:85–95.

[17] Hohdatsu T, Sasamoto T, Okada S, et al. Antigenic analysis of feline coronaviruses with monoclonal antibodies (MAbs): preparation of MAbs which discriminate between FIPV strain 79-1146 and FECV strain 79-1683. Vet Microbiol 1991;28:13–24.

[18] Corapi WV, Olsen CW, Scott FW. Monoclonal antibody analysis of neutralization and antibody-dependent enhancement of feline infectious peritonitis virus. J Virol 1992;66: 6695–705.

[19] Herrewegh AA, Vennema H, Horzinek MC, et al. The molecular genetics of feline coronaviruses: comparative sequence analysis of the ORF7a/7b transcription unit of different biotypes. Virology 1995;212:622–31.

[20] Pedersen NC. An overview of feline enteric coronavirus and infectious peritonitis virus infections. Feline Pract 1995;23:7–20.

[21] Vennema H, Poland A, Hawkins KF, et al. A comparison of the genomes of FECVs and FIPVs and what they tell us about the relationships between feline coronaviruses and their evolution. Feline Pract 1995;23:40–4.

[22] Vennema H, Poland A, Foley J, et al. Feline infectious peritonitis viruses arise by mutation from endemic feline enteric coronaviruses. Virology 1998;243:150–7.

[23] Ward JM. Morphogenesis of a virus in cats with experimental feline infectious peritonitis. Virology 1970;41:191–4.

[24] Holzworth J. Some important disorders of cats. Cornell Vet 1963;53:157–60.

[25] O'Reilly K, Fishman B, Hitchcock L. Feline infectious peritonitis: isolation of a coronavirus. Vet Rec 1979;104:348.

[26] Addie DD, Jarrett O. Feline coronavirus infections. In: Greene CE, editor. Infectious diseases of the dog and cat. Philadelphia: WB Saunders; 1990. p. 300–12.

[27] Horzinek MC, Osterhaus AD. Feline infectious peritonitis: a worldwide serosurvey. Am J Vet Res 1979;40:1487–92.

[28] Barlough JE, Jacobson RH, Downing DR, et al. Evaluation of a computer-assisted, kinetics-based enzyme-linked immunosorbent assay for detection of coronavirus antibodies in cats. J Clin Microbiol 1983;17:202–17.

[29] Pedersen NC. Feline infectious peritonitis and feline enteric coronavirus infections. Part I. Feline Pract 1983;13:13–9.

[30] McArdle F, Bennett M, Gaskell RM, et al. Canine coronavirus infection in cats; a possible role in feline infectious peritonitis. Adv Exp Med Biol 1990;276:475–9.

[31] Motokawa K, Hohdatsu T, Aizawa C, et al. Molecular cloning and sequence determination of the peplomer protein gene of feline infectious peritonitis virus type I. Arch Virol 1995; 140:469–80.

[32] Motokawa K, Hohdatsu T, Hashimoto H, et al. Comparison of the amino acid sequence and phylogenetic analysis of the peplomer, integral membrane and nucleocapsid proteins of feline, canine and porcine coronaviruses. Microbiol Immunol 1996;40:425–33.

[33] Barlough JE, Stoddart CA. Feline coronaviral infections. In: Greene CE, editor. Infectious diseases of the dog and cat. Philadelphia: WB Saunders; 1990. p. 300–12.

[34] Wege H, Siddell S, Ter Meulen V. The biology and pathogenesis of coronaviruses. Curr Top Microbiol Immunol 1982;99:165–200.

[35] McArdle F, Bennett M, Gaskell RM, et al. Induction and enhancement of feline infectious peritonitis by canine coronavirus. Am J Vet Res 1992;53:1500–6.

[36] Mochizuki M, Mitsutake Y, Miyanohara Y, et al. Antigenic and plaque variations of serotype II feline infectious peritonitis coronaviruses. J Vet Med Sci 1997;59:253–8.

[37] Hohdatsu T, Okada S, Ishizuka Y, et al. The prevalence of types I and II feline coronavirus infections in cats. J Vet Med Sci 1992;54:557–62.

[38] Benetka V, Kubber-Heiss A, Kolodziejek J, et al. Prevalence of feline coronavirus types I and II in cats with histopathologically verified feline infectious peritonitis. Vet Microbiol 2004;99:31–42.

[39] Legendre A, Luria BJ, Gorman SP, et al. Prevalence of coronavirus antibodies in feral cats in Gainesville, Florida [abstract]. In: Abstracts of the Second International Feline Coronavirus/Feline Infectious Peritonitis Symposium. Glasgow, Scotland; 2002.

[40] Pedersen NC, Sato R, Foley JE, et al. Common virus infections in cats, before and after being placed in shelters, with emphasis on feline enteric coronavirus. J Feline Med Surg 2004;6:83–8.

[41] Hartmann K, Binder C, Hirschberger J, et al. Predictive values of different tests in the diagnosis of feline infectious peritonitis [abstract]. In: Abstracts of the Second International Feline Coronavirus/Feline Infectious Peritonitis Symposium. Glasgow, Scotland; 2002.

[42] Kennedy M, Citino S, McNabb AH, et al. Detection of feline coronavirus in captive Felidae in the USA. J Vet Diagn Invest 2002;14:520–2.

[43] Kennedy M, Kania S, Stylianides E, et al. Detection of feline coronavirus infection in southern African nondomestic felids. J Wildl Dis 2003;39:529–35.

[44] Brown EW, Olmsted RA, Martenson JS. Exposure to FIV and FIPV in wild and captive cheetahs. Zoo Biol 1993;12:135–42.

[45] Weiss RC. Feline infectious peritonitis and other coronaviruses. In: Sherding RG, editor. The cat diseases and clinical management. 2nd edition. New York: Churchill Livingstone; 1994. p. 449–77.

[46] Scott FW. Update on FIP. In: Proceedings of the Kal Kann Symposium 1988;12:43–7.

[47] Pedersen NC, Addie D, Wolf A. Recommendations from working groups of the International Feline Enteric Coronavirus and Feline Infectious Peritonitis Workshop. Feline Pract 1995;23:108–11.

[48] Kass PH, Dent PH. The epidemiology of feline infectious peritonitis in catteries. Feline Pract 1995;23:27–32.

[49] Stoddart ME, Whicher JT, Harbour DA. Cats inoculated with feline infectious peritonitis virus exhibit a biphasic acute phase plasma protein response. Vet Rec 1988;123:622–4.

[50] Herrewegh AA, DeGroot RJ, Cepica A, et al. Detection of feline coronavirus RNA in feces, tissues, and body fluids of naturally infected cats by reverse transcriptase PCR. J Clin Microbiol 1995;33:684–9.

[51] Gut M, Leutenegger C, Schiller I, et al. Kinetics of FCoV infection in kittens born in catteries of high risk for FIP under different rearing conditions [abstract]. In: Abstracts of the Second International Feline Coronavirus/Feline Infectious Peritonitis Symposium. Glasgow, Scotland; 2002.

[52] Foley JE, Poland A, Carlson J, et al. Patterns of feline coronavirus infection and fecal shedding from cats in multiple-cat environments. J Am Vet Med Assoc 1997;210: 1307–12.

[53] Addie DD, Toth S, Herrewegh A, et al. Feline coronavirus in the intestinal contents of cats with feline infectious peritonitis. Vet Rec 1996;139:522–3.

[54] Goitsuka R, Hirota Y, Hasegawa A, et al. Release of interleukin 1 from peritoneal exudate cells of cats with feline infectious peritonitis. Nippon Juigaku Zasshi 1987;49:811–88.

[55] Weiss RC, Scott FW. Pathogenesis of feline infectious peritonitis: nature and development of viremia. Am J Vet Res 1981;42:382–90.

[56] Stoddart CA, Scott FW. Intrinsic resistance of feline peritoneal macrophages to coronavirus infection correlates with in vivo virulence. J Virol 1989;63:436–40.

[57] Egberink HF, Herrewegh AP, Schuurman NM, et al. FIP, easy to diagnose? Vet Q 1995;17: 24–5.

[58] Herrewegh AA, Mahler M, Hedrich HJ, et al. Persistence and evolution of feline coronavirus in a closed cat-breeding colony. Virology 1997;234:349–63.

[59] Gunn-Moore DA, Gruffydd-Jones TJ, Harbour DA. Detection of feline coronaviruses by culture and reverse transcriptase-polymerase chain reaction of blood samples from healthy cats and cats with clinical feline infectious peritonitis. Vet Microbiol 1998;62:193–205.

[60] Tresnan DB, Levis R, Holmes KV. Feline aminopeptidase N serves as a receptor for feline, canine, porcine, and human coronaviruses in serogroup I. J Virol 1996;70:8669–74.

[61] Benbacer L, Kut E, Besnardeau L, et al. Interspecies aminopeptidase-N chimeras reveal species-specific receptor recognition by canine coronavirus, feline infectious peritonitis virus, and transmissible gastroenteritis virus. J Virol 1997;71:734–7.

[62] Hegyi A, Kolb AF. Characterization of determinants involved in the feline infectious peritonitis virus receptor function of feline aminopeptidase. J Gen Virol 1998;79:1387–91.

[63] Hickman MA, Morris JG, Rogers QR, et al. Elimination of feline coronavirus infection from a large experimental specific pathogen-free cat breeding colony by serologic testing and isolation. Feline Pract 1995;3:96–102.

[64] Rottier R. The molecular dynamics of feline coronaviruses. Vet Microbiol 1999;69:117–25.

[65] Poland AM, Vennema H, Foley JE, et al. Two related strains of feline infectious peritonitis virus isolated from immunocompromised cats infected with a feline enteric coronavirus. J Clin Microbiol 1996;34:3180–4.

[66] Foley JE, Poland A, Carlson J, et al. Risk factors for feline infectious peritonitis among cats in multiple-cat environments with endemic feline enteric coronavirus. J Am Vet Med Assoc 1997;210:1313–8.

[67] Addie DD, Kennedy LJ, Ryvar R, et al. Feline leucocyte antigen class II polymorphism and susceptibility to feline infectious peritonitis. J Feline Med Surg 2004;6:59–62.

[68] Nafe LA. Topics in feline neurology. Vet Clin N Am Small Anim Pract 1984;14:1289–98.

[69] Gunn-Moore DA, Caney SM, Gruffydd-Jones TJ, et al. Antibody and cytokine responses in kittens during the development of feline infectious peritonitis (FIP). Vet Immunol Immunopathol 1998;65:221–42.

[70] Dean GA, Olivry T, Stanton C, et al. In vivo cytokine response to experimental feline infectious peritonitis virus infection. Vet Microbiol 2003;97:1–12.

[71] Kiss I, Poland AM, Pedersen NC. Disease outcome and cytokine responses in cats immunized with an avirulent feline infectious peritonitis virus (FIPV)-UCD1 and challenge-exposed with virulent FIPV-UCD8. J Feline Med Surg 2004;6:89–97.

[72] Giordano A, Spagnolo V, Colombo A, et al. Changes in some acute phase protein and immunoglobulin concentrations in cats affected by feline infectious peritonitis or exposed to feline coronavirus infection. Vet J 2004;167:38–44.

[73] Ceciliani F, Grossi C, Giordano A, et al. Decreased sialylation of the acute phase protein alpha1-acid glycoprotein in feline infectious peritonitis (FIP). Vet Immunol Immunopathol 2004;99:229–36.

[74] Paltrinieri S, Giordano A, Ceciliani F, et al. Tissue distribution of a feline AGP related protein (fAGPrP) in cats with feline infectious peritonitis (FIP). J Feline Med Surg 2004;6: 99–105.

[75] Vennema H, De Groot RJ, Harbour DA, et al. Immunogenicity of recombinant feline infectious peritonitis virus spike protein in mice and kittens. Adv Exp Med Biol 1990;276: 217–22.

[76] Olsen CW. A review of feline infectious peritonitis virus: molecular biology, immunopathogenesis, clinical aspects, and vaccination. Vet Microbiol 1993;36:1–37.

[77] Pedersen NC. The history and interpretation of feline coronavirus serology. Feline Pract 1995;23:46–51.

[78] Scott FW, Copari WV, Olsen CW. Antibody-dependent enhancement of feline infectious peritonitis. Feline Pract 1995;23:77–80.

[79] Hohdatsu T, Yamada M, Tominaga R, et al. Antibody-dependent enhancement of feline infectious peritonitis virus infection in feline alveolar macrophages and human monocyte cell line U937 by serum of cats experimentally or naturally infected with feline coronavirus. J Vet Med Sci 1998;60:49–55.

[80] Hohdatsu T, Nakamura M, Ishizuka Y, et al. A study on the mechanism of antibody-dependent enhancement of feline infectious peritonitis virus infection in feline macrophages by monoclonal antibodies. Arch Virol 1991;120:207–17.

[81] Olsen CW, Corapi WV, Ngichabe CK, et al. Monoclonal antibodies to the spike protein of feline infectious peritonitis virus mediate antibody-dependent enhancement of infection of feline macrophages. J Virol 1992;66:956–65.

[82] Olsen CW, Corapi WV, Jacobson RH, et al. Identification of antigenic sites mediating antibody-dependent enhancement of feline infectious peritonitis virus infectivity. J Gen Virol 1993;74:745–9.

[83] Corapi WV, Darteil RJ, Audonnet JC, et al. Localization of antigenic sites of the S glycoprotein of feline infectious peritonitis virus involved in neutralization and antibody-dependent enhancement. Virology 1995;5:2858–62.

[84] Hirschberger J, Hartmann K, Wilhelm N, et al. Clinical symptoms and diagnosis of feline infectious peritonitis. Tierarztl Prax 1995;23:92–9.

[85] Rush JE, Keene BW, Fox PR. Pericardial disease in the cat: a retrospective evaluation of 66 cases. J Am Anim Hosp Assoc 1990;26:39–46.

[86] Trulove SG, McCahon HA, Nichols R. Pyogranulomatous pneumonia associated with generalized noneffusive feline infectious peritonitis. Feline Pract 1992;3:25–9.

[87] Kipar A, Koehler K, Bellmann S, et al. Feline infectious peritonitis presenting as a tumour in the abdominal cavity. Vet Rec 1999;144:118–22.

[88] MacPhail C. Gastrointestinal obstruction. Clin Tech Small Anim Pract 2002;17: 178–83.

[89] Sigurdardottir OG, Kolbjornsen O, Lutz H. Orchitis in a cat associated with coronavirus infection. J Comp Pathol 2001;124:219–22.

[90] Van Kruiningen HJ, Ryan MJ, Shindel NM. The classification of feline colitis. J Comp Pathol 1983;93:275–94.

[91] Harvey CJ, Lopez JW, Hendrick MJ. An uncommon intestinal manifestation of feline infectious peritonitis: 26 cases (1986–1993). J Am Vet Med Assoc 1996;209: 1117–20.

[92] Andrew SE. Feline infectious peritonitis. Vet Clin N Am Small Anim Pract 2000;30: 987–1000.

[93] Bistner S. Allergic- and immunologic-mediated diseases of the eye and adnexae. Vet Clin N Am Small Anim Pract 1994;24:711–34.

[94] Bradshaw JM, Pearson GR, Gruffydd-Jones TJ. A retrospective study of 286 cases of neurological disorders of the cat. J Comp Pathol 2004;131:112–20.

[95] Rohrer C, Suter PF, Lutz H. The diagnosis of feline infectious peritonitis (FIP): a retrospective and prospective study. Kleintierprax 1993;38:379–89.

[96] Li Y, Kang J, Horwitz MS. Clinical, cerebrospinal fluid, and histological data from twenty-seven cats with primary inflammatory disease of the central nervous system. Can Vet J 1994; 35:103–10.

[97] Kline KL, Joseph RJ, Averdill DR. Feline infectious peritonitis with neurologic involvement: clinical and pathological findings in 24 cats. J Am Anim Hosp Assoc 1994; 30:111–8.

[98] Baroni M, Heinold Y. A review of the clinical diagnosis of feline infectious peritonitis viral meningoencephalomyelitis. Prog Vet Neurol 1995;6:88–94.

[99] Shell LG. Feline infectious peritonitis viral meningoencephalitis. Feline Pract 1997;25:24.

[100] Addie DD, Jarrett O. Use of a reverse-transcriptase polymerase chain reaction for monitoring the shedding of feline coronavirus by healthy cats. Vet Rec 2001;148:649–53.

[101] Hartmann K, Binder C, Hirschberger J, et al. Comparison of different tests to diagnose feline infectious peritonitis. J Vet Intern Med 2003;17:781–90.

[102] Paltrinieri S, Grieco V, Comazzi S, et al. Laboratory profiles in cats with different pathological and immunohistochemical findings due to feline infectious peritonitis (FIP). J Feline Med Surg 2001;3:149–59.

[103] Paltrinieri S, Ponti W, Comazzi S, et al. Shifts in circulating lymphocyte subsets in cats with feline infectious peritonitis (FIP): pathogenic role and diagnostic relevance. Vet Immunol Immunopathol 2003;96:141–8.

[104] Breuer W, Stahr K, Majzoub M, et al. Bone-marrow changes in infectious diseases and lymphohaemopoietic neoplasias in dogs and cats—a retrospective study. J Comp Pathol 1998;119:57–66.

[105] Boudreaux MK, Weiss RC, Toivio-Kinnucan M, et al. Potentiation of platelet responses in vitro by feline infectious peritonitis virus. Vet Pathol 1990;27:261–8.

[106] Paltrinieri S, Comazzi S, Spagnolo V, et al. Laboratory changes consistent with feline infectious peritonitis in cats from multicat environments. J Vet Med A 2002;49:503–10.

[107] Sparkes AH, Gruffydd Jones TJ, Harbour DA. An appraisal of the value of laboratory tests in the diagnosis of feline infectious peritonitis. J Am Anim Hosp Assoc 1994;30:345–50.

[108] Shelly SM, Scarlett Kranz J, Blue JT. Protein electrophoresis on effusions from cats as a diagnostic test for feline infectious peritonitis. J Am Anim Hosp Assoc 1988;24: 495–500.

[109] Rohrer C, Suter PF, Lutz H. The diagnosis of feline infectious peritonitis (FIP): retrospective and prospective study. European Journal of Companion Animal Practice 1994;4:23–9.

[110] Potkay S, Bacher JD, Pitts TW. Feline infectious peritonitis in a closed breeding colony. Lab Anim Sci 1974;24:279–89.

[111] Gouffaux M, Pastoret PP, Henroteaux M, et al. Feline infectious peritonitis. Proteins of plasma and ascitic fluid. Vet Pathol 1975;12:335–48.

[112] Horzinek MC, Osterhaus AD, Ellens DJ. Feline infectious peritonitis virus. Zentralbl Veterinarmed B 1977;24:398–405.

[113] Horzinek MC, Ederveen J, Egberink H, et al. Virion polypeptide specificity of immune complexes and antibodies in cats inoculated with feline infectious peritonitis virus. Am J Vet Res 1986;47:754–61.

[114] Paltrinieri S, Cammarata MP, Cammarata G, et al. Some aspects of humoral and cellular immunity in naturally occurring feline infectious peritonitis. Vet Immunol Immunopathol 1998;65:205–20.

[115] Goitsuka R, Ohashi T, Ono K, et al. IL-6 activity in feline infectious peritonitis. Immunology 1990;144:2599–603.

[116] Weiss RC. The diagnosis and clinical management of feline infectious peritonitis. Vet Med (Praha) 1991;86:308–19.

[117] Wolf A. Feline infectious peritonitis. Part 2. Feline Pract 1997;25:24–8.

[118] Duthie S, Eckersall PD, Addie DD, et al. Value of alpha 1-acid glycoprotein in the diagnosis of feline infectious peritonitis. Vet Rec 1997;141:299–303.

[119] Savary KC, Sellon RK, Law JM. Chylous abdominal effusion in a cat with feline infectious peritonitis. J Am Anim Hosp Assoc 2001;37:35–40.

[120] Hirschberger J, Koch S. Validation of the determination of the activity of adenosine deaminase in body effusions of cats. Res Vet Sci 1995;59:226–9.

[121] Berti-Bock G, Vial F, Premuda L, et al. Exudates, transudates and the Rivalta reaction (1895). Current status and historical premises. Minerva Med 1979;70:3573–80.

[122] Kasbohm C. Exudates in body cavities of the dog. Clinical and diagnostic study with special reference to punctate cytology. Tierarztl Prax 1976;4:501–5.

[123] Rand JS, Parent J, Percy D, Jacobs R. Clinical, cerebrospinal fluid, and histological data from twenty-seven cats with primary inflammatory disease of the central nervous system. Can Vet J 1994;35:103–10.

[124] Foley JE, Rand C, Leutenegger C. Inflammation and changes in cytokine levels in neurological feline infectious peritonitis. J Feline Med Surg 2003;5:313–22.

[125] Barlough JE. Serodiagnostic aids and management practice for feline retrovirus and coronavirus infections. Vet Clin N Am Small Anim Pract 1984;14:955–69.

[126] Addie DD, Dennis JM, Toth S, et al. Long-term impact on a closed household of pet cats of natural infection with feline coronavirus, feline leukaemia virus and feline immunodeficiency virus. Vet Rec 2000;146:419–24.

[127] Sparkes AH, Gruffydd Jones TJ, Harbour DA. Feline infectious peritonitis: a review of clinicopathological changes in 65 cases, and a critical assessment of their diagnostic value. Vet Rec 1991;129:209–12.

[128] Sparkes AH, Gruffydd-Jones TJ, Howard PE, et al. Coronavirus serology in healthy pedigree cats. Vet Rec 1992;131:35–6.

[129] Addie DD, McLachlan SA, Golder M, et al. Evaluation of an in-practice test for feline coronavirus antibodies. J Feline Med Surg 2004;6:63–7.

[130] Addie DD, Jarrett O. Control of feline coronavirus infections in breeding catteries by serotesting, isolation and early weaning. Feline Pract 1995;23:92–5.

[131] Blatter LA, Niggli E. Detection of feline coronaviruses in cell cultures and in fresh and fixed feline tissues using polymerase chain reaction. Vet Microbiol 1994;42:65–77.

[132] Kennedy MA, Brenneman K, Millsaps RK, et al. Correlation of genomic detection of feline coronavirus with various diagnostic assays for feline infectious peritonitis. J Vet Diagn Invest 1998;10:93–7.

[133] Soma T, Ishii H. Detection of feline coronavirus antibody, feline immunodeficiency virus antibody, and feline leukemia virus antigen in ascites from cats with effusive feline infectious peritonitis. J Vet Med Sci 2004;66:89–90.

[134] Foley JE, Lapointe JM, Koblik P, et al. Diagnostic features of clinical neurologic feline infectious peritonitis. J Vet Intern Med 1998;12:415–23.

[135] Boettcher I, Fischer A, Steinberg T, et al. Comparative evaluation of CSF anti-coronavirus titers and results of postmortem examination in cats [abstract]. In: Abstracts of the Annual Meeting of the European Society of Veterinary Neurology. Prague, Czech Republic; 2003.

[136] Fehr D, Bolla S, Herrewegh A, et al. Detection of feline coronavirus using RT-PCR: basis for the study of the pathogenesis of feline infectious peritonitis (FIP). Schweiz Arch Tierheilkd 1996;138:74–9.

[137] Witte KH, Tuch K, Dubenkropp H, et al. Antigenic relationships between feline infectious peritonitis (FIP) and transmissible gastroenteritis (TGE) viruses in swine. Berl Munch Tierarztl Wochenschr 1977;90:396–401.

[138] Toma B, Duret C, Chappuis G, Pellerin B. Echec de l'immunisation contre la peritonite infectieuse feline par injection de virus de la gastro-enterite transmissible du porc. Rec Med Vet 1979;155:799–803.

[139] Gamble DA, Lobbiani A, Gramegna M, et al. Development of a nested PCR assay for detection of feline infectious peritonitis virus in clinical specimens. J Clin Microbiol 1997; 35:673–5.

[140] Jacobse Geels HE, Daha MR, Horzinek MC. Isolation and characterization of feline C3 and evidence for the immune complex pathogenesis of feline infectious peritonitis. J Immunol 1980;125:1606–10.

[141] Parodi MC, Cammarata G, Paltrinieri S, et al. Using direct immunofluorescence to detect coronaviruses in peritoneal and pleural effusions. J Small Anim Pract 1993;34:609–13.

[142] Kipar A, Bellmann S, Kremendahl J, et al. Cellular composition, coronavirus antigen expression and production of specific antibodies in lesions in feline infectious peritonitis. Vet Immunol Immunopathol 1998;65:243–57.

[143] Tammer R, Evensen O, Lutz H, Reinacher M. Immunohistological demonstration of feline infectious peritonitis virus antigen in paraffin-embedded tissues using feline ascites or murine monoclonal antibodies. Vet Immunol Immunopathol 1995;49:177–82.

[144] Hök K. Demonstration of feline infectious peritonitis in conjunctival epithelial cells from cats. APMIS 1989;97:820–4.

[145] Haagmans BL, Egberink HF, Horzinek MC. Apoptosis and T-cell depletion during feline infectious peritonitis. J Virol 1996;70:8977–83.

[146] Kipar A, Kohler K, Leukert W, et al. A comparison of lymphatic tissues from cats with spontaneous feline infectious peritonitis (FIP), cats with FIP virus infection but no FIP, and cats with no infection. J Comp Pathol 2001;125:182–91.

[147] Li X, Scott FW. Detection of feline coronaviruses in cell cultures and in fresh and fixed feline tissues using polymerase chain reaction. Vet Microbiol 1994;42:65–77.

[148] Watari T, Kaneshima T, Tsujimoto H, et al. Effect of thromboxane synthetase inhibitor on feline infectious peritonitis in cats. J Vet Med Sci 1998;60:657–9.

[149] Weiss RC, Oostrom-Ram T. Inhibitory effects of ribavirin alone or combined with human alpha interferon on feline infectious peritonitis virus replication in vitro. Vet Microbiol 1989;20:255–65.

[150] Barlough JE, Scott FW. Effectiveness of three antiviral agents against FIP virus in vitro. Vet Rec 1990;126:556–8.

[151] Weiss RC, Cox NR, Martinez ML. Evaluation of free or liposome-encapsulated ribavirin for antiviral therapy of experimentally induced feline infectious peritonitis. Res Vet Sci 1993;55:162–72.

[152] Povey RC. In vitro antiviral efficacy of ribavirin against feline calicivirus, feline viral rhinotracheitis virus, and canine parainfluenza virus. Am J Vet Res 1978;39:175–8.

[153] Weiss RC, Cox NR, Boudreaux MK. Toxicologic effects of ribavirin in cats. J Vet Pharmacol Ther 1993;16:301–16.

[154] Zeidner NS, Myles MH, Mathiason-DuBard CK, et al. Alpha interferon (2b) in combination with zidovudine for the treatment of presymptomatic feline leukemia virus-induced immunodeficiency syndrome. Antimicrob Agents Chemother 1990;34:1749–56.

[155] Weiss RC, Cox NR, Oostrom-Ram T. Effect of interferon or Propionibacterium acnes on the course of experimentally induced feline infectious peritonitis in specific-pathogen-free and random-source cats. Am J Vet Res 1990;51:726–33.

[156] Cantell K, Pyhala L. Circulating interferon in rabbits after administration of human interferon by different routes. J Gen Virol 1973;20:97–104.

[157] Koech DK, Obel AO. Efficacy of Kemron (low dose oral natural human interferon alpha) in the management of HIV-1 infection and acquired immune deficiency syndrome (AIDS). East Afr Med J 1990;67:64–70.

[158] Tomkins WA. Immunomodulation and therapeutic effects of the oral use of interferon-α: mechanism of action. J Interferon Cytokine Res 1999;19:817–28.

[159] Schellekens H, Geelen G, Meritet J-F, et al. Oromucosal interferon therapy: relationship between antiviral activity and viral load. J Interferon Cytokine Res 2001;21:575–81.

[160] Ueda Y, Sakurai T, Yanai A. Homogeneous production of feline interferon in silkworm by replacing single amino acid code in signal peptide region in recombinant baculovirus and characterization of the product. J Vet Med Sci 1993;55:251–8.

[161] Mochizuki M, Nakatani H, Yoshida M. Inhibitory effects of recombinant feline interferon on the replication of feline enteropathogenic viruses in vitro. Vet Microbiol 1994;39:145–52.

[162] Ishida T, Shibanai A, Tanaka S, et al. Use of recombinant feline interferon and gluco-corticoid in the treatment of feline infectious peritonitis. J Feline Med Surg 2004;6:107–9.

[163] Addie DD, Schaap I, Nicolson L, et al. The persistence and transmission of type I feline coronavirus in natural infections [abstract]. In: Abstracts of the Second International Feline Coronavirus/Feline Infectious Peritonitis Symposium. Glasgow, Scotland; 2002.

[164] Addie DD, Paltrinieri S, Pedersen NC. Recommendations from workshops of the Second International Feline Coronavirus/Feline Infectious Peritonitis Symposium. J Feline Med Surg 2004;6:125–30.

[165] Addie DD, Jarrett O. Isolation of immune complexes in feline infectious peritonitis [abstract]. In: Abstracts of the IXth International Congress of Virology. 1993.

[166] Addie DD, Toth S. Feline coronavirus is not a major cause of neonatal kitten mortality. Feline Pract 1993;21:13–8.

[167] Lutz H, Gut M, Leutenegger CM, et al. Kinetics of FCoV infection in kittens born in catteries of high risk for FIP under different rearing conditions [abstract]. In: Abstracts of the Second International Feline Coronavirus/Feline Infectious Peritonitis Symposium. Glasgow, Scotland; 2002.

[168] Foley JE, Pedersen NC. The inheritance of susceptibility to feline infectious peritonitis in purebred catteries. Feline Pract 1996;1:14–22.

[169] Gonon V, Eloit M, Monteil M. Evolution de la prevalence de l'infection a coronavirus feline dans deux effectifs adoptant des conduites d'elevage differentes. Recueil Med Vet 1995;1:33–8.

[170] Horsburgh BC, Brown TD. Cloning, sequencing and expression of the S protein gene from two geographically distinct strains of canine coronavirus. Virus Res 1995;39:63–74.

[171] Glansbeek HL, Haagmans BL, Te Lintelo RG, et al. Adverse effects of feline IL-12 during DNA vaccination against feline infectious peritonitis virus. J Gen Virol 2002;83:1–10.

[172] Christianson KK, Ingersoll JD, Landon M, et al. Characterization of a temperature-sensitive feline infectious peritonitis coronavirus. Arch Virol 1989;109:185–96.

[173] Gerber JD, Ingersoll JD, Gast AM, et al. Protection against feline infectious peritonitis by intranasal inoculation of a temperature-sensitive FIPV vaccine. Vaccine 1990;8:536–42.

[174] Gerber JD, Pfeiffer NE, Ingersoll JD, et al. Characterization of an attenuated temperature sensitive feline infectious peritonitis vaccine virus. Adv Exp Med Biol 1990;276:481–9.

[175] Gerber JD. Overview of the development of a modified live temperature-sensitive FIP virus vaccine. Feline Pract 1995;23:62–6.

[176] McArdle F, Bennett M, Gaskell RM, et al. Independent evaluation of a modified live FIPV vaccine under experimental conditions (University of Liverpool experience). Feline Pract 1995;23:67–71.

[177] Scott FW, Copari WV, Olsen CW. Independent evaluation of a modified live FIPV vaccine under experimental conditions (Cornell experience). Feline Pract 1995;23:74–6.

[178] Fehr D, Holznagel E, Bolla S, et al. Evaluation of the safety and efficacy of a modified live FIPV vaccine under field conditions. Feline Pract 1995;23:83–8.

[179] Postorino-Reeves NC. Vaccination against naturally occurring FIP in a single large cat shelter. Feline Pract 1995;23:81–2.

[180] Postorino-Reeves NC, Pollock RV, Thurber ET. Long-term follow-up study of cats vaccinated with a temperature-sensitive feline infectious peritonitis vaccine. Cornell Vet 1992;82:117–23.

[181] Hoskins JD, Taylor HW, Lomax TL. Independent evaluation of a modified live feline infectious peritonitis virus vaccine under experimental conditions (Louisiana experience). Feline Pract 1995;23:72–3.

[182] Fehr D, Holznagel E, Bolla S, et al. Placebo-controlled evaluation of a modified life virus vaccine against feline infectious peritonitis: safety and efficacy under field conditions. Vaccine 1997;15:1101–9.

ELSEVIER
SAUNDERS

Vet Clin Small Anim
35 (2005) 81–88

VETERINARY
CLINICS
Small Animal Practice

Enteric Protozoal Diseases

Michael R. Lappin, DVM, PhD

*Department of Clinical Sciences, College of Veterinary Medicine and Biomedical Sciences,
Colorado State University, Fort Collins, CO 80523–1678, USA*

The most common protozoal agents infecting the gastrointestinal tract of cats are *Giardia* spp, *Cryptosporidium* spp, *Cystoisospora* spp, *Sarcocystis* spp, *Besnoitia* spp, *Hammondia* spp, *Toxoplasma gondii*, *Entamoeba histolytica*, and *Tritrichomonas fetus* [1–8]. *Giardia* spp are flagellates with trophozoite and cyst stages; *T fetus* is a flagellate that only produces trophozoites; *Cystoisospora* spp, *Sarcocystis* spp, *Besnoitia* spp, *Hammondia* spp, *T gondii*, and *Cryptosporidium* spp are coccidians that produce oocysts; and *E histolytica* is an amoeba with trophozoite and cyst stages. *Balantidium coli* is a ciliate that infects many warm-blooded vertebrates but has not been shown to infect cats [9]. *Cystoisospora* spp, *Sarcocystis* spp, *Besnoitia* spp, *Hammondia* spp, and *T gondii* only complete the intestinal cycle in one species. Some isolates of *Cryptosporidium* spp, *Giardia* spp, and *E histolytica* can infect multiple hosts and so can be zoonotic. The enteric phase of *T gondii* is blunted by immune responses to the organism; thus, enteric disease is self-limited. *T gondii* is most commonly associated with polysystemic illness [3].

Transmission and distribution

Fecal oral transmission occurs with all the enteric protozoans. *Cryptosporidium* spp oocysts are immediately infectious when passed by the host; however, *T gondii* and *Cystoisospora* spp must sporulate outside the host to be infectious. Trophozoites and cysts of *Giardia* spp are potentially infectious; however, transmission occurs most frequently after ingestion of cysts, because trophozoites are generally killed by gastric secretions. Ingestion of the organism in the tissues of transport hosts can also result in infection by *Cystoisospora* spp, *Besnoitia* spp, *Hammondia* spp, and *T gondii*. Carnivorism can result in infection by *Cryptosporidium* spp, *Giardia* spp, and *E histolytica* if the organisms are present in the intestines of the prey species. Infections can

---

E-mail address: mlappin@colostate.edu

be self-limiting for each of the agents, but with the exception of *T gondii*, fecal shedding periods are variable. After tissue cyst ingestion, infected cats rarely shed oocysts of *T gondii* for more than 2 weeks [3].

The enteric protozoans have a worldwide distribution. Because they are maintained in nature primarily by fecal oral transmission, more cases are associated with crowded and unsanitary environments. In general, *Giardia* spp, *T gondii*, *Cystoisospora* spp, *Cryptosporidium* spp, and *T fetus* infections are common in the United States; however, *E histolytica* infections are rare. Antibodies against *T gondii* (40%) and *Cryptosporidium* spp (8.3%) are commonly detected in serum from client-owned cats, suggesting that exposure is common [3,10]. Prevalence of the agents varies by region in coprologic studies [7,8].

Pathogenesis

Pathogenic mechanisms have not been ascertained for each of the enteric protozoans. *Cystoisospora* spp and *T gondii* replicate in intestinal cells and may result in clinical illness from cell destruction. *Giardia* spp, *T fetus*, and *Cryptosporidium* spp are found on the surface of enterocytes; thus, pathogenesis is unlikely secondary to direct cell damage. Some of the pathogenic mechanisms proposed for enteric pathogens include production of toxins, disruption of normal flora, induction of inflammatory bowel disease, inhibition of normal enterocyte enzymatic function, blunting of microvilli, and induction of motility disorders. *Cystoisospora* spp generally are the only pathogens resulting in clinical disease in puppies or kittens, and *Sarcocytis* spp, *Besnoitia* spp, and *Hammondia* spp are almost never pathogenic in cats; all other enteric protozoans can cause disease regardless of age. Clinical disease is more common, and duration of organism shedding into the environment may be prolonged in cats with concurrent diseases that induce immunodeficiency. Infection of cats by more than one enteric protozoan occurs in some cats. For example, cats coinfected with *Cryptosporidium* spp and *T fetus* infections had more severe clinical disease than cats infected with *T fetus* alone [11].

Clinical complaints

Primary presenting complaints in cats with enteric protozoal infections generally are vomiting, inappetence, or diarrhea; fever is uncommon. Weight loss occurs in some cats with chronic disease. *Giardia* spp, *Cryptosporidium* spp, and *T gondii* infections are most commonly associated with small bowel diarrhea; *Cystoisospora* spp, *T fetus*, and *E histolytica* infections are most commonly associated with large or mixed bowel diarrhea. Physical examination findings in cats with enteric protozoal infections are nonspecific but can include abdominal discomfort, increased gas or fluid in the intestinal tract, or thickened intestinal loops. Cats with clinical illness from *T fetus*, *Giardia* spp, or *Cystoisospora* spp infections are generally young.

Diagnosis

Enteric parasites are common in cats of all ages regardless of stool character; thus, a minimum of one fecal examination per year is indicated in all cats. All cats with diarrhea should be assessed for enteric protozoal infections. Diagnosis of gastrointestinal protozoal infection is based primarily on documentation of oocysts, trophozoites, or cysts. The American Association of Feline Practitioners recommends that all cats with diarrhea of 1 to 2 days in duration be evaluated by direct fecal examination for trophozoites of *Giardia* spp and *T fetus*; fecal flotation for eggs, cysts, and oocysts; and a *Cryptosporidium* spp screening procedure like an acid-fast stain of a fecal smear [12]. In certain cases, monoclonal antibody–based techniques (*Giardia* spp and *Cryptosporidium* spp), antigen tests (*Giardia* spp and *Cryptosporidium* spp), culture (*T fetus*), or polymerase chain reaction (PCR) assays (*Giardia* spp, *Cryptosporidium* spp, and *T fetus*) may be needed to confirm presence of infection. These techniques should not be used in lieu of routine techniques, however.

A direct smear of diarrheic stool can be used to examine for trophozoites of *T fetus*, *Giardia* spp, and *E histolytica*. More frequently, a small quantity of fresh feces or mucus is mixed with a drop of 0.9% sodium chloride on a clean microscope slide and examined at a magnification × 100 after placing a coverslip. When a motile organism is noted (http://www2.ncsu.edu/unity/lockers/project/cvmaprhome/gookin_jody.htm), structural features are assessed by examining at a magnification × 400. Application of a stain like Lugol's solution, methylene blue, or acid methyl green to the wet mount at the edge of the coverslip aids in visualizing internal structures of protozoa [13]. Trophozoites are rarely found in formed stools.

Protozoal cysts or oocysts are best demonstrated after fecal concentration; Sheather's sugar centrifugation and zinc sulfate centrifugation are two techniques commonly used in clinical practice [13]. These solutions are inexpensive and generally effective. Sugar solution is hypertonic and distorts *Giardia* spp cysts; the cytoplasm is pulled to one side and appears as a half or quarter moon. Zinc sulfate centrifugation is considered by some to be the flotation solution of choice for *Giardia* spp cysts (http://www.capcvet.org/) [12,13].

Because of their small size and limited number in feces of infected cats, *Cryptosporidium* spp oocysts are almost never seen when concentrated feces is examined at a magnification ×100. Acid-fast staining or fluorescein-labeled monoclonal antibody staining of a thin fecal smear and fecal antigen testing can aid in the diagnosis of cryptosporidiosis in cats. *Cryptosporidium* spp oocysts stain pink with modified acid-fast stain (acid-fast staining kit; Becton

Dickinson, Franklin Lakes, NJ; available at: http://catalog.bd.com/bdCat/ viewProduct.doCustomer?productNumber = 212520), and this technique can be used as an in-clinic screening procedure. A fluorescein-labeled monoclonal antibody system is available that contains monoclonal antibodies that react with *Cryptosporidium* spp oocysts and *Giardia* spp cysts (Maxiflor Crypto/Giardia IFA kit; Meridian Diagnostic Corporation, Cincinnati, OH). The assay was developed for detection of human isolates, however, and it is possible that cat isolates may not always be detected [14–18]. In addition, a fluorescence microscope is required; thus, the assay can only be performed in diagnostic laboratories. Antigens of *Giardia* spp and *Cryptosporidium* spp can be detected in feces by enzyme-linked immunosorbent assays. Most fecal antigen studies in cats have been performed with kits developed for use with human feces (ProSpectT *Giardia* Microplate Assay, ProSpectT *Cryptosporidium* Microplate Assay; Remel Microbiology Products, Lenexa, KS); thus, it is possible that cat isolates may not always be detected. Recently, an in-clinic *Giardia* spp antigen test for use with dog and cat feces was released and is currently being independently evaluated (SNAP *Giardia* Antigen Test Kit; IDEXX Laboratories, Westbrook, ME).

Feline *Giardia* isolates rarely grow in cell culture, and this technique is not practical for small animal clinics. *T fetus* readily grows in culture; the use of an in-clinic culture system for use with feline feces was recently reported (InPouchTF; BioMed Diagnostics, White City, OR) [19].

Polymerase chain reaction assays for demonstration of *Giardia* spp, *Cryptosporidium* spp, and *T fetus* DNA have been studied for use with cat feces [20–22]. In general, the assays are more sensitive than other techniques, and the amplified DNA can be studied further to determine differences in strains or species using genetic techniques. The techniques are commercially available in some laboratories but are only indicated for difficult cases (*Tritrichomonas foetus* PCR assay, North Carolina State University, Raleigh, NC, available at: http://www2.ncsu.edu/unity/lockers/project/ cvmaprhome/gookin_file1.htm; *Cryptosporidium* spp PCR assay, Colorado State University Veterinary Diagnostic Laboratory, Fort Collins, CO).

Treatment

The presence of enteric protozoans in diarrheic stool does not prove that disease was caused by the organism. Some enteric protozoans, especially *Giardia* spp, *Cryptosporidium* spp, *T fetus*, and *Cystoisospora* spp, live chronically in the intestinal tract of cats; other conditions causing gastrointestinal tract disease can induce increased levels of organism shedding. Thus, cats with enteric protozoal infections that do not respond positively to therapy should be evaluated for underlying causes of disease.

Withholding food for 24 to 48 hours is indicated in cats with acute vomiting or diarrhea. Highly digestible bland diets are used most frequently if vomiting and small bowel diarrhea are the primary manifestations of disease. High-fiber diets are generally indicated if large bowel diarrhea is occurring.

Diarrhea associated with *Giardia* spp generally resolves during or after administration of metronidazole. In a recent study, cyst shedding resolved in 26 cats after the oral administration of metronidazole benzoate at 25 mg/kg every 12 hours for 7 days [23]. Metronidazole also helps to correct the anaerobic bacterial overgrowth that commonly accompanies giardiasis. If inflammatory changes exist, metronidazole may also be beneficial because of inhibition of lymphocyte function. Central nervous system toxicity occasionally occurs with this drug; however, it is unlikely to occur if a total daily orally administered dose no more than 50 mg/kg is given [24]. Fenbendazole has not been studied extensively for treatment of giardiasis in cats. In one experiment study of cats coinfected with *Giardia* spp and *Cryptosporidium* spp, 4 of 8 cats treated with orally administered fenbendazole at a dose of 50 mg/kg daily for 5 days stopped shedding *Giardia* cysts [25]. The combination product of febantel, pyrantel, and praziquantel has been shown to have anti-*Giardia* activity in dogs [26]. When given orally at the febantel dose of approximately 56 mg/kg daily for 5 days, *Giardia* cyst shedding was eliminated in 6 of 8 treated cats [27]. Albendazole has been evaluated for treatment of giardiasis in a limited number of dogs but has been associated with neutropenia [28,29]. Furazolidone (4 mg/kg administered orally every 12 hours for 7 days) and paromomycin (appropriate dosing interval for cats is unknown) are other drugs with anti-*Giardia* effects, but they have not been evaluated extensively in cats. Lastly, because use of the commercially available *Giardia* spp vaccines as immunotherapy has resulted in variable treatment responses in dogs and cats, the use of the feline product should be reserved for resistant infections in cats (Fel-O-Vax *Giardia*; Fort Dodge Animal Health, Fort Dodge, IA) [30,31].

Multiple drugs have been evaluated for the treatment of cats with *T fetus* infections; no drug evaluated to date eliminates infection, and diarrhea rarely resolves during the treatment period [5,32]. In one small study, administration of metronidazole and enrofloxacin lessened diarrhea in kittens [33]. It is unknown if the organisms infecting those cats was *T fetus*, however. It is possible that some cats with *T fetus* have other enteric coinfections; thus, anthelmintics or drugs with activity against *Giardia* spp, *Cryptosporidium* spp, and enteric bacteria like *Campylobacter* spp are often prescribed. Paromomycin should be avoided cats with bloody stools because of the potential for being absorbed and inducing renal disease or deafness [32]. In one study, 23 of 26 cats with diarrhea and *T fetus* infection had complete resolution of diarrhea a median of 9 months after initial diagnosis [33].

Paromomycin (150 mg/kg administered orally every 12–24 hours for 5 days), tylosin (10–15 mg/kg administered orally every 12 hours for up to 21 days), and azithromycin (10 mg/kg administered orally every 24 hours for up to 21 days) have all been used by the author to lessen diarrhea in cats with cryptosporidiosis, but no treatment has consistently stopped *Cryptosporidium* spp oocyst shedding [34,35]. The most commonly prescribed drugs to treat *Cystoisospora* spp infections in cats are sulfadimethoxine (50–60 mg/kg administered orally every 24 hours for 5–20 days), trimethoprim-sulfonamide (15 mg/kg administered orally every 12 hours for 5 days), furozolidone (8–20 mg/kg administered orally every 12–24 hours for 5 days), and amprolium (60–100 mg administered orally every 24 hours for 5 days).

Prevention

Cats should be housed indoors or otherwise not be allowed to hunt. The commercially available *Giardia* vaccine was not recommended for routine use by the American Association of Feline Practitioners [36]. If recurrent infections are common in a household or cattery, however, vaccination may be beneficial in some cases.

Zoonotic considerations

Healthy cats without ectoparasites are not considered human health risks (http://www.cdc.gov/hiv/pubs/brochure/oi_pets.htm) [12]. *Cryptosporidium* spp, *T gondii*, *Giardia* spp, and *E histolytica* are potentially zoonotic, however. *E histolytica* infections of cats are extremely uncommon; thus, cats are unlikely sources of human infections. Most people are infected with *Cryptosporidium* spp or *Giardia* spp from contaminated food or water rather than from contact with pets [12,37]. It is now known that there are *Cryptosporidium* spp and *Giardia* spp that are specific to people or pets [38–40]. For example, in one recent study of *Cryptosporidium hominis* of people, the organism failed to infect dogs and cats [39]. Most cats are infected with *Giardia* assemblage F, an assemblage that has not been shown to infect people [40]. *Cryptosporidium felis* has not been detected in immunocompetent people. Thus, not all *Cryptosporidium* spp and *Giardia* spp are zoonotic. It is impossible to determine clinically if an individual strain is infectious to people, however; thus, infected cats should be managed as a potential zoonotic risk. For a more extensive discussion of feline enteric zoonoses, the reader is referred to the article on zoonotic diseases in this issue.

References

[1] Lappin MR. Protozoal diseases. In: Morgan RV, editor. Handbook of small animal practice. New York: Churchill Livingstone; 1997. p. 1169.
[2] Kirkpatrick CE, Dubey JP. Enteric coccidial infections. *Isospora, Sarcocystis, Cryptosporidium, Besnoitia*, and *Hammondia*. Vet Clin N Am Small Anim Pract 1987;17:1405.
[3] Dubey JP, Lappin MR. Toxoplasmosis and neosporosis. In: Greene CE, editor. Infectious diseases of the dog and cat. 2nd edition. Philadelphia: WB Saunders; 1998. p. 493–503.
[4] Gookin JL, Stebbins ME, Hunt E, et al. Prevalence and risk factors for feline *Tritrichomonas foetus* and *Giardia* infection. J Clin Microbiol 2004;42:2707–10.
[5] Gookin JL, Breitschwerdt EB, Levy MG, et al. Diarrhea associated with trichomonosis in cats. J Am Vet Med Assoc 1999;215:1450–4.

[6] Levy MG, Gookin JL, Poore M, et al. *Tritrichomonas foetus* and not *Pentatrichomonas hominis* is the etiologic agent of feline trichomonal diarrhea. J Parasitol 2003;89:99–104.

[7] Hill S, Lappin MR, Cheney J, et al. Prevalence of enteric zoonotic agents in cats. J Am Vet Med Assoc 2000;216:687–92.

[8] Spain CV, Scarlett JM, Wade SE, McDonough P. Prevalence of enteric zoonotic agents in cats less than 1 year old in central New York State. J Vet Intern Med 2001;15:33–8.

[9] Nkauchi K. The prevalence of *Balantidium coli* infection in fifty six mammalian species. J Vet Med Sci 1999;61:63–5.

[10] McReynolds C, Lappin MR, McReynolds L, et al. Regional seroprevalence of *Cryptosporidium parvum* IgG specific antibodies of cats in the United States. Vet Parasitol 1998;80:187–95.

[11] Gookin JL, Levy MR, Law JM, et al. Experimental infection of cats with *Tritrichomonas foetus*. Am J Vet Res 2001;62:1690–7.

[12] Brown RR, Elston TH, Evans L, Glaser C, Gulledge ML, Jarboe L, et al. American Association of Feline Practitioners 2003 report on feline zoonoses. Compend Contin Educ Pract Vet 2003;25:936–65.

[13] Lappin MR, Calpin J. Laboratory diagnosis of protozoal diseases. In: Greene CE, editor. Infectious diseases of the dog and cat. Philadelphia: WB Saunders; 1998. p. 437–41.

[14] Morgan UM, Constantine CC, Forbes DA, et al. Differentiation between human and animal isolates of *Cryptosporidium parvum* using rDNA sequencing and direct PCR analysis. J Parasitol 1997;83:825–30.

[15] Caccio S, Pinter E, Rantini R, et al. Human infection with *Cryptosporidium felis*: case report and literature review. Emerg Infect Dis 2002;8:85–6.

[16] Morgan U, Weber R, Xiao L, et al. Molecular characterization of *Cryptosporidium* isolates obtained from human immunodeficiency virus-infected individuals living in Switzerland, Kenya, and the United States. J Clin Microbiol 2000;38:1180–3.

[17] Bornay-Llinares FJ, da Silva AJ, Moura INS, et al. Identification of *Cryptosporidium felis* in a cow by morphologic and molecular methods. Appl Environ Microbiol 1999;65:1455–8.

[18] Xiao L, Morgan UM, Fayer R, et al. *Cryptosporidium* systematics and implications for public health. Parasitol Today 2000;16:287.

[19] Gookin JL, Foster DM, Poore MF. Use of a commercially available culture system for diagnosis of *Tritrichomonas foetus* infection in cats. J Am Vet Med Assoc 2003;222:1376–9.

[20] Gookin JL, Birkenheuer AJ, Breitschwerdt EB, et al. Single-tube nested PCR for detection of *Tritrichomonas foetus* in feline feces. J Clin Microbiol 2002;40:4126–30.

[21] Scorza AV, Brewer MM, Lappin MR. Polymerase chain reaction for the detection of *Cryptosporidium* spp. in cat feces. J Parasitol 2003;89:423–6.

[22] Thompson RCA, Hopkins RM, Homan WL. Nomenclature and genetic groupings of *Giardia* infecting mammals. Parasitol Today 2000;16:210–3.

[23] Scorza V, Lappin MR. Metronidazole for treatment of giardiasis in cats. J Feline Med Surg 2004;6:157–60.

[24] Caylor KB, Cassimatis MK. Metronidazole neurotoxicosis in two cats. J Am Anim Hosp Assoc 2001;37:258–62.

[25] Keith C, Lappin MR. Fenbendazole for treatment of *Giardia* spp. infection in cats concurrently infected with *Cryptosporidium parvum*. Am J Vet Res 2003;64:1027–9.

[26] Barr SC, Bowman DD, Frongillo MR, et al. Efficacy of a drug combination of praziquantel, pyrantel pamoate, and febantel against giardiasis in dogs. Am J Vet Res 1998;59:1134.

[27] Scorza V, Radecki SV, Lappin MR. Efficacy of febantel, praziquantel, and pyrantel for the treatment of giardiasis in cats. Presented at the American College of Veterinary Internal Medicine Forum. June, 2004.

[28] Barr SC, Bowman DD, Heller RL, et al. Efficacy of albendazole against giardiasis in dogs. Am J Vet Res 1993;54:926–8.

[29] Stokol T, Randoph JF, Nachbar S, et al. Development of bone marrow toxicosis after albendazole administration in a dog and cat. J Am Vet Med Assoc 1997;210:1753.

[30] Olson ME, Hannigan C, Gaviller R, et al. The use of a *Giardia* vaccine as an immuno-therapeutic agent in dogs. Can Vet J 2001;42:865.

[31] Stein JE, Radecki SV, Lappin MR. Efficacy of *Giardia* vaccination for treatment of giardiasis in cats. J Am Vet Med Assoc 2003;222:1548–51.

[32] Gookin JL, Riviere JE, Gilger BC, et al. Acute renal failure in four cats treated with paromomycin. J Am Vet Med Assoc 1999;215:1821–3.

[33] Romatowski J. *Pentatrichomonas hominis* infection in four kittens. J Am Vet Med Assoc 2000;216:1270–2.

[34] Lappin MR, Dowers K, Edsell D, et al. Cryptosporidiosis and inflammatory bowel disease in a cat. Feline Pract 1997;3:10.

[35] Barr SC, Jamrosz GF, Hornbuckle WE, et al. Use of paromomycin for treatment of cryptosporidiosis in a cat. J Am Vet Med Assoc 1994;205:1742.

[36] Richards J, Rodan I, Elston T, et al. Feline vaccine selection and administration. Compend Contin Educ Pract Vet 2001;23:71–80.

[37] Juranek DD. Cryptosporidiosis: sources of infection and guidelines for prevention. Clin Infect Dis 1995;21(Suppl):57.

[38] Thompson RCA, Hopkins RM, Homan WL. Nomenclature and genetic groupings of *Giardia* infecting mammals. Parasitol Today 2000;16:210.

[39] Monis PT, Andrews RH, Mayrhofer G, et al. Genetic diversity within the morphological species *Giardia intestinalis* and its relationship to host origin. Inf Genetics Evol 2003;3:29–38.

[40] Morgan-Ryan UM, Fall A, Ward LA, et al. *Cryptosporidium hominis* n. sp. (Apicomplexa: Cryptosporidiidae) from Homo sapiens. J Eukaryot Microbiol 2002;49:433.

ELSEVIER
SAUNDERS

Vet Clin Small Anim
35 (2005) 89–101

VETERINARY
CLINICS
Small Animal Practice

Feline Cytauxzoonosis

James H. Meinkoth, DVM, PhD*, A. Alan Kocan, PhD

*Department of Veterinary Pathobiology, College of Veterinary Medicine, 250 McElroy Hall,
Oklahoma State University, Stillwater, OK 74078–2007, USA*

Causation

Cytauxzoon felis is a protozoan hemoparasite of wild and domestic cats. In domestic cats, it causes severe clinical disease with high mortality. The genus *Cytauxzoon* was originally described in 1948 to accommodate an organism causing a fatal illness in an African duiker [1]. Organisms of the genus *Cytauxzoon* exist in two distinct tissue forms: an erythrocyte phase termed a *piroplasm* (Fig. 1) and a tissue phase known as a schizont (Figs. 2 and 3). Organisms of the genus *Cytauxzoon* are closely related to those of the genera *Babesia* and *Theileria*. *Cytauxzoon* organisms differ from *Babesia* organisms in that babesial organisms typically are exclusively intra-erythrocytic, lacking a separate phase in other tissue cells. Piroplasms of some of the "small" *Babesia spp* are morphologically indistinguishable from those of *C felis*. Theilerial organisms also have erythrocytic and non-erythrocytic phases; however, the tissue phase of *Theileria spp* occurs as numerous distinct schizonts within lymphocytes, whereas in *Cytauxzoon spp*, a single large schizont occurs within macrophages.

Because they are easily seen (and photographed) in peripheral blood smears, the erythrocytic phase of *C felis* is probably the more easily recognized form of this parasite, and cytauxzoonosis is often discussed in textbooks as a cause of anemia or hemolytic anemia. The piroplasm itself is relatively innocuous, however, and does not cause severe clinical signs in cats. Infection with only the piroplasms of *C felis* typically results in asymptomatic parasitemia [2]. The schizogonous phase of the organism is responsible for the marked clinical signs of disease. Schizont-laden macrophages can be found in virtually any tissue in the body, being particularly numerous in the lungs, spleen, and liver. These parasitized cells become greatly enlarged and are typically found within the lumen of vessels or in a subendothelial location

---

* Corresponding author.
E-mail address: jhm@cvm.okstate.edu (J.H. Meinkoth).

doi:10.1016/j.cvsm.2004.08.003
vetsmall.theclinics.com

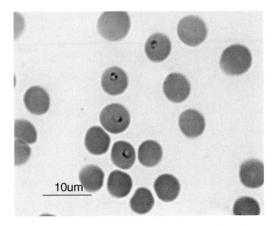

Fig. 1. Peripheral blood from a cat with cytauxzoonosis. Four piroplasms are present within erythrocytes. Two of the piroplasms (*top*) contain two nuclear areas each. Two of the erythrocytes (*bottom*) contain small particulate stain precipitate that must be differentiated from organisms (Wright's-Giemsa stain).

(see Fig. 3). Vessels are often nearly or totally occluded by parasitized cells, and vascular obstruction is thought to be one of the major pathophysiologic mechanisms in this disease [3].

Epizootiology

The emergence and evolution of cytauxzoonosis as a disease of cats in the United States are interesting. *C felis* was first recognized relatively recently, in a report published by Wagner [4] in 1976. This and subsequent reports described a previously unrecognized parasite in cats from heavily wooded areas of southwestern Missouri that resulted in an acute febrile illness, which proved to be uniformly fatal. Some of the early cases of cytauxzoonosis were initially suspected to represent *Hemobartonella felis* infection, because the cats were anemic and icteric and had detectable erythroparasites [4]. On postmortem examination, however, the recognition of the tissue phase of the organism clearly differentiated this disease from hemobartonellosis.

Within 6 years, this previously unrecognized disease had been reported in numerous southeastern states, including Arkansas, Oklahoma, Texas, Mississippi, Georgia, Louisiana, and Florida [5]. The question remains as to whether the disease was simply previously unrecognized, had been recently introduced to the country, or represented new exposure of pet cats to wildlife parasites because of encroachment into wildlife habitats or a change in pathogenicity of a previously less virulent parasite. The rapid and uniformly fatal course of the clinical disease described in these early reports and prominent nature of tissue forms of the parasite on

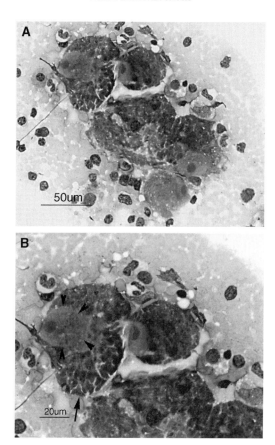

Fig. 2. (*A*) Impression smear of spleen from a cat with cytauxzoonosis. Five large schizont-containing macrophages are present. Scattered myeloid cells and plasma cells are also present. (*B*) Higher magnification of the area shown in A. The nucleus of a host cell is outlined by arrowheads. Note that each of the host cell nuclei contains a greatly enlarged nucleolus. The schizont completely fills the cells' cytoplasm, often being indistinct. In portions of the cells, multiple merozoites are seen forming within the schizont, giving the cytoplasm a "packeted" appearance (*arrow*) (Wright's-Giemsa stain).

histopathologic examination would make it unlikely that this disease would go unrecognized if it had been occurring with any significant prevalence [6].

Because no *Cytauxzoon* species had been previously recognized in the United States and the only known members of this genus in Africa were pathogens of ruminants, there was concern as to whether this disease represented a possible threat to food animals [6,7]. Because of this, a significant amount of work was done early on concerning the host range and pathogenicity of this parasite. Kier et al [7] exposed a variety of farm, wildlife, and laboratory animals to this organism via inoculation with whole blood from cats with terminal cytauxzoonosis. The organism was found to parasitize only domestic and wild cats, specifically bobcats. Results of

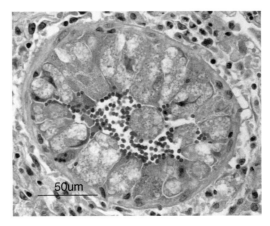

Fig. 3. Section of lung from a cat with cytauxzoonosis. A vessel is shown that is almost completely occluded by the presence of schizont-containing macrophages. These macrophages often appear to be adherent to the endothelium. Other vessels within this section were completely occluded (hematoxylin-eosin stain).

several studies revealed that the manifestations of infection varied greatly between these species. Infection of domestic cats typically resulted in an acute febrile illness and death in approximately 19 to 21 days [3]. Domestic cats developed erythroparasitemia and massive numbers of schizonts in various tissues. Infection in healthy bobcats is most often asymptomatic, resulting only in long-lasting erythroparasitemia [2,5,7]. In naturally infected and persistently parasitemic bobcats, no schizogonous forms were found in tissues [2]. Sometimes, infection of bobcats would result in systemic illness and death, and there would be marked tissue schizont development similar to that seen in domestic cats [8,9]. It was suspected that bobcats were the natural host for *C felis* and that the rapidly fatal infection seen in domestic cats represented an aberrant infection of an unnatural host. This was further substantiated by a study in which 13 of 21 apparently healthy wild-trapped bobcats in two counties in Oklahoma were found to be parasitemic [5].

Most of the initial transmission studies were done by inoculating animals with peripheral blood or homogenates of the spleen, lung, or lymph node from infected animals [3]. Because ticks serve as the natural vector for transmission of most closely related organisms, they were suspected to be involved in the natural transmission of *C felis* as well. Blouin et al [10] showed that *Dermacentor variabilis* was a competent vector by feeding nymphs on parasitemic bobcats and then successfully transmitting disease to two domestic cats after the ticks had molted to adults. Cats exposed to *C felis* via this mechanism died on days 13 and 17 after tick engorgement, respectively. Postmortem examination revealed widespread presence of schizont containing macrophages in tissues [10].

Using *D variabilis* to transmit the disease between bobcats, Blouin et al [8] showed that bobcats do undergo schizogonous development after infection but that it seems to be transient and self-limiting. *C felis*–infected *D variabilis* adults were fed on two bobcats. Eleven days after tick attachment, sections of surgically removed lymph nodes from these animals showed numerous schizont-laden macrophages. One bobcat died at day 19, with clinical signs and microscopic lesions typical of cytauxzoonosis. Subsequent examination of lymph node tissue from the surviving bobcat at 30 days showed no evidence of schizogonous tissue phases despite a persistent parasitemia. Inoculation of domestic cats with homogenates of the bobcat lymph node tissue taken at 11 days produced fatal disease, whereas homogenates of lymph node tissue taken at 30 days induced only erythroparasitemia in the recipient cats. These findings support the presence of schizogonous phases in bobcat tissue shortly after tick exposure but not after 30 days. Although some bobcats succumb to cytauxzoonosis in this acute period, schizogony in this species is presumably typically self-limiting and most animals survive to become persistently erythroparasitemic. These surviving animals serve as reservoirs of this organism.

The clinical outcome of experimental infection by inoculation in domestic cats depends on the method of exposure and is ultimately dependent on whether cats are exposed to schizogonous tissue phases or only to erythrocytic piroplasms. Inoculation of domestic cats with schizont-containing tissue homogenates (usually spleen obtained from other domestic cats succumbing to cytauxzoonosis) consistently produces a predictable fatal clinical disease [3]. Developing schizonts are first detected in tissue by 12 days. Erythroparasitemia also develops. The parasitemia is low at first but generally increases as the disease progresses, being of greatest magnitude terminally. Clinical signs are typically first noted by days 5 through 14, and cats succumb to disease approximately 8 to 20 days after exposure [3,6,11,12].

Inoculation of domestic cats with peripheral blood of cats dying of cytauxzoonosis produces a similar course of disease, because schizont-containing macrophages are often present in the circulation in cats with advanced disease. Conversely, inoculation of cats with peripheral blood of persistently parasitemic bobcats typically results in development of only erythroparasitemia with no schizont development or overt clinical signs of disease. Presumably, because bobcats undergo only transient schizogony (at least at detectable levels), inoculation of blood from these animals transfers only erythrocytic piroplasms, which cannot progress through their natural life cycle without passing through the tick host.

Cats exposed by this mechanism remain parasitemic indefinitely (although the parasitemia may decrease to low levels) but do not develop a protective immunity. If these cats are subsequently challenged via inoculation with tissue homogenates, they succumb to disease, as do naive cats. In the initial studies with transmission of *C felis*, rare cats ($\sim$4 of >500 cats) were reported to survive infection via exposure to tissue homogenates

[6,13]. These cats presumably survived the schizogonous development of the organism in a similar fashion to the course of disease in bobcats. In contrast to the blood-inoculated cats, domestic cats that have survived infection in this manner are solidly immune to re-exposure [6,13]. Thus, it seems that development of the tissue phases of the organism is essential to inducing protective immunity.

In contrast to blood inoculation from bobcats, infection of domestic cats using ticks that have fed on parasitemic bobcats produces schizogonous phases and erythroparasitemia and results in full manifestation of clinical disease. These findings demonstrate that ticks are more than a mechanical vector and are integral to completing a portion of the life cycle of *C felis*.

Cytauxzoonosis has also been reported in other wild cats. A survey of Florida panthers and Texas cougars showed erythroparasitemia in approximately 36% of apparently healthy free-ranging animals [14]. There were no differences in the results of hemograms from infected and noninfected animals, suggesting that the infection in these animals is similar to that in bobcats. No studies have been published concerning experimental infections in this species, so it is not known if any morbidity or mortality occurs in the acute phases of infection and the animals detected simply represent those that recovered. Organisms from one Florida panther were transferred to a domestic cat via inoculation with peripheral blood mononuclear cells and resulted in fatal disease in the recipient cat [15]. This would suggest that low levels of schizonts are present and circulating in chronically infected animals.

An asymptomatic parasitemia has been reported in two cheetahs; however, the identity of the organism was never clearly established [16]. The cheetahs, diagnosed in California, had been born in Oregon and spent time in Africa. Cytauxzoonosis is not endemic in any of those areas, although morphologically similar *Babesia spp* have been reported in Africa. Inoculation of whole blood from one of these cheetahs into a domestic cat failed to produce parasitemia or disease in the domestic cat.

Fatal cytauxzoonosis has been reported in a 7-year-old female White Tiger born in a private breeding facility in Florida [17]. Similarly, we have observed two cases of fatal cytauxzoonosis in tigers (Corr M et al, unpublished observations, 2001). These cats were part of a privately owned collection of exotic cats in Oklahoma and were housed in proximity to other species of Felidae, including bobcats. Samples from the affected animals demonstrated marked erythroparasitemia and numerous schizont-containing macrophages in impression smears of splenic tissue. Fatal disease has also been reported in a Bengal tiger from a German zoo [18]. This case was unusual in that feline cytauxzoonosis had not previously been reported outside the United States. Three young bobcats had been imported from the United States and introduced into the zoo approximately 14 months before the animal in this report became ill, however. Thus, cytauxzoonosis is a potential concern for exotic cats in areas with the appropriate reservoir and tick vectors.

We have reported the presence of a *Cytauxzoon*-like piroplasm in the blood of Pallas' cats imported from Mongolia [19]. The organisms were found in samples of peripheral blood collected from these animals within 10 days of their importation; thus, the cats were probably infected at their point of origin rather than acquiring the infection in the United States. Sequencing of the small subunit ribosomal RNA (ssrRNA) gene of this organism suggested it to be a distinct species of *Cytauxzoon*. Sequence variation within this gene is commonly used to determine the phylogenetic relations between various organisms. Inoculation of whole blood from these animals demonstrated that the organism is capable of replicating in domestic cats (Joyner P et al, unpublished observations, 2002). No clinical signs were noted in the recipient cats, although this is not unusual, given the method of exposure (blood inoculation of virulent *C felis* from bobcats does not result in clinical signs in the recipient cats). It is not known if there is a competent tick vector for this organism in the United States, but this underscores the potential dangers associated with importation of exotic animals.

Clinical features

There is tremendous variability in the incidence of this disease between different locations. Even within "endemic areas," the incidence of disease seems to vary greatly between relatively short distances. The incidence of cytauxzoonosis is highly seasonal, correlated with tick activity. In these authors' region of the country, the incidence is highest in spring to early summer. The number of new cases significantly declines during the hot dry periods of summer and then increases again in the early fall. Most affected cats have significant outdoor exposure, usually with access to wooded environments, and are often reported to have been missing for 1 to 2 days before being found profoundly ill [20,21].

The disease follows an acute course. Based on experimental exposures, clinical signs are first seen approximately 5 to 14 days after exposure via inoculation with blood or infected tissue [3,6,11]. Cats become profoundly depressed, dehydrated, and anorexic [3]. Many become reluctant to move or be touched and act as if they have generalized pain [3,6,20]. Fever is a prominent finding, with body temperature commonly exceeding 106°F [3]. Many cats become icteric. Miscellaneous signs noted in some cats include abnormal vocalization, ataxia, and nystagmus. Terminally, cats become moribund, hypothermic, and dyspneic [6].

Laboratory findings

Results of a complete blood cell count (CBC) from cats with cytauxzoonosis may show any combination of cytopenias. Anemia is a common finding. Anemia develops late relatively late in the course of disease but may become profound near death [11]. Unlike many other hemoparasites, there is no evidence of a bone marrow response to the anemia. Reticulocyte counts are not increased, and there are few to no polychromatophilic red blood cells in circulation [11,12]. Anemia probably results, at least in part, from phagocytosis of red blood cells, because erythrophagocytosis is a prominent finding in many organs [6,11,22]. The lack of bone marrow response may be the result of insufficient time for a regenerative response to occur and marrow suppression from inflammatory disease.

Leukopenia, often profound, with toxic changes of neutrophils is also a common finding in cytauxzoonosis [12,22,23]. Bone marrow examination may show depletion of mature myeloid cells and toxic change [22]. Aside from the morphology of the parasites, profound leukopenia and the lack of a bone marrow regenerative response to anemia are two major differences readily apparent on blood smear examination between cytauxzoonosis and hemobartonellosis, two diseases that can present with anemia and icterus.

Thrombocytopenia is seen in many cats with cytauxzoonosis [23]. This may result from increased consumption of platelets [17]. Activated partial thromboplastin time (APTT) is prolonged in some cats [23].

Many clinical chemistry changes have been described; most of them are nonspecific and vary from animal to animal. Hyperbilirubinemia and hypoalbuminemia are fairly consistent findings, particularly late in disease [21,23].

Diagnostic procedures

Although clinical signs and some laboratory findings are suggestive of cytauxzoonosis, definitive diagnosis typically requires identification of the organism. Examination of blood smears is the most common method of diagnosing cytauxzoonosis, but it is associated with several biologic and technical limitations.

The biologic limitation is that cats may not have circulating piroplasms at the time of initial presentation. Clinical signs of disease result from the development of schizogonous phases in tissues and often precede detectable erythroparasitemia. When parasitemia does occur, the magnitude is initially low. At this stage of disease, piroplasms can easily be missed, especially when performing routine examination of a smear as part of a CBC. If cytauxzoonosis is suspected, the laboratory should be alerted so that specific attention can be directed to examining erythrocytes for the presence of organisms. Dramatic increases in the number of circulating organisms can occur in as little as 24 hours. Thus, a negative smear should be repeated if there is strong clinical suspicion of disease. Typically, the magnitude of parasitemia continues to increase as the disease progresses.

Technical limitations relate to the fact that the organism is extremely small and pleomorphic, and artifacts (eg, stain precipitate, Howell-Jolly bodies) are often mistakenly identified as parasites. False diagnoses of cytauxzoonosis are frustratingly common. The organism may assume several different shapes. The characteristic shape that is most easily differentiated from artifact is the signet-ring shape. This classic form of *C felis* is a small ring (~1–3 μm in diameter, feline red blood cells are 6–7 μm in diameter) with a thick round nuclear area at one point of the ring (see Fig. 1). Sometimes, the nuclear area is a linear thickening of a portion of the ring rather than being round. The central area within the ring stains somewhat lighter than the remainder of the red blood cell. Sometimes, elongated "safety-pin" forms that have two nuclear structures on opposite sides are seen. Small comma-shaped or linear forms can also be seen. These forms can lack a distinct nuclear thickening and are more difficult to differentiate from artifact.

Cytauxzoon organisms must be differentiated from Howell-Jolly bodies, stain precipitate, and water artifact. Howell-Jolly bodies are variably sized, round, dark dots representing nuclear remnants. They do not have the ring form typical of *C felis*. Stain precipitate is usually abundant and is usually present between the cells as well as overlying the cells. *Hemobartonella* organisms are smaller and usually form dots and chains. They can be small rings, but they do not have the nuclear area (thick "dot" on the ring) that is typical of *C felis*. Diagnosis should never be based on the identification of one presumed organism.

Because of the difficultly associated with identifying this relatively small parasite, it is critical that that sample be appropriate. It is essential to have a thin well-made blood smear so that cells have an opportunity to spread out sufficiently. It is also important that slides be thoroughly air-dried before staining to prevent the development of water artifact, which can resemble intraerythrocytic structures. Wright's stain and Diff-Quik stain *Cytauxzoon* well; thus, either may be used. Diff-Quik often produces less stain precipitate and is sometimes preferable.

In cases in which the animal has died before samples can be collected or in which cytauxzoonosis is strongly suspected clinically but erythroparasites are not seen on peripheral blood smears, the schizogonous phases of the organism can be identified in impression smears of many tissues. Lung and spleen tissues are particularly useful, although the organisms can also be found in the liver, lymph nodes, and bone marrow. Parasitized macrophages become greatly enlarged and contain an extremely large prominent nucleolus (see Fig. 2). The cytoplasm is distended with the developing schizont. Initially, the schizont is a small, lobulated, ill-defined blue structure within the cytoplasm. Later, it can fill the entire cytoplasm and become even more indistinct. As the schizont matures, numerous small purple nuclear areas can be seen within the blue schizont. Ultimately, hundreds of individual merozoites are formed. These are seen as tightly packed, small, circular blue structures with a purple nucleus. Identification of schizonts is easiest in the lung and spleen, where the large schizont-containing cells stand out against the relative small tissue cells. In the liver, schizont-laden macrophages are often similar in size to hepatocytes and are more difficult to differentiate.

Although serologic methods have been used in research settings, they are not commercially available. Fortunately, serology is not needed in most clinical settings. Like serology, polymerase chain reaction (PCR) amplification of the organism's ssrRNA gene has been used in research settings but is not typically needed in a clinical setting. PCR amplification using general primers and subsequent sequencing can be used to confirm the identity of a piroplasm, because the piroplasms of some *Theileria spp* and *Babesia spp* can be morphologically identical to those of *C felis*. Fortunately, no *Theileria* or *Babesia* species have yet been reported in domestic cats in the United States.

Postmortem findings

Consistent with the rapid course of disease, cats are usually in good nutritional condition with adequate adipose tissue [21]. Pallor and icterus are common necropsy findings and correlate with the degree of anemia and hyperbilirubinemia, respectively [21]. Most animals have splenomegaly, enlarged reddened lymph nodes, and diffusely congested edematous lungs [6,12,21]. Petechial and ecchymotic hemorrhage is found in many tissues, including the lungs, urinary bladder, kidneys, heart, and meninges [15]. Abdominal veins are often distended two to three times their normal diameter as a result of vascular obstruction [12]. Pleural, pericardial, and abdominal effusions are present in some animals [12,15,20].

Histologically, there are accumulations of large schizont-containing macrophages in the lumens of veins and sinusoids of many tissues. In severely affected tissues, these cells may totally occlude the lumen of the vessel [6]. Thrombosis of affected vessels is common, and histologic changes consistent with ischemia are seen in many tissues, including the brain and heart [3]. The lungs, spleen, and liver are usually the most severely affected organs, but almost any parenchymatous organs can be involved.

Treatment and prognosis

The prognosis for cats with cytauxzoonosis has historically been grave. The mortality rate has been nearly 100%. In early studies, specific therapy was attempted using a variety of agents, including numerous antibiotics as well as antiprotozoal agents known to be effective in bovine theileriosis [6,13]. None of these agents proved to be effective. There are sporadic reports of cats surviving experimental or natural infection, but these are rare cases and often considered to be unrelated to therapeutic attempts [6,13,24]. Supportive care can prolong the course of disease by a few days but typically does not alter the outcome.

A study by Greene et al [23] reported the successful treatment of five cats utilizing diminazine aceturate, a drug used to treat babesiosis and other protozoal diseases, and of one cat utilizing imidocarb dipropionate. Intensive supportive therapy and heparinization to prevent disseminated intravascular coagulation (DIC) were also considered to be important components of therapy in this report. Unfortunately, diminazine (Ganaseg, Berenil) is not marketed in the United States, although it is available in other countries. Imidocarb (Imizol) is available in the United States for the treatment of canine babesiosis. Experience with imidocarb in our area has not been rewarding. One cat survived infection when treated with imidocarb as well as intensive supportive therapy and heparinization. Use of this drug in several other cases has not been effective. It is possible that the strain of cytauxzoonosis involved, time of treatment within the course of infection, and degree of ancillary therapy affect the clinical outcome. The authors do not have experience with the use of diminazine aceturate in clinical cases.

Recently, cats infected with *C felis* in one area have been reported to recover seemingly unrelated to treatment [25]. These cats have shown clinical signs compatible with cytauxzoonosis and had organisms within erythrocytes at the time of presentation. These cats recovered with no treatment or with supportive care in the absence of specific antiprotozoal therapy. Most of these cases have been limited to areas of western Arkansas and eastern Oklahoma. The number of cats that have survived has increased in this area, consistent with perpetuation of a less virulent strain. Infected cats are persistently parasitemic (some for >6 years) but, once recovered, have not shown recurrence of clinical disease. Similar findings may occur in other areas as well.

Prevention and client education

Transmission cannot occur directly from cat to cat without passing through the tick vector, even when animals are housed in close proximity throughout the course of disease [3]. This is a common owner concern when cytauxzoonosis is diagnosed in one animal from a multicat household. Although cat-to-cat transmission does not occur, it is likely that all cats in a household have had similar exposure to infected ticks and it is common for owners to lose several cats to this disease within a short period.

Currently, no vaccine for cytauxzoonosis exists. Because ticks are the only known mechanisms of transmission, prevention is based solely on limiting exposure to the tick vector. Studies determining the length of time that a tick must be attached to transmit disease have not been performed. With other related organisms, ticks must typically be attached for several hours for transmission to occur; thus, application of products that kill ticks within a few hours of attachment is likely to be beneficial. Cases of cytauxzoonosis have occurred in cats with reportedly diligent application of current tick control products, however. The most effective prevention is totally limiting outdoor exposure.

References

[1] Neitz WO, Thomas AD. *Cytauxzoon sylvicaprae* gen. nov., spec. nov., a protozoan responsible for a hitherto undescribed disease in the duiker [*Sylvicapra grimmia* (Linné)]. Onderstepoort J Vet Sci Anim Ind 1948;23(1/2):63–76.

[2] Glenn BL, Kocan AA, Blouin EF. Cytauxzoonosis in bobcats. J Am Vet Med Assoc 1983; 183(11):1155–8.

[3] Wagner JE, Ferris DH, Kier AB, Wightman SR, Maring E, Morehouse LG, et al. Experimentally induced cytauxzoonosis-like disease in domestic cats. Vet Parasitol 1980;6: 305–11.

[4] Wagner JE. A fatal cytauxzoonosis-like disease in cats. J Am Vet Med Assoc 1976;168(7): 585–8.

[5] Glenn BL, Rolley RE, Kocan AA. *Cytauxzoon*-like piroplasms in erythrocytes of wild-trapped bobcats in Oklahoma. J Am Vet Med Assoc 1982;181(11):1251–3.

[6] Ferris DH. A progress report on the status of a new disease of American cats: cytauxzoonosis. Comp Immun Microbiol Infect Dis 1979;1:269–76.

[7] Kier AB, Wightman SR, Wagner JE. Interspecies transmission of *Cytauxzoon felis*. Am J Vet Res 1982;43(1):102–5.

[8] Blouin EF, Kocan AA, Kocan KM, Hair J. Evidence of a limited schizogenous cycle for *Cytauxzoon felis* in bobcats following exposure to infected ticks. J Wildl Dis 1987;23(3): 499–501.

[9] Nietfeld JC, Pollock C. Fatal cytauxzoonosis in a free-ranging bobcat (*Lynx rufus*). J Wildl Dis 2002;38(3):607–10.

[10] Blouin EF, Kocan AA, Glenn BL, Kocan KM. Transmission of *Cytauxzoon felis* Kier, 1979 from bobcats, *Felis rufus* (Schreber), to domestic cats by *Dermacentor variabilis* (Say). J Wildl Dis 1984;20(3):241–2.

[11] Franks PT, Harvey JW, Shields RP, Lawman MJP. Hematologic findings in experimental feline cytauxzoonosis. J Am Anim Hosp Assoc 1988;24:395–401.

[12] Kier AB, Wagner JE, Kinden DA. The pathology of experimental cytauxzoonosis. J Comp Pathol 1987;97:415–29.

[13] Motzel SL, Wagner JE. Treatment of experimentally induced cytauxzoonosis in cats with parvaquone and buparvaquone. Vet Parasitol 1990;35:131–8.

[14] Rotstein DS, Taylor SK, Harvey JW, Bean J. Hematologic effects of cytauxzoonosis in Florida panthers and Texas cougars in Florida. J Wildl Dis 1999;35(3):613–7.

[15] Butt MT, Bowman D, Barr MC, Roelke ME. Iatrogenic transmission of *Cytauxzoon felis* from a Florida panther (*Felis concolor coryi*) to a domestic cat. J Wildl Dis 1991;27(2):342–7.

[16] Zinkl JG, McDonald SE. *Cytauxzoon*-like organisms in erythrocytes of two cheetahs. J Am Vet Med Assoc 1981;179(11):1261–2.

[17] Garner MM, Lung NP, Citino S, Greiner EC, Harvey JW, Homer BL. Fatal cytauxzoonosis in a captive-treated White Tiger (*Panthera tigris*). Vet Pathol 1996;33(1):82–6.

[18] Jakob W, Wesemeier HH. A fatal infection in a Bengal Tiger resembling cytauxzoonosis in domestic cats. J Comp Pathol 1996;114:439–44.

[19] Ketz-Riley CJ, Reichard MV, Van Den Bussche RA, Hoover JP, Meinkoth JH, Kocan AA. An intraerythrocytic small piroplasm in wild-caught Pallas' cats (Otocolobus manul) from Mongolia. J Wildl Dis 2003;39(2):424–30.

[20] Wightman SR, Kier AB, Wagner JE. Feline cytauxzoonosis: clinical features of a newly described blood parasite disease. Feline Pract 1977;7:23–6.

[21] Hoover JP, Walker BD, Hedges JD. Cytauxzoonosis in cats: eight cases (1985–1992). J Am Vet Med Assoc 1994;205(3):455–60.

[22] Meinkoth JH, Cowell RL, Cowell AK. What is your diagnosis? 10-year-old vomiting, anorexic cat. Vet Clin Pathol 1996;25(2):48, 59–60.

[23] Greene CE, Latimer K, Hopper E, Shoeffler G, Lower K, Cullens F. Administration of diminazine aceturate or imidocarb dipropionate for treatment of cytauxzoonosis in cats. J Am Vet Med Assoc 1999;215(4):497–500.

[24] Walker DB, Cowell RL. Survival of a domestic cat with naturally acquired cytauxzoonosis. J Am Vet Med Assoc 1995;206(9):1363–5.

[25] Meinkoth JH, Kocan AA, Whitworth L, Murphy G, Fox JC, Woods JP. Cats surviving natural infection with *Cytauxzoon felis*: 18 cases (1997–1998). J Vet Intern Med 2000;14: 521–5.

ELSEVIER
SAUNDERS

Vet Clin Small Anim
35 (2005) 103–128

VETERINARY
CLINICS
Small Animal Practice

Infectious Diseases of the Central Nervous System

Danièlle Gunn-Moore, BVM&S, PhD, ILTM, MACVSc, MRCVS, RCVS

*Feline Clinic, University of Edinburgh Hospital for Small Animals,
Easter Bush Veterinary Clinics, Midlothian, Scotland EH25 9RG*

Prevalence of neurologic disease in cats and the preponderance of cases with no known cause

Neurologic disease is seen commonly in cats. For example, neurologic cases make up approximately 10% of the case load of two separate feline medicine referral clinics (D.A. Gunn-Moore, BVM&S, PhD, Edinburgh University Feline Clinic data, 2004) [1]. There are many well-documented causes of neurologic disorder in cats [2,3], and infectious causes are believed to account for 30% to 45% of cases [1,4]. It is important to realize that a specific cause cannot be identified in 12% to 40% of cases, however. This holds true when looking at clinical cases [2,5,6] and histopathologic data (Table 1) [1,4]. In addition, although there are many known infectious causes (Box 1), a large number of cases (35%–40%) are found to have histopathologic changes suggestive of viral infection (that is not consistent with feline infectious peritonitis [FIP]), but no causal agent can be identified (Table 2) [1,4]. This group becomes even more significant if you consider cats with particular clinical signs. For example, of 30 cats that were investigated for having recurrent seizures, all were found to have structural brain disease and 14 (47%) had nonsuppurative meningoencephalitis suggestive of a viral infection, but no infectious agent could be found [5].

From this, we can see that infectious disease is a common cause of central nervous system (CNS) disorders in cats. In addition, the most common infectious agents are feline coronaviruses (FCoV, which can cause FIP) and some other, as yet unidentified, infectious agent(s), which are probably

The author received funding support for her lectureship from Nestlé Purina Petcare.
E-mail address: Danielle.Gunn-Moore@ed.ac.uk

Table 1
Histopathologic diagnoses in 286 feline neurology cases (University of Bristol 1975–1998)

Cause	Number	Percent
Inflammatory/infectious	92	32
No abnormalities detected	51	18
Degenerative	42	15
Neoplasia	38	13
Feline dysautonomia	27	9
Feline spongiform encephalopathy (FSE)	24	8
Congenital	12	4

Data from Bradshaw JM, Pearson GR, Gruffydd-Jones TJ. A retrospective study of 286 cases of neurological disorders of the cat. J Comp Pathol 2004;131:112–20.

viruses [1,5]. Unfortunately, because we cannot identify the cause, we do not know how best to treat these cases, nor do we know how to prevent them. It is therefore essential that we try harder to identify the etiology behind the pathologic findings. This means performing more detailed diagnostics on individual clinical cases, such as looking for potential infectious organisms by serology, cerebrospinal fluid (CSF) IgG quotient, and IgG index [6]; CSF polymerase chain reaction (PCR) assays to detect the infectious organism's DNA or RNA [7]; and immunohistochemistry or PCR on brain samples collected postmortem. In addition, it underlines the need for further experimental investigation into potential pathogens. It is only by adopting a more questioning approach to disease pathogenesis that we can hope to determine what may be causing neurologic disease in many of our pet cats.

Reasons for the increased recognition of infectious central nervous system disease in cats

Improved diagnostics and changing concepts in disease pathogenesis

Over the past 10 years, there has been a dramatic increase in the recognition and understanding of many different infectious diseases and of how they can affect the CNS. Advances in molecular technology have enabled the detection of pathogens within the CNS (eg, by using PCR assays), led to the recognition of new infectious diseases, and expanded our understanding of the etiopathogenesis of these infections.

With the changing understanding of etiopathogenesis, we have had to redefine our concept of "infectious disease." No longer can we think that infectious agents can only cause acute disease that classically fulfills Koch's postulates of cause and effect. For example, the acute disease that is seen when a bacterial infection spreads from otitis media to cause suppurative meningoencephalitis [8]. We now know that some diseases result from chronic insidious infections and that this is particularly true within the relatively protected confines of the CNS. In addition, progressively more

Box 1. Naturally occurring infectious causes of central nervous system disease in domestic cats

Viral
    Feline coronavirus (FCoV)[a]
    Feline panleukopenia virus (FPV)
    Feline immunodeficiency virus (FIV)
    Feline leukemia virus (FeLV)
    Rabies virus
    Aujeszky's disease virus
    Feline herpesvirus-1 (FHV-1)
    Borna disease virus (BDV)
    Certain arboviruses (see text)
Bacterial
    Pasturella
    Staphylococcus
    Other aerobic organisms
    Anaerobic organisms
    Mycobacteria
Protozoal
    Toxoplasmosis[a]
Rickettsial
    Ehrlichiosis
Fungal
    Cryptococcosis[a]
    Blastomycosis
    Histoplasmosis
    Aspergillosis
    Dematiaceous fungi
Parasitic
    Cuterebra larval myiasis
    Visceral larva migrans (eg, *Toxocara*)
    Sarcocystis
    Dirofilaria immitis
Probable and other
    Feline spongiform encephalopathy (FSE)
    Feline polioencephalomyelitis and miscellaneous
        nonsuppurative (meningo)encephalitides[a]

---

[a] Most common causes of encephalitis in cats. Others are sporadic and rare. *Data from* Refs. [8,24,36,37,44,167].

Table 2
Diagnoses in 92 feline neurologic cases found to have central nervous system histopathology
consistent with inflammation and/or infection (University of Bristol 1975–1998)

Cause	Number	Percent
Feline infectious peritonitis (FIP)[a]	47	51
Viral (non-FIP)[b]	32	35
Protozoal cysts (eg, toxoplasmosis)	8	9
Bacterial infection	3	3
Feline immunodeficiency virus (FIV)	1	1
Cryptococcosis	1	1

[a] One of the cats with FIP was also found to have an incidental nematode larvae (*Toxocara*)
within its lateral ventricle.
[b] Nonsuppurative meningitis and/or encephalitis was present, but no cause could be found.
Five of these cats also had changes consistent with feline spongiform encephalopathy.
Data from Bradshaw JM, Pearson GR, Gruffydd-Jones TJ. A retrospective study of 286
cases of neurological disorders of the cat. J Comp Pathol 2004;131:112–20.

diseases are being identified that, although being associated with the presence of a particular pathogen, require a number of other factors to occur
concurrently before disease becomes apparent. For these diseases to develop, there has to be a specific interaction between the infectious organism,
host factors (especially genetics affecting the immune system), and the
environment.

Unfortunately, establishing a causal relation can be difficult, particularly
when the prevalence of the infection is high in the general population but
only a few individuals have the necessary factors required for clinical signs
to develop. Serologic surveys have been largely responsible for recognizing
the role of infectious organisms in this type of disease. After detecting a
serologic relation, it is then possible to use more complex molecular biology
techniques to detect the pathogen within a particular individual or particular pathologic lesion. It is highly likely that it will be by using this type of
approach that the causes for many feline CNS disorders will be found (eg,
Borna disease [BD]).

Changing population dynamics

Populations are changing; people are living in progressively larger urban
groups, and international travel is now commonplace. This allows for rapid
spread of disease, not only among human beings but from human beings to
other species. In addition, as the global human population increases, the
demand for housing means that previously unexplored habitats are being
developed, new pathogens are being exposed, and old pathogens are finding
new hosts. There are a number of examples of infections that have crossed
between species because of altered population dynamics, and many of them
involve feline species. Examples include canine distemper virus (CDV),
which is now causing disease in a number of large feline species, particularly
lions in the Serengeti [9], but has not yet been detected in domestic cats [10];

severe acute respiratory syndrome (SARS), which is caused by a coronavirus that seems to have been passed from civet cats in China to human beings (although the civet cat is not actually a feline species) [11,12]; avian influenza virus (H5N1), which has killed domestic and captive wild felids in Thailand [13]; and West Nile virus (WNV), which is now present in the United States, being spread by mosquitoes to many wild and captive birds as well as to horses and humans beings [14].

WNV is a particularly interesting infection to consider. This is because experimental studies have shown that it is relatively easy to transmit WNV to cats by a mosquito bite or orally via consumption of infected prey [15]. Experimental cats in one study showed only mild nonneurologic signs [15]. This does not mean that WNV cannot cause neurologic disease in cats, however. This is because dogs in the same study remained perfectly healthy [15] but have been shown to develop encephalitis and myocarditis in a separate study [16]. To date, domestic cats tested in New York City have not been found to be seropositive for WNV [17]. Seropositive cats have been identified in the United States, however, and several cases demonstrated seroconversion coincident with neurologic illness (A. Glaser, DVM, PhD, Cornell University Animal Health Diagnostic Laboratory, personal communication, 2004). The potential role that WNV may play in feline neurologic disease requires further investigation.

Increasing demand for inexpensive food

An increasing demand for inexpensive food has resulted in a growing number of food-related infections. In addition to classic types of food poisoning, the transmission of the transmissible spongiform encephalopathies (TSEs) should be considered in this group.

Increasing awareness of zoonotic infections

It is perhaps of some concern that there has been a particular increase in the recognition of zoonotic conditions (diseases that can be spread from animals to people). In fact, three quarters of all emerging human pathogens are zoonotic [18]. Because of this, it is important that we raise our general awareness of this type of disease and monitor closely for any evidence of interspecies transfer of infections.

By studying the genetic relation between pathogens and performing infectivity studies, a number of infectious agents have already been identified that can cross species barriers and raise the possibility of zoonotic infection. Two such diseases are feline spongiform encephalopathy (FSE) and BD. In both cases, the infectious agents can infect a number of mammalian species, including cats and people. In addition, both infections have a poorly understood etiopathogenesis and may result in terminal neurologic disease.

Known causes of central nervous system infection in cats

From the data shown in Tables 1 and 2, we can see that FIP and nonsuppurative encephalitides (also called viral non-FIP encephalitides) are the only two commonly recognized potentially infectious causes of CNS disease in the cat. Other infections, for example, toxoplasmosis, feline leukemia virus (FeLV), feline immunodeficiency virus (FIV), feline panleukopenia (FPV), and fungal and parasitic infections, are seen only rarely. Detailed summaries of the pathogenesis, clinical signs, diagnostic approach, treatment, and neuropathologic findings of these specific infections are readily available [1,4,6,7,19–24]. The rest of this article therefore adds only selected comments in relation to these organisms and focuses on the nonsuppurative encephalitides and the more unusual infections for which information is less readily available.

Feline infectious peritonitis

FIP is the most commonly detected infectious cause of neurologic disease in cats. It accounts for 45% to 50% of all cases associated with inflammatory changes, which equates to 15% to 20% of all feline neurologic cases [1,4]. It is essential to realize just how common this infection is and that although most clinical cases are seen in young pedigree cats, usually with obvious systemic involvement, this is not always the case.

As with many viral infections affecting the CNS, histopathologic examination reveals nonsuppurative meningoencephalomyelitis, with perivascular cuffing and meningeal infiltration with mononuclear cells, gliosis, and variable neuronal degeneration. The inflammation is often pyogranulomatous, is located around the lateral ventricles or in the meninges, or may affect the choroid plexus. In addition, vasculitis or acquired hydrocephalus may be present, and systemic changes are usually apparent [1,25,26].

Feline immunodeficiency virus

FIV can cause neurologic disease as a direct primary neurotropic effect of the virus or via secondary opportunistic infections, such as FIP, toxoplasmosis, or cryptococcosis [27–32]. It is important to note that this virus cannot be excluded on the basis of negative serology. This is because several studies have failed to detect antibody in some virus-positive individuals [27,33], and in one report, approximately 20% of cats naturally infected with FIV were antibody-negative [33]. Although the reason for this is unknown, it has been suggested that some cats were tested early in the course of infection, before the development of an antibody response. These cats are unlikely to show CNS disease. Alternatively, some cats may have been tested late in the disease, once antibody levels had fallen, along with the terminal decline of the immune system [27]. Other factors may also play a role, because some cats fail to produce a detectable antibody response to

FIV at any time during infection [33]. Therefore, to confirm that a cat is not infected with FIV, it may be necessary to perform PCR on a blood or CSF sample or PCR or immunohistochemistry on brain sections collected postmortem [32].

Rare or experimental infectious causes of central nervous system disease in cats

Naturally occurring and clinically significant CNS infections have occasionally been seen in cats, resulting from a wide range of organisms. These include feline herpesvirus-1 (FHV-1) [34], feline calicivirus (FCV) [35], dematiaceous fungi (*Cladophialophora bantiana*) [36], and nematodes (eg, *Sarcocystis neurona*) [37].

It is also prudent to consider clinically significant CNS infections that have been produced experimentally in cats. These include *Bartonella henselae* [38], which typically causes cat scratch disease in people [39]; equine herpesvirus-9 [40]; Newcastle disease virus [41]; human poliovirus [42]; and simian cytomegalovirus-related stealth virus (which was taken from a human being with chronic fatigue syndrome) [43].

Much speculation has concerned the arboviruses (the arthropod-borne encephalomyelitis group) and whether or not they may be responsible for significant natural CNS infection in cats [44]. Many of these viruses have been shown to cause natural or experimental infection in cats. For example, natural infections have been seen in cats with BD virus (BDV), which can be subclinical or clinically significant. Antibodies to St. Louis encephalitis virus, Japanese encephalitis virus, yellow fever virus, Tenshaw virus, Snowshoe hare virus, Jamestown Canyon virus, and Powassan virus have been found in free-living cats, indicating previous subclinical infections [45–47]. Experimental infections have been documented with Near Eastern equine encephalitis virus [48,49], Powassan virus [46], and Rift Valley fever virus in kittens [47]. Many of these viruses have a wide geographic distribution, including the United States and Europe, and some are endemically present in wild mammal populations to which free-living cats may become exposed [50]. Although these studies show that cats are potentially at risk of becoming infected with these organisms, their role in causing a significant incidence of naturally arising feline neurologic disease remains to be determined.

Borna disease virus

Epizootiology

Classical BD is a severe neurologic disease that is seen predominantly in horses and sheep in endemic areas of Germany and Switzerland. Natural infections have also been seen in cats and ostriches and, occasionally, in rabbits, cattle, goats, deer, foxes, and dogs [51–59]. Experimentally, BDV can also be transmitted to birds, rodents, and monkeys, and it is likely that the host range includes all warm-blooded animals and birds [52,58,60,61]. The exact geographic distribution of the virus is uncertain, but serologic evidence has documented infection in Europe, the United States, and Asia [62–70].

BD in cats is also known as "staggering disease." It was first described in Sweden [71] and later shown to be caused by BDV [72]. Based on serologic surveys or surveys looking for BDV RNA in peripheral blood samples, it is clear that BDV infection is usually asymptomatic. The prevalence of seropositivity increases steadily with age in cats [72,73] and, interestingly, seems to be higher in cats that are also FIV antibody-positive [68,74]. In the United Kingdom, 6% of cats with no evidence of CNS disease have antibodies against BDV [65], as do 9% of ill cats submitted for FIV, FeLV, and FIP virus testing (D.A. Harbour, PhD, unpublished results from 654 cat blood samples, 1999). In Japan, 13% to 22% of healthy randomly selected cats are seropositive for BDV [62,75]. Antibodies against BDV or BDV RNA are seen most frequently in cats with neurologic disease, however. When cats with undefined neurologic disorders were investigated, 13% were found to be BDV antibody-positive in Germany [76] compared with 35% in the United Kingdom [65] and 67% in Japan [77]. Although most documented cases of feline BD have originated from northern and central Europe, probable cases have been seen in many other countries [65] (see section on nonsuppurative encephalomyelitis of unknown cause). Given the difficulty in making a premortem diagnosis (and even a postmortem diagnosis) and the low index of suspicion, it is likely that BD is underdiagnosed.

Pathogenesis

The source of BDV infection is rarely known. Infected cats usually, but not always, have outdoors access, particularly to rural or woodland areas, however [78–80]. This has led to the suggestion that rodents or wild birds may be viral carriers [80–82]. Natural infections are believed to be transmitted via saliva or nasal secretions [52,73,83].

BDV is a neurotropic RNA virus [84,85] that is genetically stable [86,87]. It is ubiquitously distributed and seems to have many well-adapted species-specific biotypes [54,72,88–90]; in most cases, infection causes little or no sign of disease. It is currently believed that clinical signs only develop when a host is exposed to a particular strain of BDV [57,62,73,91] or is particularly susceptible and mounts an abnormal immune response to the virus (ie, disease seems to result from a T-cell–dependent immune mechanism) [60,91–93].

Clinical signs

Natural BD has been reported in more than 100 cats [54,78–80,94]. It is seen most frequently in male cats, with no particular breed predisposition.

Although a wide age range of cats may be affected (from 5 months to 11 years of age), young adults seem to be most at risk [54,78,79]. Disease is characterized by behavioral and motor disturbances resulting from meningoencephalomyelitis. In experimental infections, clinical signs included protrusion of the third eyelid, behavioral changes, circling, ataxia, and tremors [72]. Natural infections may present with progressive hind limb ataxia, loss of appetite, fever, increased affection toward the owner, unusual staring expression, apparent pain over the sacrum, increased salivation, aggression, an inability to retract claws, seizures, focal or generalized pruritus, hypersensitivity to light and sound, or constipation [76,78,79]. Occasional atypical cases have been seen, for example, causing muscle fasciculation and proprioceptive defects (without evidence of encephalitis) [95]. Disease is usually progressive, and mortality rates are high because affected cats usually warrant euthanasia within a week to 6 months [78,79]. Cats that survive the initial episode may remain chronically infected or may experience recurrent episodes of disease [72]. Although fatal BD is seen most commonly as a rare isolated event, it can occasionally occur as a large outbreak, where as many as 30 to 40 cases may be seen in a week [78].

Diagnosis

Premortem diagnosis is difficult. In most cases, typical clinical signs in a cat from an endemic area result in a presumptive diagnosis of BD. Unfortunately, detection of serum antibodies is not reliable. This is because although raised serum antibodies are present in some cats with BD (~40%) [76], particularly those with acute disease, others may be antibody-negative, particularly if they have subacute or chronic disease [54,62,65,72,79]. Although clinical signs of BD tend to develop at the same time that BDV RNA can be detected within the peripheral blood [89], this does not necessarily reflect the extent of the viral load in the CNS [60], and asymptomatic cats can also be positive [75]. Routine serum biochemistry and hematology are generally unremarkable, although some cats may show a leukopenia, and mild elevations in glucose or alanine aminotransferase (ALT) levels may also occur [72,78]. CSF analysis may show a leukocytosis with mononuclear cells predominating, protein levels may be increased (Table 3) [78], and antibodies to BDV may be detected [92].

Histopathologically, BD usually results in nonsuppurative meningoencephalomyelitis, with neuronophagia, microgliosis, and heavy perivascular cuffing by mononuclear cells [10,72,78]. Occasional cases seem to result in neurologic signs without evidence of associated inflammation [95]. In most cases, lesions are particularly evident in the gray matter of the cerebral hemispheres, the limbic system, and the brain stem [10,54,78]. The cerebellum and spinal cord are less frequently affected [79].

Confirmation that BDV is the cause of this disease has been demonstrated by experimental transmission studies to cats and rabbits [72,79]. In

Table 3
Infectious disease and typical cerebrospinal fluid changes

Disease	CSF Pressure	CSF Appearance	WBC Count[a]	WBC Type	Total Protein concentration[b]	Albumin	Globulin	CSF Antibodies detectable	Organisms visible
Feline infectious peritonitis (FIP)	WNL or ↑	Clear or turbid	+++ (WNL- ++)	PMN-mono-mixed	+++ (WNL-+)	++	++	Yes	No
Other viral encephalitis (eg, Borna disease)[c]	WNL	Clear (turbid)	+ (++)	Mono	+ (++)	WNL	?	No	No
Protozoal meningoencephalitis (eg, toxoplasmosis)	WNL or ↑	Xanthochromic	+ (++)	Mixed-PMN, eos, mono	+ (++)	+	+	Variable	Rarely
Fungal meningoencephalitis (eg, cryptococcosis)	↑ or viscous	Turbid, xanthochromic	++	Mixed-PMN, mono, eos	++	++	+(+)	Varies	Varies
Bacterial meningitis	WNL or ↑	Turbid	++ (+++)	PMN (mixed)	++ (+++)	++	++	Varies	Yes (varies)

Abbreviations: CSF, cerebrospinal fluid; eos, eosinophils predominate; FIP, feline infectious peritonitis; mono, mononuclear cells (ie, lymphocytes, monocytes, macrophages) predominate; PMN, polymorphonuclear cells (neutrophils) predominate; WBC, white blood cell; WNL, within normal limits; ↑ = increased.

[a] Reference range for WBC count = <4 per microliter; + = 5–80 per microliter; ++ = 81–500 per microliter; +++ = >500 per microliter.

[b] Reference range for total protein concentration = <25 mg/dL; + = 25–100 mg/dL; ++ = 100–300 mg/dL; +++ = >300mg/dL.

[c] Some viral infections cause neuropathologic changes without inflammation, and these may alter the CSF little [43].

Symbols in parentheses indicate less frequently seen variations.

Data from Refs. [4,10,20,72,167].

addition, BDV antigen may be detected by immunohistochemistry or enzyme-linked immunosorbent assay (ELISA) [54], and BDV RNA may be detected by PCR; all three methodologies can be performed on brain samples. Clinical cases are most easily confirmed by detecting BDV RNA within the inflamed areas of the brain using PCR [54,65,72,96,97].

Treatment

There is no specific treatment for BD. Supportive care and corticosteroids may help in some cases. Prednisolone may be given orally at a rate of 1 to 2 mg/kg every 24 hours until clinical signs regress, after which it should be reduced gradually over several weeks or months.

Zoonotic risk

It is currently unclear what role BDV may play in the induction of human disease. Antibodies against BDV, BD viral proteins, and BDV RNA have been found in people in Europe, the United States, and Asia. A higher prevalence of infection is seen in patients with neurologic or psychiatric disorders, particularly schizophrenia and uni- or bipolar disorders [61,70,98–106]. Because the virus has also been detected in clinically normal patients [67,101,107], however, its role in the development of these complex psychiatric disorders has still to be proven [61,63].

The presence of BDV infection in many domestic species as well as evidence of cross-species transfer raises the possibility of zoonotic spread. Although animal species may pose a potential risk to people, finding BDV RNA in blood from normal human blood donors suggests that people may also be at risk from horizontal spread from person to person [64]. Considerably more investigation needs to be performed before the zoonotic potential of BDV can be determined.

Nonsuppurative encephalitides of unknown cause

Introduction and geographic distribution

A number of other nonsuppurative encephalitides have also been described in cats. These seem to comprise a group of diseases that are possibly related, and the histopathologic changes suggest a viral origin. They are geographically widespread and have been reported in Australia [108], the United States [109], Canada [4,5,23], Sweden [10,71,78], Norway [110], Switzerland [44], and the United Kingdom [1,111,112]; other potential cases have been seen as widely distributed as Morocco [113] and Sri Lanka [114]. A similar condition has been found in a number of large cats, including lions and tigers [115–118]. In all cases, the reports state an unknown cause but comment that the histopathologic changes are suggestive of viral infection. Unfortunately, early studies performed few diagnostic investigations to try to determine the possible cause. Later studies usually assessed for FIV, FeLV, FIP, and *Toxoplasma gondii* and, in some cases, for FHV-1, FCV, FPV, and *Borrelia burgdorferi*. In almost all cases, the cats have been found to be negative for all these agents [1,4,5,10,23,44,112].

Reviewing the data available on these cases suggests that although these diseases generally affect cats of a similar age and sex and cause a range of rather similar clinical signs, they seem to separate into two groups based on histopathologic changes:

Group I: CNS histopathologic examination reveals nonsuppurative encephalomyelitis [44,78,79,110]
Group II: CNS histopathology reveals polioencephalomyelitis or polio-encephalitis [44,108,109,112,119]

Group I: nonsuppurative encephalomyelitis

Clinical signs

These cats are of a wide age range (from a few months to >18 years), but young adults seem to be overrepresented. They show no sex or breed predisposition. They tend to have an acute duration of illness and typically develop ataxia, nystagmus, seizures, head tremor, anorexia, apathy, fever, and, occasionally, preceding vomiting and diarrhea (although not all cats show all signs) [4,6,10,71,78].

Diagnosis

A premortem diagnosis is typically based on the presence of suggestive clinical signs and typical CSF changes (see Table 3) [4,6]. Some cats show leukopenia or a mildly increased ALT concentration [4,78]. Neuroimaging of the brain may reveal multifocal areas of contrast enhancement suggestive of inflammatory disease.

Histopathologic examination reveals mild to severe nonsuppurative meningoencephalomyelitis characterized by mononuclear perivascular cuffing, inflammatory nodules of lymphocytes and macrophages, and neuronal degeneration. Changes can occur throughout the brain and spinal cord but are most prominent in the thalamocortex and brain stem [4,78]. Lesions may be diffuse or focal [4].

Treatment

There is no curative treatment, but supportive therapies include anticonvulsants to control the seizures and, possibly, corticosteroids to reduce CNS inflammation. Because the disease is often self-limiting, the prognosis is quite good for those cats in which neurologic signs are not too severe [6].

Potential causes

Interestingly, when blood samples from affected Swedish and Austrian cats [10,71,78,79] were retrospectively assessed by serologic testing for the organisms listed previously, they were found to be negative, as were their brain sections when assessed by immunohistochemistry for *T gondii,* CDV, FHV-1, tick-borne encephalitis, and Aujeszky's disease virus [10,79]. After finding that the cats were seropositive for BDV and then performing experimental transmission studies, however, subsequent publications from the same authors determined that these cases had actually been caused by BDV [72,79]. It has therefore been suggested that BDV may be responsible for more of these cases. Although this remains a possibility, it is also possible that there are a number of other previously unrecognized viruses. For this reason, it is important that these cases be fully studied before any causal relation can be proven (for diagnostic methods, see section on prevalence of neurological disease in cats and the preponderance of cases with no known cause) [6,7]. In addition, because BDV can be found in the CNS of some clinically normal individuals [65], its presence, per se, within the CNS of a cat showing neurologic disease does not prove that it is the cause of the disorder.

Group II: polioencephalomyelitis or polioencephalitis

Clinical signs

These diseases also tend to affect younger cats (from a few months old to middle-aged), and there is no sex or breed predisposition. Affected individuals tend to have a subacute to chronic course that may last for months. Partial recovery may be seen in some cats, which can go on to live for many years [44,109,112]. Disease is most commonly sporadic [44,109,119]; however, there are also reports describing what seems to be the chronic form of this condition within large groups of research cats in the United Kingdom [111,112].

Cats with polioencephalomyelitis or polioencephalitis present with problems of locomotion, including ataxia, paresis, and depressed postural reaction in all four limbs. Affected cats may occasionally show hyperesthesia or even lower motor neuron signs (muscle atrophy and decreased tendon reflexes). They can also show tremors, pupillary abnormalities, defective vision, nystagmus, and seizures [44,109,111,112,119]. When seizures occur, they do so as episodes of multiple short seizures [109]. Affected cats rarely show any other signs of systemic disease [109].

Diagnosis

A premortem diagnosis is typically based on the presence of suggestive clinical signs and typical CSF changes (see Table 3) [4,6]. Some affected cats may be leukopenic or anemic (with myeloid hypoplasia) [109].

Early on in the disease, histopathologic examination reveals disseminated inflammatory lesions in the brain and spinal cord, with the spinal cord and medulla oblongata being most severely affected. The changes are those of polioencephalomyelitis or polioencephalitis. The lesions consist of perivascular mononuclear cuffing, gliosis, and neuronal degeneration, with the latter being most obvious in the ventral horns of the spinal cord [44,109,119].

In chronic cases, little inflammation remains. There is extensive neuronal loss and intense astrogliosis, however, particularly in the spinal cord. Wallerian degeneration arises secondary to the neuronal damage and is particularly evident in the lateral and ventral columns, where it may resemble a primary degenerative disorder [112,119]. In addition, some cats have multifocal areas of Purkinje cell degeneration and gliosis in the cerebellar cortex [109,112]. The changes are similar to those seen in human [120] and porcine poliomyelitis [121].

Treatment

There is no curative treatment. Supportive therapies are as previously discussed and include anticonvulsants to control seizures and, possibly, corticosteroids to reduce CNS inflammation. The prognosis can be good for those cats in which neurologic signs are not too severe.

Potential causes

The cause remains unknown. Genetic and nutritional causes seem unlikely [112], and a viral cause has been suggested by most authors [109,112,119]. Transmission studies have only been attempted occasionally and have been unsuccessful [108]. A number of infectious agents are known to be able to cause poliomyelitis or demyelination in cats. Some of these, including rabies virus, Aujeszky's disease virus, and Newcastle disease virus, have been ruled out on the basis of somewhat differing pathologic findings [109]. It has also been suggested that the condition may be an unusual manifestation of FPV infection [109,112]. Although FPV classically causes cerebellar hypoplasia in kittens, with degeneration of the germinal and Purkinje cells [122,123], it has occasionally been associated with inflammatory lesions within the brain, leukodystrophic lesions, neuronal degeneration, and gliosis of the spinal cord gray matter or spinal cord demyelination [124]. In addition, in FPV-vaccinated cats, FPV infection can still cause leukopenia and nonregenerative anemia [125]. Interestingly, 2 of 33 cases of clinical BD were seen in kittens that came from litters in which the rest of the litter had died of FPV [78]. Other suggested causes include FeLV [126] and arboviruses (see section on rare or experimental infectious causes of CNS disease in cats).

Although the pattern of disease is clinically and histopathologically distinct from that known to be caused by BDV, the author can find no evidence that this possibility has been investigated. Interestingly, the clinical signs and histopathologic findings of the chronic cases are somewhat similar to those of a case report in which the disease was attributed to an unusual case of BDV. It was an interesting case because it was found to have massive neuronal infection with BDV but lacked inflammatory change [95]. This poses an intriguing question as to whether this case was incorrectly attributed to BDV (with the BDV representing a striking but clinically insignificant finding), while also raising the possibility that most of the rest of the cases could actually be attributable to a second variant of BDV infection.

Central nervous system neuropathologic findings without inflammatory changes

Based on the histopathologic changes seen in the chronic cases of polioencephalomyelitis, it is important to realize that viral infections do not necessarily need to be associated with inflammatory changes within the CNS to cause clinically significant neurologic disease.

Neuropathologic changes, without inflammation, may be seen for a number of reasons. It may be that the inflammatory phase has passed and has been missed. Alternately, some viruses can induce direct neuropathic effects while hiding from the immune system within neurons or glial cells (eg, FIV [28]; CDV [127]; human stealth viruses [43]; many herpes viruses, such as chickenpox [128] and varicella zoster virus [129]). In addition, some perinatal infections can result in lasting CNS infection without the development of antibodies (circulating within the blood stream or within the CNS) or encephalitis, but they can still be associated with neurologic disease [95]. This has been seen with BDV infection of some rodents, where infected individuals develop subtle behavioral changes and defects in memory and learning [130,131]. It is therefore possible that BDV infection or other viral infections could result in a number of different disease patterns, depending on differences in viral pathogenicity as well as on as yet unidentified host-specific factors.

Realizing that viral infections can cause CNS disease without obvious inflammatory change and recognizing that the changes can consist mainly of degenerative changes raise the possibility that a viral cause may be responsible for an even higher proportion of CNS disease in cats. Because approximately 35% of feline neurology cases are currently found to result from infectious or inflammatory causes and approximately 15% are degenerative, this could suggest that up to approximately 50% of all feline neurologic disease may potentially be caused by CNS infection (see Table 1) [1].

Unusual patterns of seizure activity

When seizures have been reported as part of the clinical syndromes described previously, the seizure pattern is rather striking; they occur in episodes of multiple short seizures [109]. When looking at studies focusing on all causes of recurrent seizures in cats, it is fascinating to see that they all result from structural brain disease and that the most common cause (~50%) seems to be a result of nonsuppurative encephalitides [4,5,23]. Although the seizure pattern is similar, the cats in these studies were presented primarily for seizures rather than for ataxia, and despite the onset of seizures being rather dramatic, the prognosis was reasonably good [5].

Whether or not the same virus (or group of viruses) results in all forms of seizure-associated nonsuppurative encephalitides remains to be proven. Interestingly, experimental studies have shown that this pattern of seizure results from lesions in the periaqueductal gray matter of the midbrain [120]. It is therefore possible that it may simply be that this area is preferentially targeted by a number of different infectious agents in cats.

Feline spongiform encephalopathy

Epizootiology

FSE was first recognized in 1990 during the bovine spongiform encephalopathy (BSE) epidemic in the United Kingdom [132–134]. FSE is one of a group of naturally occurring TSEs. TSEs occur in many mammalian species [135], including scrapie in sheep and goats; BSE in cattle and captive exotic ungulates [136,137]; FSE in domestic cats and captive exotic feline species, including the cheetah [137–139], puma [137,140], and lion (A.L. Meredith, MA, VetMB, MRCVS, University of Edinburgh, personal communication, 1999); chronic wasting disease (CWD) of deer and elk [141]; transmissible mink encephalopathy (TME) in mink [142]; and Creutzfeldt-Jakob disease (CJD), variant CJD (vCJD), Gerstmann-Sträussler-Scheinker disease, and kuru in human beings [143]. Experimentally, TSEs can be transmitted to an even wider range of species, including rodents and nonhuman primates [144–146]. Although the widespread interest in TSEs developed only fairly recently, associated with the BSE epidemic and the recognition of vCJD, this type of disease is far from new. Historical records show that scrapie was first recognized approximately 300 years ago [147].

TSEs have been seen throughout the world. Although scrapie and human TSEs have a widespread distribution, BSE has been seen mainly in Europe, particularly in the United Kingdom. The situation is similar with FSE, with almost all cases having been seen in Britain; occasional cases have been seen in animals that had previously lived in the United Kingdom [148] or been fed on tissue from British cattle [135–141].

To understand FSE, it is necessary to know how BSE is believed to have originated. BSE was first reported in 1987 [149]. It is believed to have resulted from the inclusion of scrapie-infected sheep carcasses into feedstuffs for cattle [150]. This resulted in a change to the agent's pathogenicity, making it more infectious to cattle (and cats). Cattle succumbing to BSE were then included in cattle feed, thereby amplifying the transmission and spreading the infection [150,151]. Once this epidemiologic pattern had been determined, the feeding of meat and bonemeal to ruminants was banned. Since then, the incidence of BSE first plateaued and then fell [152,153].

The agent responsible for FSE is believed to be the same as for BSE [146]. It probably entered the feline population of the United Kingdom in contaminated pet food, and the temporal distribution of cases supports this hypothesis. Since its recognition in 1990, approximately 90 cases of FSE have been confirmed, mostly between 1990 and 1994 (J.W. Wilesmith, BVSc, PhD, J. Spriopoulos, DVM, PhD, Veterinary Laboratories Agency, Weybridge, UK, personal communication on confirmed cases up to the end of 2001, 2004) (Fig. 1). In addition, retrospective study of brain tissue from cats with neurologic disease failed to find cases of FSE before 1990 [1,154]. Although, like BSE, the peak of FSE seems to have passed, occasional cases are still seen (see Fig. 1) [153]. Because few domestic cats are subject to routine postmortem examination, it is likely that the total number of FSE cases has been underestimated.

Most TSEs, like FSE and BSE, seem to be transmitted by ingestion. Although maternal and even genetic transmission may occur in some species [135,143,155], there is no evidence of it occurring in cats or cattle [150,152].

Pathogenesis

The TSE agents are unlike any other microorganisms. All TSE diseases are characterized by the accumulation of an abnormal isoform of a host-coded protein, the prion protein (PrP). PrP is found in all animals; it is a cell surface glycoprotein of unknown significance. Although the PrP isolated from normal individuals (PrPc) and the PrP isolated from TSE-infected individuals (PrP-res) have the same amino acid sequence and secondary structure, PrPc is totally degraded by proteinase K, whereas PrP-res resists digestion. Once present, PrP-res is believed to induce additional copies of

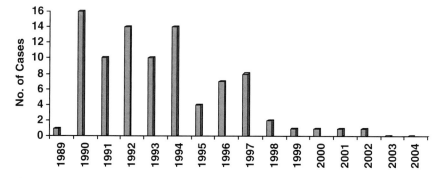

Fig. 1. Graph showing the incidence of feline spongiform encephalopathy cases in cats by year of onset of clinical signs (cases confirmed to mid 2004; J.W. Wilesmith, BVSc, PhD, J. Spriopoulos, DVM, PhD, Veterinary Laboratories Agency, Weybridge, UK, personal communication).

itself by interacting with normal PrPc. In doing this, PrP-res acts as an infectious agent [156]. Once the host-coded PrPc has been transformed to PrP-res, it accumulates in fibrils (scrapie-associated fibrils [SAFs]), and this eventually leads to disease [135]. Because the process is slow, however, all TSEs have prolonged incubation periods. More detailed information on TSE pathogenesis is reviewed elsewhere [157–159]. Because PrP is host-coded, the accumulation of SAFs induces no immune response [160,161].

Clinical signs

FSE shows no breed predisposition, and cats from all types of households have been affected. There seems to be a slight male predisposition [154]. The mean age at onset is approximately 5 to 7 years (range: 2–12 years) [132–134,148].

FSE is characterized by progressive behavioral and motor disturbances. Affected cats present with progressive hind limb ataxia; increased aggression or affection; hyperesthesia to touch, sound, or light; altered grooming patterns; increased salivation; dilated pupils with an unusual staring expression; polyphagia or polydipsia; abnormal head posture; muscle fasciculations; or an inability to retract their claws [132–134,148,154]. Behavioral changes have usually been noted first, followed by progressive locomotor dysfunction. The cats tend to show ataxia, with dysmetria or hypermetria, which often leads to an erratic crouching gait [134,148]. They also show an inability to judge distances. The disease is generally progressive, warranting euthanasia within 8 to 12 weeks of the onset of clinical signs [134].

Diagnosis

Premortem diagnosis is rarely possible. Although clinical signs may be suggestive of FSE, and nonspecific tests, such as electroencephalography (EEG) or MRI, may indicate the presence of diffuse CNS disease, specific tests are currently lacking. Significant abnormalities have not been detected on serum biochemistry, hematology, or CSF analysis [154]. Diagnosis of FSE is usually made by histopathologic examination of the brain (formalin-fixed tissue) and ultrastructural detection of SAFs in brain extracts (fresh-frozen brain or spinal cord) [162]. After euthanasia, any animal suspected of having FSE should have a full postmortem examination, which should be performed by a trained veterinary pathologist.

Pathologic changes are confined to the CNS and consist of variable degrees of neurophil vacuolation, vacuolation of the neuronal parenchyma, and an astrocytic response. Changes are particularly evident in the gray matter of the thalamus, basal ganglia, and cerebral and cerebellar cortices. More advanced cases may show neuronal loss and more striking gliosis. There are no inflammatory changes. Fibrils analogous to SAFs can be seen on electron microscopy [134,163,164].

Treatment

There is no effective treatment for FSE.

Zoonotic risk

Although it is generally difficult to transmit a TSE agent from one species to another by mouth, BSE seems to have been transmitted naturally, not only to cats, captive exotic felids, and captive exotic ungulates but to human beings, in the form of vCJD [137,165]. Thankfully, with the introduction of strict laws regulating the slaughter and rendering of ruminants and the overall decline in the incidence of BSE, the possibility of the BSE agent continuing to be included in the food chain is extremely small. Because the incubation period is long and variable, however, we are likely to continue to see new cases of vCJD in the United Kingdom for a few years yet to come. That said, the increasing prevalence of CWD in deer and elk in the United States is of concern, and the potential for this TSE to be transmitted to human beings (or cats) is still to be determined [141].

It is unlikely that cats present a zoonotic risk. This is because the disease is now extremely rare (it was never common) and the likelihood of FSE-infected brain or spinal cord entering the human food chain is almost nonexistent. Although there has been one case of CJD and FSE occurring within the same household, the strain of TSE with which both individuals were affected seems to have been a variant more typically associated with spontaneous CJD rather than with BSE [166], and even that diagnosis has been questioned. The method of transmission in this case is not known.

References

[1] Bradshaw JM, Pearson GR, Gruffydd-Jones TJ. A retrospective study of 286 cases of neurological disorders of the cat. J Comp Pathol 2004;131:112–20.

[2] Hopkins A. Feline neurology. Part 1. Intracranial disorders. In Pract 1992;14:59–65.

[3] Summers BA, Cummings JF, deLahunta A. Veterinary neuropathology. St. Louis: Mosby-Year Book; 1995.

[4] Rand JS, Parent J, Percy D, et al. Clinical, cerebrospinal fluid, and histological data from twenty-seven cats with primary inflammatory disease of the central nervous system. Can Vet J 1994;35:103–10.

[5] Quesnel AD, Parent JM, McDonell W, et al. Diagnostic evaluation of cats with seizure disorders: 30 cases(1991–1993). J Am Vet Med Assoc 1997;210:65–71.

[6] Munana KR. Inflammatory disorders of the central nervous system. In: August JR, editor. Consultations in feline internal medicine, vol. 4. Philadelphia: WB Saunders; 2001. p. 425–33.

[7] Schatzberg SJ, Haley NJ, Barr SC, et al. Use of a multiplex polymerase chain reaction assay in the antemortem diagnosis of toxoplasmosis and Neospora in the central nervous system of cats and dogs. Am J Vet Res 2003;64(12):1507–13.

[8] Cook LB, Bergman RL, Bahr A, et al. Inflammatory polyp in the middle ear with secondary suppurative meningoencephalitis in a cat. Vet Radiol Ultrasound 2003;44(6):648–51.

[9] Cleaveland S, Appel MGJ, Chalmers WSK, et al. Serological and demographic evidence for domestic dogs as a source of canine distemper virus infection for Serengeti wildlife. Vet Microbiol 2000;72:217–27.

[10] Lundgren AL. Feline non-suppurative meningoencephalomyelitis. A clinical and pathological study. J Comp Pathol 1992;107:411–25.

[11] Guan Y, Zheng BJ, He YQ, et al. Isolation and characterization of viruses related to the SARS coronavirus from animals in southern China. Science 2003;302(5643):276–8.

[12] Martina BE, Haagmans BL, Kuiken T, et al. Virology: SARS virus infection of cats and ferrets. Nature 2003;425:915.

[13] Kuiken T, Rimmelzwaan G, Van Riel D, et al. Avian H5N1 influenza in cats. Science 2004; 306:241.

[14] Lanciotti RS, Roehrig JT, Deubel V, et al. Origin of the West Nile virus responsible for an outbreak of encephalitis in the northeastern United States. Science 1999;286(5448):2333–7.

[15] Austgen LE, Bowen RA, Bunning ML, et al. Experimental infection of cat and dogs with West Nile virus. Emerg Infect Dis 2004;10(1):82–6.

[16] Lichtensteiger CA, Heinz-Taheny K, Osborne TS, et al. West Nile virus encephalitis and myocarditis in wolf and dog. Emerg Infect Dis 2003;9(10):1303–6.

[17] Komar N, Panella NA, Boyce E. Exposure of domestic mammals to West Nile virus during an outbreak of human encephalitis, New York City, 1999. Emerg Infect Dis 2001;7(4):736–8.

[18] Woolhouse MEJ. Population biology of emerging and re-emerging pathogens. Trends Microbiol 2002;10(Suppl 10):s3–7.

[19] Luttgen PJ. Inflammatory disease of the central nervous system. Vet Clin N Am Small Anim Pract 1988;18(3):623–40.

[20] Chrisman CL, editor. Problems in small animal neurology. 2nd edition. Philadelphia: Lea & Febiger; 1991.

[21] Skerritt GC. Brain disorders in dogs and cats. In: Wheeler SJ, editor. Manual of small animal neurology. Cheltenham, UK: BSAVA; 1992. p. 127–39.

[22] Parent JM, Quesnel AD. Seizures in cats. Vet Clin N Am Small Anim Pract 1996;26(4): 811–25.

[23] Munana KR. Encephalitis and meningitis. Vet Clin N Am Small Anim Pract 1996;26(4): 857–76.

[24] Greene CE, editor. Infectious diseases of the dog and cat. 2nd edition. Philadelphia: WB Saunders; 1998.

[25] Foley JE, Leutenegger C. A review of coronavirus infection in the central nervous system of cats and mice. J Vet Intern Med 2001;15:438–44.

[26] Foley JE, Rand C, Leutenegger C. Inflammation and changes in cytokine levels in neurological feline infectious peritonitis. J Feline Med Surg 2003;5(6):313–22.

[27] Pedersen NC, Yamamoto JK, Ishida T, et al. Feline immunodeficiency virus infection. Vet Immunol Immunopathol 1989;21:111–29.

[28] Dow SW, Poss ML, Hoover EA. Feline immunodeficiency virus: a neurotropic lentivirus. J Acquir Immune Defic Hum Retrovirol 1990;3:658–68.

[29] Dow SW, Dreitz MJ, Hoover EA. Exploring the link between feline immunodeficiency virus infection and neurologic disease in cats. Vet Med 1992;87:1181–4.

[30] Hurtrel M, Ganiere JP, Guelfi JF, et al. Comparison of early and late feline immunodeficiency virus encephalopathies. AIDS 1992;6:399–406.

[31] Henriksen SJ, Prospero-Garcia O, Phillips TR, et al. Feline immunodeficiency virus as a model for study of lentivirus infection of the central nervous system. Curr Top Microbiol Immunol 1995;202:167–86.

[32] Gunn-Moore D, Pearson G, Harbour D, et al. Encephalitis with giant cells in a cat with naturally occurring feline immunodeficiency virus infection demonstrated by in situ hybridization. Vet Pathol 1996;33:699–703.

[33] Hopper CD, Sparkes AH, Gruffydd-Jones TJ, et al. Clinical and laboratory findings in cats infected with feline immunodeficiency virus. Vet Rec 1989;125:341–6.

[34] Karpas A, Routledge JK. Feline herpes virus: isolation and experimental studies. Zentralbl Veterinaermed 1968;15:599–606.

[35] Love DN, Baker KD. Sudden death in a kitten associated with a feline Picorna virus. Aust Vet J 1972;48:643.

[36] Bouljihad M, Lindeman CJ, Hayden DW. Pyogranulomatous meningoencephalitis associated with dematiaceous fungal (Cladophialophora bantiana) infection in a domestic cat. J Vet Diagn Invest 2002;14(1):70–2.

[37] Dubey JP, Benson J, Larson MA. Clinical Sarcocystis neurona encephalomyelitis in a domestic cat following routine surgery. Vet Parasitol 2003;112(4):261–7.

[38] Kordick DL, Breitschwerdt EB. Relapsing bacteremia after blood transmission of Bartonella henselae to cats. Am J Vet Res 1997;58(5):492–7.

[39] Marra CM. Neurologic complications of Bartonella henselae infection. Curr Opin Neurol 1995;8(3):164–9.

[40] Yanai T, Tujioka S, Sakai H, et al. Experimental infection with equine herpesvirus 9 (EHV-9) in cats. J Comp Pathol 2003;128(2–3):113–8.

[41] Luttrell CN, Bang FB. Newcastle disease encephalomyelitis in cats. I. Clinical and pathological features. Arch Neurol Psychiatr 1958;79:647–57.

[42] Salvioli G, Gotti D, Sternini G. Effetti polimorfi nel gatto da inoculazione di materiale poliomielitico. Riv Ist Sieroter Ital 1952;27:225–45.

[43] Martin WJ, Glass RT. Acute encephalopathy induced in cats with a stealth virus isolated from a patient with chronic fatigue syndrome. Pathobiology 1995;63(3):115–8.

[44] Hoff EJ, Vandevelde M. Non-suppurative encephalomyelitis in cats suggestive of a viral origin. Vet Pathol 1981;18:170–80.

[45] Wilson MS, Wherrett BA, Mahdy MS. Powassan virus meningoencephalitis: a case report. Can Med Assoc J 1979;121(3):320–3.

[46] Keane DP, Parent J, Little PB. Californian subgroup: Powassan virus infection of cats. Can J Microbiol 1987;33:693–7.

[47] Greene CE, Baldwin CA. Arboviral infections. In: Greene CE, editor. Infectious diseases of the dog and cat. 2nd edition. Philadelphia: WB Saunders; 1998. p. 131–3.

[48] Daubney R. Viral encephalitis of equines and domestic ruminants in the Near East. Part II. Res Vet Sci 1967;8:419–39.

[49] Daubney R, Mahlau EA. Viral encephalitis of equines and domestic ruminants in the Near East. Part I. Res Vet Sci 1967;8:375–97.

[50] Artsob H, Spence L, Th'ng C, et al. Arbovirus infections in several Ontario mammals, 1975–1980. Can J Vet Res 1986;50(1):42–6.

[51] Nicolau S, Galloway IA. Borna disease and enzootic encephalomyelitis of sheep and cattle. Special Reports Series. Medical Research Council 1928;121:7–90.

[52] Ludwig H, Bode L, Gosztonyi G. Borna disease: a persistent virus infection of the central nervous system. Prog Med Virol 1988;35:107–51.

[53] Lundgren AL, Czech G, Bode L, Ludwig H. Natural Borna disease in domestic animals other than horses and sheep. J Vet Med 1993;B40:298–303.

[54] Lundgren AL, Zimmermann W, Bode L, et al. Staggering disease in cats: isolation and characterization of the feline Borna virus. J Gen Virol 1995;76(9):2215–22.

[55] Malkinson M, Weisman Y, Ashash E, et al. Borna disease in ostriches. Vet Rec 1993;133:304.

[56] Malkinson M, Weisman Y, Perl S, et al. A Borna-like disease of ostriches in Israel. Curr Top Microbiol Immunol 1995;190:31–8.

[57] Bode L, Durrwald R, Ludwig H. Borna virus infections in cattle associated with fatal neurological disease. Vet Rec 1994;135:283–4.

[58] Rott R, Becht H. Natural and experimental Borna disease in animals. Curr Top Microbiol Immunol 1995;190:15–30.

[59] Weissenbock H, Nowotny N, Caplazi P, et al. Borna disease in a dog with lethal meningoencephalitis. J Clin Microbiol 1998;36:2127–30.

[60] Narayan O, Herzog S, Frese K, et al. Pathogenesis of Borna disease in rats: immune-mediated viral ophthalmoencephalopathy causing blindness and behavioural abnormalities. J Infect Dis 1983;148:305–15.

[61] Hatalski CG, Lewis AJ, Lipkin WI. Borna disease. Emerg Infect Dis 1997;3:129–35.

[62] Nakamura Y, Asahi S, Nakaya T, et al. Demonstration of Borna disease virus RNA in peripheral blood mononuclear cells derived from domestic cats in Japan. J Clin Microbiol 1996;34:188–98.

[63] Richt JA, Pfeuffer I, Christ M, et al. Borna disease virus infection in animals and humans. Emerg Infect Dis 1997;3:343–52.

[64] Takahashi H, Nakaya T, Nakamura Y, et al. Higher prevalence of Borna disease virus infection in blood donors living near thoroughbred horse farms. J Med Virol 1997;52: 330–5.

[65] Reeves NA, Helps CR, Gunn-Moore DA, et al. Natural Borna disease virus infection in cats in the United Kingdom. Vet Rec 1998;143:523–6.

[66] Weissenbock H, Suchy A, Caplazi P, et al. Borna disease in Austrian horses. Vet Rec 1998; 143:21–2.

[67] Cotto E, Neau D, Cransac-Neau M, et al. Borna disease virus RNA in immunocompro-mised patients in southwestern France. J Clin Microbiol 2003;41(12):5577–81.

[68] Helps CR, Turan N, Bilal T, et al. Detection of antibodies to Borna disease virus in Turkish cats by using recombinant p40. Vet Rec 2001;149:647–50.

[69] Dauphin G, Legay V, Pitel P-H, et al. Borna disease: current knowledge and virus detection in France. Vet Res 2002;33:127–38.

[70] Terayama H, Nishino Y, Kishi M, et al. Detection of anti-Borna disease virus (BDV) antibodies from patients with schizophrenia and mood disorders in Japan. Psychiatry Res 2003;120(2):201–6.

[71] Kronevi T, Nordstrom M, Moreno W, et al. Feline ataxia due to non-suppurative meningoencephalomyelitis of unknown aetiology. Nord Veterinmed 1974;26:720–5.

[72] Lundgren AL, Johannisson A, Zimmermann W, et al. Neurological disease and encephalitis in cats experimentally infected with Borna virus. Acta Neuropathol (Berl) 1997;93:391–401.

[73] Ludwig H, Bode L. The neuropathogenesis of Borna disease virus infections. Intervirology 1997;40:185–97.

[74] Huebner J, Bode L, Ludwig H. Borna disease virus infection in FIV-positive cats in Germany. Vet Rec 2001;149:152.

[75] Nishino Y, Funaba M, Fukushima R, et al. Borna disease virus infection in domestic cats: evaluation by RNA and antibody detection. J Vet Med Sci 1999;61(10):1167–70.

[76] Lundgren AL, Ludwig H. Clinically diseased cats with non-suppurative meningoencepha-lomyelitis have Borna disease virus-specific antibodies. Acta Vet Scand 1993;34:101–3.

[77] Nakamura Y, Watanabe M, Kamitani W, et al. High prevalence of Borna disease virus in domestic cats with neurological disorders in Japan. Vet Microbiol 1999;70(3–4):153–69.

[78] Strom B, Andren B, Lundgren AL. Idiopathic non-suppurative meningoencephalo-myelitis (Staggering disease) in the Swedish cat: a study of 33 cases. Svensk Veterinar Tindning 1992; 44(1):19–24 (translation published in the European Journal of Companion Animal Practice 1992;3(1):9–13).

[79] Nowotny N, Weissenbock H. Description of feline nonsuppurative meningoencephalo-myelitis ("Staggering Disease") and studies of its etiology. J Clin Microbiol 1995;33: 1668–9.

[80] Berg AL, Reid-Smith R, Larsson M, et al. Case control study of feline Borna disease in Sweden. Vet Rec 1998;142:715–7.

[81] Staeheli P, Sauder C, Hausmann J, et al. Epidemiology of Borna disease virus. J Gen Virol 2000;81:2123–35.

[82] Berg M, Johansson M, Montell H, et al. Wild birds as possible natural reservoirs of Borna disease virus. Epidemiol Infect 2001;127:173–8.

[83] Richt JA, Herzog S, Haberzettl K, Rott R. Demonstration of Borna disease virus-specific RNA in secretions of naturally infected horses by the polymerase chain reaction. Med Microbiol Immunol (Berl) 1993;182:293–304.

[84] Binz T, Lebelt J, Niemann H, et al. Sequence analysis of the p24 gene of Borna disease virus in naturally infected horse, donkey and sheep. Vet Res 1994;34:281–9.

[85] Schneider PA, Briese T, Zimmermann W, et al. Sequence conservation in field and experimental isolates of Borna disease virus. J Virol 1994;68:63–8.

[86] Briese T, Lipkin WI, de la Torre JC. Molecular biology of Borna disease virus. Curr Top Microbiol Immunol 1995;190:1–16.

[87] Cubitt B, de la Torre JC. Borna disease virus (BDV), a nonsegmented RNA virus, replicates in the nucleus of infected cells where infectious BDV ribonucleoproteins are present. J Virol 1994;68:1371–81.

[88] Gonzalez-Dunia D, Sauder C, de la Torre JC. Borna disease virus and the brain. Brain Res Bull 1997;44(6):647–64.

[89] Bode L, Ludwig H. Clinical similarities and close genetic relationship of human and animal Borna disease virus. Arch Virol 1997;(Suppl 13):167–82.

[90] Cubitt B, Oldstone C, de la Torre JC. Sequence and genome organisation of Borna disease virus. J Virol 1994;68:1382–96.

[91] Stitz L, Dietzschold B, Carbone KM. Immunopathogenesis of Borna disease. Curr Top Microbiol Virol 1995;190:75–92.

[92] Narayan O, Herzog S, Frese K, et al. Behavioral disease in rats caused by immunopathological responses to persistent Borna virus in the brain. Science 1983;220:1401–3.

[93] Berg AL, Johansson A, Johansson M, et al. Peripheral and intracerebral T cell immune response in cats naturally infected with Borna disease virus. Vet Immunol Immunopathol 1999;68(2–4):241–53.

[94] Weissenböck H, Nowotny N, Zoher J. Feline meningoencephalo-myelitis ("Staggering Disease"). Osterr Wien Tierarztl Mschr 1994;81:195–201.

[95] Berg AL, Berg M. A variant form of feline Borna disease. J Comp Pathol 1998;119:323–31.

[96] Lundgren AL, Lindberg R, Ludwig H, et al. Immunoreactivity of the central nervous system in cats with a Borna disease-like meningoencephalomyelitis (staggering disease). Acta Neuropathol (Berl) 1995;90:184–93.

[97] Lundgren AL. Borna disease in cats. Vet Rec 1999;145:87.

[98] Bode L, Riegel S, Ludwig H, et al. Borna disease virus-specific antibodies in patients with HIV and with mental disorders. Lancet 1988;2:689.

[99] Bode L, Zimmermann W, Ferszt R, et al. Borna disease virus genome transcribed and expressed in psychiatric patients. Nat Med 1995;1:232–6.

[100] Waltrip RW, Buchanan RW, Carpenter WT, et al. Borna disease antibodies and the deficit syndrome of schizophrenia. Schizophr Res 1997;23:253–7.

[101] Bode L, Ludwig H. Borna disease virus infection, a human mental-health risk. Clin Microbiol Rev 2003;16(3):534–45.

[102] Rott R, Herzog S, Fleischer B, et al. Detection of serum antibodies to Borna disease virus in patients with psychiatric disorders. Science 1985;228:755–6.

[103] Bode L, Riegel S, Lange W, et al. Human infection with Borna disease virus: seroprevalence in patients with chronic diseases and healthy individuals. J Med Virol 1992;36:309–15.

[104] Bode L, Durrwald R, Rantam FA, et al. First isolates of infectious human Borna disease virus from patients with mood disorders. Mol Psychiatry 1996;1:200–12.

[105] Salvatore M, Morzunov S, Schwemmle M, et al. Borna disease virus in brains of North American and European people with schizophrenia and bipolar disorder. Lancet 1997;349:1813–4.

[106] Iwahashi K, Watanabe M, Nakamura K, et al. Clinical investigation of the relationship between Borna disease virus (BDV) infection and schizophrenia in 67 patients in Japan. Acta Psychiatr Scand 1997;96(6):412–5.

[107] Haga S, Yoshimura M, Motoi Y, et al. Detection of Borna disease virus genome in normal human brain tissue. Brain Res 1997;770:307–9.

[108] Borland R, McDonald N. Feline encephalomyelitis. Br Vet J 1965;121:479–83.

[109] Vandevelde M, Braund KG. Polioencephalomyelitis in cats. Vet Pathol 1979;16:420–7.

[110] Kronevi T, Nordström M, Moreno W, et al. Feline ataxia due to nonsuppurative meningoencephalomyelitis of unknown aetiology. Nord Vet Med 1974;26:720–5.

[111] Bleby J, Brierley JB. An idiopathic demyelination in SPF cats [abstract]. Vet Rec 1972; 91(Suppl):10.

[112] Palmer AC, Cavanagh JB. Encephalomyelopathy in young cats. J Soc Adm Pharm 1995;36: 57–64.

[113] Martin LA, Hintermann J. Une malade non décrite du chat; la myélite infectieuse. Bull de Arch Inst Pasteur Maroc 1955;5:64–73.

[114] McGaughey CA. Infectious myelitis of cats: preliminary communication. Ceylon Veterinary Journal 1953;1:34–40.

[115] Flir K. Encephalomyelitis bei Grosskatzen. Dtsch Tierarztl Wochenschr 1973;80:401–4.

[116] Melchior G. Meningo-enzephalitis beim löwen and tiger. In: Ippen, Schröder, editors. Erkrankungen der Zootiere, Verhandlungsbericht des XV. Internationalen Symposiums uber die Erkrankungen der Zootiere. Berlin: Akademie-Verlag; 1973. p. 245–54.

[117] Gutter A, Wells S, Baskin G. Neurological disease in three cats at the Audubon Park Zoo. In: Proceedings of the Annual Meeting of the American Association of Zoo Veterinarians. Tampa; 1983. p. 21–6.

[118] Truyen U, Stockhofe-Zurwieden N, Kaaden OR, et al. A case report: encephalitis in lions. Pathological and virological findings. Dtsch Tierarztl Wochenschr 1990;97:89–91.

[119] Vandevelde M. Neurologic diseases of suspected infectious origin. In: Greene CD, editor. Infectious diseases of the dog and cat. Philadelphia: WB Saunders; 1998. p. 530–9.

[120] Greenfield JG. Neuropathology. 3rd edition. London: Edward Arnold; 1976. p. 306–8.

[121] Innes JRM, Saunders LZ. Comparative neuropathology. New York: Academic Press; 1962. p. 361–4.

[122] Kilham L, Margolis G. Viral etiology of spontaneous ataxia in cats. Am J Pathol 1966;48: 991–1011.

[123] Csiza CK, deLahunta A, Scott FW, et al. Spontaneous feline ataxia. Cornell Vet 1972;62: 300–22.

[124] Csiza CK, Scott FW, deLahunta A, et al. Respiratory signs and central nervous system lesions in cats infected with panleukopenia virus. A case report. Cornell Vet 1972;62:192–5.

[125] Carlson JH. Feline panleukopenia. In: Kirk RW, editor. Current veterinary therapy, vol. VI. Philadelphia: WB Saunders; 1977. p. 1292–6.

[126] Mesfin GM, Kusewitt D, Parker A. Degenerative myelopathy in a cat. J Am Vet Med Assoc 1980;176:62–4.

[127] Bollo E, Zurbriggen A, Vandevelde M, et al. Canine distemper virus clearance in chronic inflammatory demyelination. Acta Neuropathol (Berl) 1986;72(1):69–73.

[128] Shope TC. Chickenpox encephalitis and encephalopathy: evidence for differing pathogenesis. Yale J Biol Med 1982;55(3–4):321–7.

[129] Gray F, Mohr M, Rozenberg F, et al. Varicella-zoster virus encephalitis in acquired immunodeficiency syndrome: report of four cases. Neuropathol Appl Neurobiol 1992; 18(5):502–14.

[130] Dittrich W, Bode L, Ludwig H, et al. Learning deficiencies in Borna disease virus-infected but clinically healthy rats. Biol Psychiatry 1989;26:818–28.

[131] Bautista JR, Schwartz GJ, de la Torre JC, et al. Early and persistent abnormalities in rats with neonatally acquired Borna virus infection. Brain Res Bull 1994;34:31–40.

[132] Leggett MM, Dukes J, Pirie HM. A spongiform encephalopathy in a cat. Vet Rec 1990;127: 586–8.

[133] Wyatt JM, Pearson GR, Smerdon TN, et al. Spongiform encephalopathy in a cat. Vet Rec 1990;126:513.

[134] Wyatt JM, Pearson GR, Smerdon TN, et al. Naturally occurring scrapie-like spongiform encephalopathy in five domestic cats. Vet Rec 1991;129:233–6.

[135] Kimberlin RH. Transmissible spongiform encephalopathies in animals. Can J Vet Res 1990;54:30–7.

[136] Wells GAH, McGill IS. Recently described scrapie-like encephalopathies in animals: case descriptions. In: Bradley R, Savey M, Marchant B, editors. Sub-acute spongiform encephalopathies. Current topics in veterinary medicine and animal science, vol. 55. Dordrecht: Kluwer Academic Publishers; 1991. p. 11–24.

[137] Kirkwood JK, Cunningham AA. Epidemiological observations on spongiform encephalopathies in captive wild animals in the British Isles. Vet Rec 1994;135:296–303.

[138] Kirkwood JK, Cunningham AA, Flach EJ, et al. Spongiform encephalopathy in another captive cheetah (Acinonyx jubatus): evidence for variation in susceptibility or incubation periods between species? J Zoo Wildl Med 1995;24:577–82.

[139] Baron T, Belli P, Madec JY, et al. Spongiform encephalopathy in an imported cheetah in France. Vet Rec 1997;141:270–1.

[140] Willoughby K, Kelly DF, Lyon DG, et al. Spongiform encephalopathy in a captive puma (Felis concolor). Vet Rec 1992;131:431–4.

[141] Miller MW, Willians ES, Hobbs NT, et al. Environmental sources of prion transmission in mule deer. Emerg Infect Dis 2004;10(6):1003–6.

[142] Hartsough GR, Burger D. Encephalopathy of mink I. Epizootiology and clinical observations. J Infect Dis 1965;115:387–92.

[143] Brown P. Transmissible spongiform encephalopathies in humans: kuru, Creutzfeldt-Jakob disease, Gerstmann-Sträussler-Scheinker disease. Can J Vet Res 1990;54:38–41.

[144] Gibbs CJ, Gajdusek DC. Experimental subacute spongiform virus encephalopathies in primates and other laboratory animals. Science 1973;182:67–9.

[145] Baker HF, Ridley RM, Wells GAH. Experimental transmission of BSE and scrapie to the common marmoset. Vet Rec 1993;132:403–6.

[146] Fraser H, Pearson GR, McConnell I, et al. Transmission of feline spongiform encephalopathy to mice. Vet Rec 1994;134:449.

[147] Parry HB. Scrapie disease in sheep. In: Oppenheimer DR, editor. London: Academic Press; 1983. p. 31.

[148] Bratberg B, Ueland K, Wells GAH. Feline spongiform encephalopathy in a cat in Norway. Vet Rec 1995;136:444.

[149] Wells GAH, Scott AC, Johnson CT, et al. A novel progressive spongiform encephalopathy in cattle. Vet Rec 1987;121:419–20.

[150] Wilesmith JW, Wells GAH, Cranwell MP, et al. Bovine spongiform encephalopathy: epidemiological studies. Vet Rec 1988;123:638–44.

[151] Wilesmith JW, Ryan JB, Atkinson MJ. Bovine spongiform encephalopathy: epidemiological studies on the origin. Vet Rec 1991;128:199–203.

[152] Hoinville LJ. Decline in the incidence of BSE in cattle born after the introduction of the 'feed ban'. Vet Rec 1994;134:274–5.

[153] Wilesmith JW, Ryan JB. Bovine spongiform encephalopathy: observations on incidence during 1992. Vet Rec 1993;132:300–1.

[154] Gruffydd-Jones TJ, Galloway PE, Pearson GR. Feline spongiform encephalopathy. J Soc Adm Pharm 1991;33:471–6.

[155] Donnelly CA. Maternal transmission of BSE: interpretation of the data on the offspring of BSE-affected pedigree suckler cows. Vet Rec 1998;142:579–80.

[156] Prusiner SB. Genetic and infectious prion diseases. Arch Virol 1993;50:1129–53.

[157] Gunn-Moore DA, Harbour DA. Feline spongiform encephalopathy and Borna disease. In: August JR, editor. Consultations in feline internal medicine, vol. 4. Philadelphia: WB Saunders; 2001. p. 62–70.

[158] Schreuder BEC, van Keulen LJM, Vromans MEW, et al. Tonsillar biopsy and PrP^{Sc} detection in the preclinical diagnosis of scrapie. Vet Rec 1998;142:564–8.

[159] Hadlow WJ, Kennedy RC, Race RE. Natural infection of Suffolk sheep with scrapie virus. J Infect Dis 1982;146:657–64.

[160] Bolton DC, McKinley MP, Prusiner SB. Identification of a protein that purifies with scrapie prion. Science 1982;218:1309–11.

[161] Chesebro B, Race R, Wehrly K, et al. Identification of scrapie prion protein-specific mRNA in scrapie-infected and uninfected brain. Nature 1985;315:331–3.

[162] Gibson PH, Somerville RA, Fraser H, et al. Scrapie associated fibrils in the diagnosis of scrapie in sheep. Vet Rec 1987;120:125–7.

[163] Pearson GR, Gruffydd-Jones TJ, Wyatt JM, et al. Feline spongiform encephalopathy. Vet Rec 1991;128:532.

[164] Pearson GR, Wyatt JM, Gruffydd-Jones TJ, et al. Feline spongiform encephalopathy: fibril and PrP studies. Vet Rec 1992;131:307–10.

[165] Collinge J, Sidle KCL, Meads J, et al. Molecular analysis of prion strain variation and the etiology of new variant CJD. Nature 1996;383:685–90.

[166] Zanusso G, Nardelli E, Zosati A, et al. Simultaneous occurrence of spongiform encephalopathy in a man and his cat in Italy. Lancet 1998;352:1116–7.

[167] Fenner WR. Central nervous system infections. In: Greene CE, editor. Infectious diseases of the dog and cat. 2nd edition. Philadelphia: WB Saunders; 1998. p. 647–57.

ELSEVIER
SAUNDERS

Vet Clin Small Anim
35 (2005) 129–146

VETERINARY
CLINICS
Small Animal Practice

Managing Pain in Feline Patients

Sheilah A. Robertson, BVMS, PhD, MRCVS

Department of Large Animal Clinical Sciences, College of Veterinary Medicine, University of Florida, PO Box 100136, Gainesville, FL 32610–0136, USA

Pet-owning households in the United States increased from 56% to 62% between 1988 and 2002, and recent statistics show that the 77.7 million pet cats outnumber dogs by almost 13 million [1]. Despite this, our understanding and treatment of pain in this species have lagged behind what is available for dogs. When questioned, veterinarians considered surgical procedures in dogs and cats to be equally painful but treated cats less often [2]. The undertreatment of surgical, traumatic, and chronic pain resulted from the difficulty in recognizing and assessing pain, lack of species-specific data on analgesic agents, fear of side effects, and lack of licensed products for cats.

The need for perioperative pain management is great, because most pet cats are spayed or castrated, and in the United States, many are also declawed. The incidence of chronic pain in cats is not well documented, but osteoarthritis is more prevalent than previously thought [3], challenging us to find safe and effective ways to make these animals comfortable.

Over the past few years, a better understanding of the cat's unique metabolism, combined with research and clinical studies, has led to more rational and effective drug choices for our feline patients.

Pain assessment

The benefits of pain management are numerous; however, to treat pain, we must first recognize it. Assessment of pain in animals is not an easy task but is essential for successful pain management. Pain is a complex multidimensional experience involving sensory and affective (emotional) components. It is now accepted that animals do experience pain even if they cannot communicate it in the same way that human beings do. Pain is a subjective and individual experience. We cannot "feel" another person's

---

E-mail address: robertsons@mail.vemted.ufl.edu

pain, and it is well documented that after identical surgical procedures, different people do not experience the same quality and intensity of pain. In animals, pain is what the observer says it is; because all judgments are subjective, if we "get it wrong," the animals suffer.

There is no "gold standard" for assessing pain in animals. Many different scoring methods have been published, but few have been validated. It is now clear that each species exhibits pain differently and that we must take into account the different types and sources of pain, such as acute versus chronic pain and visceral compared with somatic pain. There is no question that as more studies focus on species-specific pain behaviors and the different types of pain, our ability to recognize pain in animals will improve, but we must accept that it is currently a subjective and inaccurate science. Ignoring pain simply because it is difficult to measure is not an option, however.

Most pain assessment studies have focused on acute postoperative pain, and more has been published about dogs than about cats. Investigators have failed to find a good correlation between physiologic variables (eg, heart rate, blood pressure) or plasma cortisol levels and pain scores in cats [4–6]. Conversely, changes in wound sensitivity have correlated well with visual analog pain scores in cats [7], suggesting that this simple clinically applicable technique is a valuable tool and should be incorporated into an overall assessment protocol. Recent adaptations of gait analysis platforms and pressure mats to suit cats show great promise for studying acute musculoskeletal [8] and arthritis pain [9].

Any pain-scoring system that is adopted for use must be valid, reliable, and sensitive as well as simple and quick to perform in a busy clinical setting. There are many to choose from (for a review, see the article by Robertson [10]), including simple descriptive scales, numeric rating scales, and visual analog scales, which are faulted for large interobserver variability [11]. It is now accepted that systems including behavior assessments and observation and interaction with the animal are most reliable. Knowledge of normal behavior of the individual animal evaluated is essential, and, often, the owner and technicians who spend a lot of time with the animal are the best judges. Deviations from normal behavior suggest pain, anxiety, or some combination of stressors.

Pain assessment after surgery should be an integral part of care just as temperature, pulse, and respiration are. In general, the more frequent the observations, the more likely it is that subtle signs of pain will be detected, but this must be weighed against what is practical.

Signs that suggest pain in cats include a hunched posture with the head held low, squinted eyes, sitting quietly and seeking no attention, trying to hide, or resentment at being handled. Excessive licking or biting at a surgical incision should initiate a prompt reassessment for pain. A cat sitting quietly in the back of the cage after surgery may be in pain and ignored by caretakers; interacting with the cat is essential. Once the effects of anesthesia have worn off, cats should perform normal tasks, such as grooming and climbing into a litter box, if they are comfortable. Most cats dislike bandages, even the tape used to secure intravenous catheters, and respond by shaking their legs, biting at the bandage, or throwing themselves around. These reactions could indicate pain or dislike of the bandage, so it is important to differentiate between the two by palpation.

Cats may experience chronic pain associated with dental and gum disease, cancer, interstitial cystitis, chronic wounds, dermatitis, or osteoarthritis. Compared with dogs, little is known about degenerative joint disease in cats, but radiographic evidence in geriatric cats suggests the incidence may be as high as 90% [3]. The behavioral changes that accompany osteoarthritis may be insidious and easily missed or assumed to be inevitable with advancing age. Because of their lifestyle, lameness in cats is not a common owner complaint, but changes in behavior, including decreased grooming, reluctance to jump up on favorite places, and soiling outside the litter box, should prompt the veterinarian to look for sources of chronic pain. Other changes that owners report are altered sleeping habits (an increase or decrease), withdrawing from human interaction, hiding, and dislike of being stroked or brushed.

Drug metabolism

Cats have a low capacity to handle drugs that require hepatic glucuronidation, which has recently been explained by molecular genetic studies [12–14]. Domestic cats have fewer hepatic UDP-glucuroninosyl-transferase (UGT) isoforms, which represent major phase II drug-metabolizing enzymes, as a result of mutations of UGT and the presence of pseudogenes. It is suggested that because cats are carnivores, they had no evolutionary need to develop systems that metabolized the phytoalexins, a group of compounds found in cruciferous plants. The clinical consequence of this is twofold: toxic side effects may occur if doses and dosing intervals are not adjusted, or, alternatively, if the parent compound is metabolized to an active component via this pathway, the drug may be less effective. The cat's susceptibility to toxic side effects of phenolic drugs, such as acetaminophen (paracetamol), and the long half-life of aspirin can be explained by the deficient glucuronidation pathway.

Analgesic drugs

The "classic" analgesic drug categories include the opioids, nonsteroidal anti-inflammatory drugs (NSAIDs), and local anesthetics. The α_2-agonists, such as xylazine and medetomidine, provide analgesia in addition to sedation and muscle relaxation. Other drugs with potential as analgesic agents in cats include ketamine and other N-methyl-D-aspartate (NMDA) inhibitors, such as amantadine; the tricyclic antidepressants amitriptyline and clomipramine; gabapentin, an anticonvulsant agent; and tramadol.

Opioids

In this section, some general features of opioids unique to cats are discussed, and individual drugs and different routes of administration are also covered.

Opioids are the mainstay of analgesic protocols in most species but have historically been avoided in cats because of a fear of producing excitement. Using expressions like morphine or opioid "mania" is unjustified and stems from the early literature when excessive doses were administered [15,16]. More recent studies show that at appropriate doses, opioids can have beneficial analgesic effects and that behavioral effects usually include euphoria, with purring, rolling, and kneading with the front paws [17–19]. Meperidine, methadone, morphine, oxymorphone, hydromorphone, buprenorphine, butorphanol, and fentanyl are now commonly used in cats alone or in conjunction with acepromazine, benzodiazepines, or α_2-agonists in clinical practice [20].

It is now apparent that individuals are unique with respect to number, morphology, and distribution of opioid receptors and that these differences are genetically determined [21]. This is proposed as the reason for the marked variability in response of human beings to opioids, with some individuals experiencing excellent pain relief and others only little. The morphology and sequencing of feline opioid receptors have not been extensively studied [22] compared with other species, but in controlled research environments, marked variation in analgesic response to opioids has been reported [23], suggesting that cats also express genetic variability. This underscores the importance of careful assessment of pain in cats, because one analgesic at a set dose is unlikely to be equally effective in all patients.

Elevation in body temperature after a medical or surgical procedure may be caused by infection, administration of certain drugs, or overzealous warming, and the cause must be identified so that appropriate treatment can be initiated. In cats, opioid-related hyperthermia is something the practitioner should be aware of. At doses of morphine greater than 1 mg/kg, cats may experience hyperthermia [24], and meperidine (Demerol, pethidine) at three times clinically recommended doses resulted in temperatures as high as 41.7°C (107°F) [25].

Although this phenomenon seems to be dose related, commonly used opioids at clinical doses may result in elevated body temperature. In cats that underwent onychectomy, the use of transdermal fentanyl (TDF) patches was associated with higher rectal temperatures (1.0°C above baseline) 4 to 12 hours after patch application compared with cats that received butorphanol [26]. Newer and more potent opioids, including alfentanil, produce elevated rectal temperatures in cats anesthetized with isoflurane [27]. In a retrospective study comparing the use of buprenorphine or hydromorphone in a clinical setting (Niedfeldt R, DVM; Robertson S, BVMS, PhD, unpublished data, 2004), there was a strong association between the use of hydromorphone and hyperthermia. There was no change in mean rectal temperature in cats treated with buprenorphine in the 20-hour postanesthetic period, and only a few cats had temperatures higher than 40°C (104°F), but none exceeded 40.8°C (105.5°F). In contrast, those cats that received hydromorphone had elevated temperatures from 1 to 5 hours after anesthesia, with temperatures higher than 40°C (104°F) being recorded in 75% of the 74 cats and a peak temperature of 42.5°C (108.5°F) occurring in 1 cat. Administration of the NSAID ketoprofen had no impact on the incidence of hyperthermia (Niedfeldt R, DVM; Robertson S, BVMS, PhD, unpublished data, 2004).

Research studies support these clinical findings: hydromorphone at doses of 0.025 and 0.05 mg/kg (intravenous) was not associated with changes in skin temperature, but 0.1 mg/kg produced an increase of 1.0°C to 2.0°C in skin temperature (K. Wegner, DVM; S.A. Robertson, BVMS, PhD, unpublished data, 2004) [28].

In contrast to many other species, opioids cause marked mydriasis in cats. Resultant effects on their vision may cause them to bump into objects, and they may not see a handler approaching. For these reasons, they should be approached slowly, while being spoken to, so that they are not startled. They should also be kept away from bright light while their pupils are dilated. In research models, opioid-induced mydriasis does not correlate with the duration of analgesia.

When used alone for premedication in pain-free cats, some opioids may cause nausea, vomiting, and salivation; this is common after morphine and hydromorphone but not after buprenorphine, meperidine, or butorphanol [17,18,29]. The incidence of nausea and vomiting also depends on the route of administration; subcutaneous hydromorphone results in a higher incidence of vomiting than the intravenous or intramuscular route [29]. When administered with acepromazine, the incidence of vomiting is considerably less.

Little is known about opioid dependence in cats, and if this group of drugs is used for chronic pain management, this could be an issue if treatment were suddenly withdrawn. In this author's experience, cats frequently become inappetent after 2 to 3 days of opioid treatment, and this may be a result of decreased gastrointestinal motility.

Specific opioids and their actions in cats

The pure μ-agonist opioids (morphine, meperidine, oxymorphone, hydromorphone, and fentanyl) are subject to stringent regulatory controls (US Drug Enforcement Administration schedule II). Opioids not subject to such tight controls, for example, butorphanol, are popular for veterinary use because of their convenience, and this drug is licensed for use in cats. Butorphanol is a μ-antagonist and produces analgesia through its κ-agonist activity. It is the most commonly used opioid in cats in North America and is generally given at doses from 0.1 to 0.4 mg/kg [30]. More recently its analgesic properties have been questioned in dogs and cats [31]. Agonist-antagonist opioids, such as butorphanol, exhibit a "ceiling" effect, after which increasing doses do not produce any further analgesia [23]. Butorphanol seems to be an effective visceral but poor somatic analgesic [32]. Clinical studies and experimental investigations indicate that butorphanol is short acting (<90 minutes) [18,23] and requires frequent dosing to be effective. In addition to an injectable formulation, butorphanol is available as a tablet. These produced better analgesia than placebo when used for several days after declawing surgery [33]. Butorphanol is a poor analgesic choice for surgical patients in which there will be somatic and visceral pain, but it would be a reasonable choice for acute visceral pain, such as that associated with interstitial cystitis. Its ceiling effect limits its use to minor procedures, and frequent dosing is inconvenient and expensive.

Meperidine is licensed for use in cats in the United Kingdom, where it is widely used. This drug is only given by the intramuscular or subcutaneous route because of reports of excitement after intravenous dosing. In clinical studies (3.3–10 mg/kg administered intramuscularly) it seems to have a fast onset but short duration of action [34,35]. Research studies that used a thermal stimulus to assess analgesia suggest that at a dose of 5 mg/kg, its duration of action is less that 1 hour [17]. Methadone is widely used in Europe and is said to produce good sedation and short-lived analgesia in cats, although there are few published data about this drug in cats. Clinical doses are generally 0.1 to 0.5 mg/kg administered intramuscularly or subcutaneously. Neither methadone nor meperidine is commonly used in cats in the United States.

Morphine has been widely used in cats, and doses of 0.1 to 0.2 mg/kg are effective in clinical cases and do not cause excitement [36]. In thermal threshold models, morphine produces significant hypoalgesia [18,37]. Clinically [36] and in research models [18], onset of action is slow. Morphine seems to be less effective in cats compared with dogs, and this may be related to cats' limited production of morphine metabolites [38]. Cats produce little of the metabolite morphine-6-glucuronide (see section on drug metabolism), which may contribute significantly to morphine's overall analgesic effect in human beings [39].

Oxymorphone has been a popular analgesic for many years in the United States [19,40]. Oxymorphone is up to 10 times more potent than morphine, but its duration of action is not well documented. Using a visceral pain model, Briggs et al [41] reported that a combination of oxymorphone and butorphanol produced a greater degree of analgesia than either drug used alone and that this could be further enhanced by adding acepromazine.

Hydromorphone has become popular in veterinary medicine and has replaced oxymorphone to a great extent because it is less expensive [42].

Doses of 0.05 to 0.2 mg/kg are generally recommended, and hydromorphone combined with acepromazine (0.05–0.2 mg/kg) produces excellent sedation and chemical restraint [42].

In our laboratory, we examined the relation between dose, thermal antinociception (a measure of analgesia), and change in body temperature after administering hydromorphone to cats. At doses of 0.025 and 0.05 mg/kg (intravenous), there was a small increase in thermal antinociception of short duration and no change in skin temperature. An intravenous dose of 0.1 mg/kg produced a substantial increase in thermal antinociception for up to 5 hours but was accompanied by a 1.0°C to 2.0°C increase in skin temperature [28] and has been implicated in postanesthetic hyperthermia in a clinical setting (Niedfeldt R, DVM; Robertson S, BVMS, PhD, unpublished data, 2004). Route of administration has a significant effect on the quality and duration of analgesia and side effects. When doses of 0.1 mg/kg given by the intravenous, intramuscular, or subcutaneous route were compared, the intravenous route produced the greatest intensity and duration of antinociceptive effect, with the least incidence of vomiting and salivation [29]. In contrast to the study by Briggs et al [41], a combination of hydromorphone and butorphanol did not have additive effects on thermal antinociception but instead produced a longer lasting (up to 9 hours) but less intense effect than hydromorphone alone [43].

Buprenorphine is a partial μ-agonist and is a US Drug Enforcement Administration schedule III drug. Buprenorphine is the most popular opioid used in small animal practice in the United Kingdom [2] and is also widely used in the rest of Europe, Australia, and South Africa [44,45]. In research cats, it has been studied after intramuscular [18], intravenous, and buccal [46] administration. Intramuscular doses of 0.01 mg/kg resulted in a slow onset (2 hours) of analgesia, but once established, this lasted at least 6 hours [18]. Buprenorphine was almost 100% bioavailable after buccal administration [47], which is much higher than in human beings. The effectiveness of this route in cats is thought to be a result of the alkaline (pH 8–9) environment of the cat's mouth [47]. The buccal route (0.02 mg/kg) was also shown to be as effective as the intravenous route, providing analgesia for more than 6 hours in research cats [46]. In a clinical setting, buccal administration has proved to be simple, effective, and well accepted by cats and can be mastered by owners for at-home treatment. In clinical studies, buprenorphine has produced better analgesia than morphine [48], oxymorphone [19], and pethidine [49]. Buprenorphine rarely causes vomiting or dysphoria and has not been associated with hyperthermia; these features, combined with ease of administration, efficacy, and long duration of action, make it an ideal drug for perioperative use in cats.

A transdermal delivery system for buprenorphine is now available for use in human beings in several European countries (Buprenorphine TDS, Transtec; Gruenenthal GmbH, Aachen, Germany). Radbruch [50] reported that 81% of more than 3000 patients with chronic pain received good pain relief. Murrell and colleagues [51] reported systemic uptake after application of a 35-μg/h patch in cats, which was not associated with significant increases in thermal threshold. A 52.5-μg/h patch and 70-μg/h patch are available, but they have not been tested in cats.

Fentanyl is a potent, short-acting, pure μ-agonist that is most commonly used to supplement general anesthesia, where it can be given as intermittent boluses or by infusion [20].

A more popular formulation is TDF patch that releases fentanyl over several days. These are intended for treatment of cancer-related pain in people [52] but have been used for acute perioperative pain in cats [26,53,54]. They provide a "hands-off" approach to pain management that is especially attractive in cats that are difficult to medicate. The plasma concentrations associated with analgesia are reported to be greater than 1 ng/mL in dogs [55] and people [56], and recent work would suggest that this is also true in cats [57]. Plasma fentanyl concentrations are variable after patch placement in cats [26,53], and in one study [58], two of six cats never achieved plasma fentanyl concentrations above 1 ng/mL.

Factors affecting plasma levels include the size of the patch compared with the weight of the cat, skin permeability, and body temperature. Mean serum levels in normothermic (38°C) cats were 1.83 ± 0.63 ng/mL compared with 0.59 ± 0.30 ng/mL in hypothermic (35°C) animals during isoflurane anesthesia [59]. In cats weighing less than 4 kg, placement of a 25-μg/h patch with full exposure of the adhesive layer resulted in a steady-state plasma concentration of 1.78 ± 0.92 ng/mL compared with 1.14 ± 0.86 ng/mL when only half of the adhesive was exposed [60]. In general, cats achieve steady-state plasma concentration faster than dogs (6–12 hours compared with 18–24 hours, respectively) [61], and this persists longer after patch removal in cats (up to 18–20 hours) [58] compared with the rapid decline seen in dogs [62]. TDF patches have proved useful in a clinical setting for routine ovariohysterectomy [54] and were at least as good or better than butorphanol for onychectomy [26,53]. The dangers of accidental or deliberate human ingestion must be considered, and TDF patches should not be placed on cats that are being discharged to a home with young children.

The use of various drugs, including fentanyl, compounded in transdermal creams has become popular in veterinary medicine but is only based on empiric information [63]. The American Veterinary Medical Association has stated that "no published scientific data exist to document the proper regimen of a gel product necessary to deliver a safe, yet effective, dose of any drug in any species." For instance, although widely used for treatment of hyperthyroidism, methimazole in pluronic lecithin organogel (PLO) applied to the inner pinnae of cats produces no measurable plasma drug levels [64]. In our laboratory, fentanyl compounded in PLO cream failed to be absorbed through the skin of the inner pinnae or dorsum of the shaved neck even after a dose of 30 μg/kg; measurable plasma levels were obtained in one cat after it was observed licking the application site [57].

Although not classified as an opioid, tramadol has weak binding affinity at μ-receptors and is thought to activate monoaminergic spinal inhibition of pain. In dogs, this drug shows promise for acute [65] and chronic [66] pain. A dose of 1 to 2 mg/kg administered intravenously has been suggested for cats, but there are as yet no published reports of controlled clinical studies.

Epidural administration of opioids

Opioids exert their major analgesic effect in the dorsal horn of the spinal cord, and intrathecal or epidural administration provides long-lasting analgesia with fewer systemic side effects. Morphine (0.1 mg/kg), fentanyl (4 μg/kg), pethidine, and methadone have been used successfully via the epidural route in cats [67–72]. Morphine is probably the most appropriate opioid with regard to duration of action and quality of analgesia combined with the fewest systemic effects. Epidural injection is technically more challenging in cats because of their small size, and because the spinal cord ends more caudally, entering the subarachnoid space is more likely. If this occurs, half of the epidural dose may still be administered [20].

Nonsteroidal anti-inflammatory drugs

The NSAIDs have the advantage of being long acting, providing up to 24 hours of analgesia, and they are not subject to the regulations of opioids. NSAIDs have not been widely used in cats, however, primarily because of the fear of toxicity. NSAIDs inhibit the cyclooxygenase enzymes COX-1 and COX-2 that are responsible for prostaglandin synthesis. In general, COX-1 is responsible for normal homeostatic functions, such as maintenance of gastric mucosal integrity, platelet function, and renal autoregulation, whereas COX-2 is generally associated with inflammation. The development of COX-2–selective NSAIDs was hailed as a breakthrough in preventing toxicity from these drugs, but continued reports of problems associated with their use suggest that the simple COX-1/COX-2 concept is flawed. It is now known that some constitutive COX-2 is produced in the kidney and central nervous system and is required for normal function. There is considerable species variation in COX expression, so that safety in one species cannot be assumed in another, a fact particularly relevant to the cat, where few pharmacokinetic and pharmacodynamic studies have been performed.

There is considerable potential for NSAID toxicity in cats. Their deficiency and variability of glucuronidation pathways result in slow metabolism of several NSAIDs, leading to prolonged duration of effect and drug accumulation. For example, the mean half-life of carprofen in cats is approximately 20 hours, twice that of the dog, but can vary from 9 to 49 hours [73,74]. More recently, newer NSAIDs have become available for veterinary use, and based on reports of their pharmacokinetic profiles and efficacy, carprofen, meloxicam, and ketoprofen are now being used in cats [34,35,49,75,76]. Although licensed for use in cats in some countries, this is restricted to short-term use only, and no drugs in this class are labeled for feline use in the United States.

Carprofen was one of the first "newer" NSAIDs to be studied in cats, and this drug has a long history in the United Kingdom, where the injectable formulation (4 mg/kg) is licensed. Carprofen causes limited COX inhibition [73], which may explain its good safety record in widespread clinical use in cats. Renal autoregulation may be particularly important during anesthesia, where hypotension is common, and NSAIDs that affect renal autoregulation through COX inhibition are often avoided. Because of its limited potential for COX inhibition, carprofen is used before surgery but is only approved for a single dose.

There have been reports of gastrointestinal toxicity, which has generally been associated with concurrent disease and prolonged administration of the oral formulation [77]. Problems with repeated dosing are likely a result of individual variation in pharmacokinetics.

Meloxicam is a COX-2–selective NSAID that is available as an injectable and oral formulation. In the United Kingdom only, the injectable formulation (0.3 mg/kg) is approved for cats; preoperative administration is permitted and may be continued for a maximum of 3 days. The honey-flavored oral liquid marketed for dogs is widely used (off label) in cats because it is palatable.

Ketoprofen has been used as an analgesic in cats for some years, but because it is a potent COX-1 inhibitor, it is not licensed for preoperative use. The pharmacokinetics and clinical efficacy of ketoprofen are well documented [69,75,78].

There seems to be little difference in the efficacy of the NSAIDs described previously in the acute perioperative setting [75]. Comparison of three injectable NSAIDs given subcutaneously at extubation after ovariohysterectomy (carprofen, 4 mg/kg; ketoprofen, 2 mg/kg; and meloxicam, 0.2 mg/kg) resulted in 9 of 10 cats in each group having desirable overall clinical assessment scores for 18 hours. Despite the cats' apparent comfort, none of the NSAIDs prevented postoperative wound tenderness [75]. Choice of agent depends on personal preference, convenience of dosing, and intended duration of use.

There is only one clinical report on the use of NSAIDs for onychectomy in cats [19]. Those authors concluded that for declawing surgery, with or without sterilization, buprenorphine resulted in lower cumulative pain scores than ketoprofen.

Comparison of opioids and nonsteroidal anti-inflammatory drugs for surgical pain

Carprofen and meperidine have been compared when given subcutaneously at the end of surgery. Two hours after ovariohysterectomy, meperidine (10 mg/kg administered intramuscularly) provided better analgesia than carprofen, but from 2 to 20 hours, carprofen was superior, and the cats that received carprofen required less "rescue analgesia" [35]. Injection of carprofen before castration or ovariohysterectomy was found to be more effective than meperidine given at the end of surgery [34] and seemed to offer good analgesia for 24 hours. A single dose of ketoprofen (2 mg/kg administered subcutaneously) given at the end of anesthesia outperformed a single dose of buprenorphine or meperidine [49].

The combined use of an opioid and an NSAID has not been critically evaluated, and a multimodal approach may produce better results than a single agent, because each drug works at a different part of the pain pathway.

Long-term use of nonsteroidal anti-inflammatory drugs in cats

In dogs and people, NSAIDs form the basis for managing chronic pain. Pharmacokinetic data are only available for single doses of NSAIDs in cats, and no studies have examined the metabolism or safety of chronic administration. As noted previously, most NSAIDs have a relatively long half-life in cats, and repeated dosing must be done carefully to avoid toxicity. Even when NSAIDs are approved for cats, none carries a label for more that 5 days of use, although long-term off-label dosing is now common. The key to successful chronic NSAID administration in cats is to use the lowest effective dose.

As in dogs, cats receiving NSAIDs for chronic pain should be monitored for side effects related to renal and hepatic function and gastrointestinal erosions. There are no accepted monitoring guidelines, but a biochemistry panel, packed cell volume, and total protein measurement before initiating treatment and repeated at 1 and 4 weeks and then every 4 to 6 weeks are recommended. Continual reassessment of the patient by the veterinarian and owner is important so that the dose can be tapered to the smallest effective amount.

Only one published study has evaluated the use of NSAIDs for musculoskeletal pain in cats. Sixty-nine cats with acute or chronic locomotor disorders were randomly assigned to receive meloxicam (liquid formulation, 0.3 mg/kg orally on day 1 and then 0.1 mg/kg for 4 more days) or ketoprofen (tablet formulation, 1 mg/kg orally for 5 days) [79]. Based on general attitude, appetite, weight bearing, lameness, and pain on manipulation, both drugs were equally effective, but meloxicam was more palatable and easier to administer. With care, meloxicam can be used long term in cats, and doses as low as 0.025 mg/kg administered three to four times a week can markedly improve the comfort of cats with cancer-related pain or osteoarthritis (author's personal experience).

Local anesthetic drugs

Local anesthetic blocks provide excellent analgesia in cats, but these techniques are underused. Local and regional blockade inhibits pain transmission, which decreases anesthetic requirements and may limit central sensitization. A review of techniques is outside the scope of this article and is available elsewhere [20].

Newer formulations and routes of administration of local anesthetic drugs show promise. Phospholipid-encapsulated bupivacaine has a long residence time at the site of application and has provided effective analgesia after onychectomy in cats [80]. Two topical anesthetic creams are available: an over-the-counter liposome-encapsulated formulation of lidocaine (ELA-Max) and a prescription-only eutectic mixture of lidocaine and prilocaine (EMLA cream). These are applied to shaved skin to provide analgesia in advance of venipuncture, catheter placement, or skin biopsies. Transdermal absorption did occur after application ELA-Max at a dose of 15 mg/kg, but plasma concentrations remained significantly below toxic values [81]. A lidocaine patch (Lidoderm) is marketed for topical analgesia in people with postherpetic neuralgia. Horses with musculoskeletal pain showed clinical improvement after local patch application, and plasma levels were undetectable [82]. Currently, there are no reports on the safety or efficacy of this technique in cats.

α_2-Adrenoceptor agonists

This group of drugs, which includes xylazine, medetomidine, and, more recently, dexmedetomidine, provides sedation, muscle relaxation, and analgesia in cats. They are not commonly used for their analgesic effect alone because of the profound sedation and cardiovascular depression that accompanies their use. The vasoconstriction and decrease in cardiac output associated with α_2-agonists precludes their use in cats with cardiovascular disease or preexisting hypovolemia.

These drugs are excellent when used as part of the anesthetic protocol for healthy surgical patients because they make cats easier to handle, decrease anesthetic requirements, and provide analgesia. After ovariohysterectomy, medetomidine at a dose of 15 µg/kg provided similar pain relief as butorphanol at a dose of 0.1 mg/kg and was better than placebo treatment [83]. In painful and fractious cats, oral administration of medetomidine, which likely results in transmucosal uptake, is a useful technique [84].

Epidural administration of medetomidine (10 µg/kg) was found it to be superior to fentanyl (4 µg/kg) [70], and systemic effects were mild and short-lived [69]. This technique may be an option for cats undergoing caudal abdominal, pelvic, or hind limb surgery.

Ketamine

Ketamine has traditionally been viewed as a dissociative anesthetic used for chemical restraint in cats. More recently, ketamine, an NMDA antagonist, has been studied for its analgesic properties, because spinal

NMDA receptors are involved in the process of central sensitization and "wind-up" [85].

In a research model, a weak visceral analgesic effect of ketamine was reported [86]. Anesthetic protocols incorporating ketamine provide better postoperative analgesia in cats after ovariohysterectomy [87]. Ketamine (2 mg/kg administered intravenously) resulted in a brief increase in thermal antinociception, followed by a later period of significant hyperalgesia [88]. It should be noted that cats did not undergo any painful procedures in the latter study and that the effect of ketamine may be different when used for sedation alone compared with its use in surgical patients. Although popular and effective in dogs undergoing major surgery, low-dose ketamine infusions have not been critically evaluated in cats.

Other NMDA antagonists, such as amantadine at a dose of 3 to 5 mg/kg administered orally [89], have been suggested for treating chronic pain in cats, and there are anecdotal reports of its success.

Other analgesic agents and treatment modalities

Tricyclic antidepressants, including amitriptyline, clomipramine, and imipramine, can provide relief in human beings with chronic neuropathic pain. Amitriptyline (2.5–12.5 mg/kg administered orally once daily) has been used to treat feline interstitial cystitis with few side effects [90], and it may be effective for other chronic pain syndromes, including osteoarthritis.

The anticonvulsant gabapentin is clinically effective in diabetic-induced neuropathic pain in people, although the mechanism of action is not clear [91]. Based on individual case reports, this drug shows promise in cats [92], and suggested doses have been published [89].

Combinations of chondroitin sulfate, glucosamine hydrochloride, and manganese ascorbate are being used with some success in cats with osteoarthritis and cancer as part of a multimodal approach to pain relief (Duncan Lascelles, BVSc, PhD, personal communication, January 2004).

Many cats tolerate acupuncture and massage surprisingly well, and these treatment modalities can provide significant pain relief. It is difficult to document the efficacy of acupuncture, because each patient is unique and is treated differently even if the underlying cause (eg, osteoarthritis) is the same. Large-scale prospective trials of complimentary therapies should be undertaken in veterinary medicine as they have been in human medicine.

Summary

In the past 10 years, great strides have been made in the field of feline analgesia. A better understanding of the cat's unique metabolism has led researchers to realize that extrapolation across species boundaries is unwise, and this has resulted in feline-specific studies. The opioids are now used more commonly in cats, with good analgesic effect and few side effects. Excellent acute pain management is achievable in cats by using opioids, NSAIDs, α_2-agonists, and local anesthetics. Although much of the research data has compared the use of single drugs, a multimodal approach using agents that work at different parts of the pain pathway is commonly used in clinical settings, with added benefit. Compared with dogs, few pain-scoring systems have been developed for cats, and this remains an important goal.

Management of chronic pain in cats is a challenge because of the potential problems with long-term NSAID use; however, reports of low doses given at extended intervals are encouraging. As we gain experience with less traditional analgesics, such as amitriptyline, amantadine, and gabapentin, and critically evaluate complimentary therapies, our ability to provide comfort to this population of cats will improve.

References

[1] Wise JK, Heathcott BL, Gonzalez ML. Results of the AVMA survey on companion animal ownership in US pet-owning households. J Am Vet Med Assoc 2002;221(11):1572–3.

[2] Lascelles B, Capner C, Waterman-Pearson AE. A survey of current British Veterinary attitudes to peri-operative analgesia for cats and small mammals. Vet Rec 1999;145(21): 601–4.

[3] Hardie EM, Roe SC, Martin FR. Radiographic evidence of degenerative joint disease in geriatric cats: 100 cases (1994–1997). J Am Vet Med Assoc 2002;220(5):628–32.

[4] Cambridge A, Tobias K, Newberry R, Sarkar D. Subjective and objective measurements of postoperative pain in cats. J Am Vet Med Assoc 2000;217(5):685–90.

[5] Smith J, Allen S, Quandt J, Tackett R. Indicators of postoperative pain in cats and correlation with clinical criteria. Am J Vet Res 1996;57(11):1674–8.

[6] Smith J, Allen S, Quandt J. Changes in cortisol concentration in response to stress and postoperative pain in client-owned cats and correlation with objective clinical variables. Am J Vet Res 1999;60(4):432–6.

[7] Slingsby L, Jones A, Waterman-Pearson AE. Use of a new finger-mounted device to compare mechanical nociceptive thresholds in cats given pethidine or no medication after castration. Res Vet Sci 2001;70(3):243–6.

[8] Conzemius M, Horstman C, Gordon W, Evans R. Non-invasive, objective determination of limb function in cats using pressure platform gait analysis. In: Abstracts of the 30th Annual Conference, Veterinary Orthopedic Society, Steamboat Springs. Okemos (MI): Veterinary Orthopedic Society; 2003. p. 84.

[9] Carroll G, Taylor L, Kerwin S, Narbe R, Petersen K. Evaluation of sodium urate synovitis as a reversible model for arthritis in cats. In: Abstracts of the Veterinary Midwest Anesthesia and Analgesia Conference, Indianapolis. Midwest Veterinary Anesthesia Society; 2004. p. 8.

[10] Robertson S. How do we know if they hurt? Pain assessment in small animal. Vet Med 2003; 98(8):700–9.

[11] Holton LL, Scott EM, Nolan AM, Reid J, Welsh E, Flaherty D. Comparison of three methods used for assessment of pain in dogs. J Am Vet Med Assoc 1998;212(1):61–6.

[12] Court M, Greenblatt D. Molecular basis for deficient acetaminophen glucuronidation in cats. An interspecies comparison of enzyme kinetics in liver microsomes. Biochem Pharmacol 1997;53(7):1041–7.

[13] Court M, Greenblatt D. Biochemical basis for deficient paracetamol glucuronidation in cats: an interspecies comparison of enzyme constraint in liver microsomes. J Pharm Pharmacol 1997;49(4):446–9.

[14] Court M, Greenblatt D. Molecular genetic basis for deficient acetaminophen glucuronidation by cats: UGT1A6 is a pseudogene, and evidence for reduced diversity of expressed hepatic UGT1A isoforms. Pharmacogenetics 2000;10(4):355–69.

[15] Joel E, Arndts F. Beitrange zur Pharmakologie der Koperstellung und der Labyrinthreflexe. XIX Mitteilung: Morphin. Arch Ges Physiol 1925;210:280–93.

[16] Fertziger A, Stein E, Lynch J. Suppression of morphine-induced mania in cats. Psychopharmacologia 1974;36:185–7.

[17] Dixon MJ, Robertson SA, Taylor PM. A thermal threshold testing device for evaluation of analgesics in cats. Res Vet Sci 2002;72(3):205–10.

[18] Robertson SA, Taylor PM, Lascelles BD, Dixon MJ. Changes in thermal threshold response in eight cats after administration of buprenorphine, butorphanol and morphine. Vet Rec 2003;153(15):462–5.

[19] Dobbins S, Brown NO, Shofer FS. Comparison of the effects of buprenorphine, oxymorphone hydrochloride, and ketoprofen for postoperative analgesia after onychectomy or onychectomy and sterilization in cats. J Am Anim Hosp Assoc 2002;38(6):507–14.

[20] Lamont LA. Feline perioperative pain management. Vet Clin North Am Small Anim Pract 2002;32(4):747–63.

[21] Mogil JS. The genetic mediation of individual differences in sensitivity to pain and its inhibition. Proc Natl Acad Sci USA 1999;96(14):7744–51.

[22] Billet O, Billaud J, Phillips T. Partial characterization and tissue distribution of the feline mu opiate receptor. Drug Alcohol Depend 2001;62(2):125–9.

[23] Lascelles B, Robertson S. Use of thermal threshold response to evaluate the antinociceptive effects of butorphanol in cats. Am J Vet Res 2004;65:1085–9.

[24] Clark WG, Cumby HR. Hyperthermic responses to central and peripheral injections of morphine sulphate in the cat. Br J Pharmacol 1978;63(1):65–71.

[25] Booth N, Rankin A. Evaluation of meperidine hydrochloride in the cat. Vet Med (Praha) 1954;49(6):249–52.

[26] Gellasch KL, Kruse-Elliott KT, Osmond CS, Shih AN, Bjorling DE. Comparison of transdermal administration of fentanyl versus intramuscular administration of butorphanol for analgesia after onychectomy in cats. J Am Vet Med Assoc 2002;220(7): 1020–4.

[27] Ilkiw J, Pascoe P, Fisher L. Effect of alfentanil on the minimum alveolar concentration of isoflurane in cats. Am J Vet Res 1997;58(11):1274–9.

[28] Wegner K, Robertson SA. Evaluation of the side effects and thermal threshold antinociceptive effects of intravenous hydromorphone in cats. Vet Anaesth Analg 2003; 30(2):101.

[29] Robertson S, Wegner K, Lascelles B. Effect of route of administration on the thermal antinociceptive actions of hydromorphone in cats. In: Abstracts from the 8th World Congress of Veterinary Anesthesia. Knoxville; 2003. p. 106.

[30] Dohoo S, Dohoo I. Postoperative use of analgesics in dogs and cats by Canadian veterinarians. Can Vet J 1996;37(9):546–51.

[31] Wagner AE. Is butorphanol analgesic in dogs and cats? Vet Med 1999;94:346–51.

[32] Sawyer D, Rech R. Analgesia and behavioral effects of butorphanol, nalbuphine, and pentazocine in the cat. J Am Anim Hosp Assoc 1987;23:438–46.

[33] Carroll G, Howe L, Slater M, Haughn L, Martinez EA, Hartsfield SM. Evaluation of analgesia provided by postoperative administration of butorphanol to cats undergoing onychectomy. J Am Vet Med Assoc 1998;213(2):246–50.

[34] Balmer T, Irvine D, Jones R, Roberts MJ, Slingsby L, Taylor PM, et al. Comparison of carprofen and pethidine as postoperative analgesics in the cat. J Small Anim Pract 1998; 39(4):158–64.

[35] Lascelles B, Cripps P, Mirchandani S, Waterman A. Carprofen as an analgesic for postoperative pain in cats: dose titration and assessment of efficacy in comparison to pethidine hydrochloride. J Small Anim Pract 1995;36(12):535–41.

[36] Lascelles D, Waterman A. Analgesia in Cats. In Practice 1997:203–13.

[37] Davis LE, Donnelly EJ. Analgesic drugs in the cat. J Am Vet Med Assoc 1968;153(9):1161–7.

[38] Taylor PM, Robertson SA, Dixon MJ, Ruprah M, Sear JW, Lascelles BD, et al. Morphine, pethidine and buprenorphine disposition in the cat. J Vet Pharmacol Ther 2001;24(6):391–8.

[39] Murthy BR, Pollack GM, Brouwer KL. Contribution of morphine-6-glucuronide to antinociception following intravenous administration of morphine to healthy volunteers. J Clin Pharmacol 2002;42(5):569–76.

[40] Palminteri A. Oxymorphone, an effective analgesic in dogs and cats. J Am Vet Med Assoc 1963;143:160–3.

[41] Briggs SL, Sneed K, Sawyer DC. Antinociceptive effects of oxymorphone-butorphanol-acepromazine combination in cats. Vet Surg 1998;27(5):466–72.

[42] Pettifer G, Dyson D. Hydromorphone: a cost-effective alternative to the use of oxymorphone. Can Vet J 2000;41(2):135–7.

[43] Lascelles BD, Robertson SA, Taylor PM, Hauptman JG. Thermal antinociceptive pharmacodynamics of 0.1 mg/kg hydromorphone administered intramuscularly in cats, and effect of concurrent butorphanol administration. Vet Anaesth Analg 2003;30(2):108–9.

[44] Watson A, Nicholson A, Church D, Pearson M. Use of anti-inflammatory and analgesic drugs in dogs and cats. Aust Vet J 1996;74(3):203–10.

[45] Joubert K. The use of analgesic drugs by South African veterinarians. J S Afr Vet Assoc 2001;72(1):57–60.

[46] Lascelles B, Robertson S, Taylor P, Hauptman J. Comparison of the pharmacokinetics and thermal antinociceptive pharmacodynamics of 20 μg/kg buprenorphine administered sublingually or intravenously in cats. In: Abstracts from the 27th Annual Meeting of the American College of Veterinary Anesthesiologists, Orlando. American College of Veterinary Anesthesiologists; 2002. p. 31.

[47] Robertson SA, Taylor PM, Sear JW. Systemic uptake of buprenorphine by cats after oral mucosal administration. Vet Rec 2003;152(22):675–8.

[48] Stanway G, Taylor P, Brodbelt D. A preliminary investigation comparing pre-operative morphine and buprenorphine for postoperative analgesia and sedation in cats. Vet Anaesth Analg 2002;29:29–35.

[49] Slingsby L, Waterman-Pearson A. Comparison of pethidine, buprenorphine and ketoprofen for postoperative analgesia after ovariohysterectomy in the cat. Vet Rec 1998;143(7):185–9.

[50] Radbruch L. Buprenorphine TDS: use in daily practice, benefits for patients. Int J Clin Pract Suppl 2003;133:19–24.

[51] Murrell JC, Demers J, Davies W, Taylor PM, Robertson SA. Evaluation of the side effects and thermal antinociceptive effects of transdermal buprenorphine in cats. In: Abstracts from the Association of Veterinary Anaesthetists Spring Meeting, London. Association of Veterinary Anaesthetists; 2004. p. 47.

[52] Muijsers RB, Wagstaff AJ. Transdermal fentanyl: an updated review of its pharmacological properties and therapeutic efficacy in chronic cancer pain control. Drugs 2001;61(15): 2289–307.

[53] Franks JN, Boothe HW, Taylor L, Geller S, Carroll GL, Cracas V, et al. Evaluation of transdermal fentanyl patches for analgesia in cats undergoing onychectomy. J Am Vet Med Assoc 2000;217(7):1013–20.

[54] Glerum LE, Egger CM, Allen SW, Haag M. Analgesic effect of the transdermal fentanyl patch during and after feline ovariohysterectomy. Vet Surg 2001;30(4):351–8.

[55] Robinson T, Kruse-Elliott K, Markel M, Pluhar G, Massa K, Bjorling D. A comparison of transdermal fentanyl versus epidural morphine for analgesia in dogs undergoing major orthopedic surgery. J Am Anim Hosp Assoc 1999;35(2):95–100.

[56] Gourlay GK, Kowalski SR, Plummer JL, Cousins MJ, Armstrong PJ. Fentanyl blood concentration-analgesic response relationship in the treatment of postoperative pain. Anesth Analg 1988;67(4):329–37.

[57] Robertson SA, Taylor PM, Sear JW, Pettifer G, Keuhnel G. Fentanyl in cats: pharmacokinetics and pharmacodynamics with intravenous dosing and disposition after alternative routes of administration. J Vet Pharmacol Ther, in press.

[58] Lee D, Papich M, Hardie E. Comparison of pharmacokinetics of fentanyl after intravenous and transdermal administration in cats. Am J Vet Res 2000;61(6):672–7.

[59] Pettifer GR, Hosgood G. The effect of rectal temperature on perianesthetic serum concentrations of transdermally administered fentanyl in cats anesthetized with isoflurane. Am J Vet Res 2003;64(12):1557–61.

[60] Davidson CD, Pettifer GR, Henry JD. Plasma fentanyl concentrations and analgesic effects during full or partial exposure to transdermal fentanyl patches in cats. J Am Vet Med Assoc 2004;224(5):700–5.

[61] Riviere J, Papich M. Potential and problems of developing transdermal patches for veterinary applications. Adv Drug Deliv Rev 2001;50(3):175–203.

[62] Kyles AE, Papich M, Hardie EM. Disposition of transdermally administered fentanyl in dogs. Am J Vet Res 1996;57(5):715–9.

[63] Marks SL, Taboada J. Transdermal therapeutics. J Am Anim Hosp Assoc 2003;39(1):19–21.

[64] Hoffman SB, Yoder AR, Trepanier LA. Bioavailability of transdermal methimazole in a pluronic lecithin organogel (PLO) in healthy cats. J Vet Pharmacol Ther 2002;25(3): 189–93.

[65] Mastrocinque S, Fantoni DT. A comparison of preoperative tramadol and morphine for the control of early postoperative pain in canine ovariohysterectomy. Vet Anaesth Analg 2003; 30(4):220–8.

[66] Lambert C, Bianchi E, Keroack S, Genevois JP, Soldani G, Troncy E. Reduced dosage of ketoprofen alone or with tramadol for long-term treatment of osteoarthritis in dogs. In: Abstracts from the 8th World Congress of Veterinary Anesthesia, Knoxville. American College of Veterinary Anesthesiologists; 2003. p. 157.

[67] Tung A, Yaksh T. The antinociceptive effects of epidural opiates in the cat: studies of the pharmacology and the effects of lipophilicity in spinal analgesia. Pain 1982;12(4):343–56.

[68] Golder F, Pascoe P, Bailey C, Ilkiw J, Tripp L. The effect of epidural morphine on the minimum alveolar concentration of isoflurane in cats. J Vet Anaesth 1998;25(1):52–6.

[69] Duke T, Cox AM, Remedios AM, Cribb PH. The cardiopulmonary effects of placing fentanyl or medetomidine in the lumbosacral epidural space of isoflurane-anesthetized cats. Vet Surg 1994;23(2):149–55.

[70] Duke T, Cox AM, Remedios AM, Cribb PH. The analgesic effects of administering fentanyl or medetomidine in the lumbosacral epidural space of cats. Vet Surg 1994;23(2):143–8.

[71] Jones RS. Epidural analgesia in the dog and cat. Vet J 2001;161(2):123–31.

[72] Troncy E, Junot S, Keroack S, Sammut V, Pibarot P, Genevois JP, et al. Results of preemptive epidural administration of morphine with or without bupivacaine in dogs and cats undergoing surgery: 265 cases (1997–1999). J Am Vet Med Assoc 2002;221(5): 666–72.

[73] Taylor PM, Delatour P, Landoni FM, Deal C, Pickett C, Shojaee Aliabadi F, et al. Pharmacodynamics and enantioselective pharmacokinetics of carprofen in the cat. Res Vet Sci 1996;60(2):144–51.

[74] Parton K, Balmer TV, Boyle J, Whittem T, MacHon R. The pharmacokinetics and effects of intravenously administered carprofen and salicylate on gastrointestinal mucosa and selected biochemical measurements in healthy cats. J Vet Pharmacol Ther 2000;23(2):73–9.

[75] Slingsby L, Waterman-Pearson AE. Postoperative analgesia in the cat after ovariohyster-ectomy by use of carprofen, ketoprofen, meloxicam or tolfenamic acid. J Small Anim Pract 2000;41:447–50.

[76] Slingsby L, Waterman-Pearson AE. Comparison between meloxicam and carprofen for postoperative analgesia after feline ovariohysterectomy. J Small Anim Pract 2002;43(7): 286–9.

[77] Runk A, Kyles A, Downs M. Duodenal perforation in a cat following the administration of
      nonsteroidal anti-inflammatory medication. J Am Anim Hosp Assoc 1999;35(1):52–5.
[78] Lees P, Taylor PM, Landoni FM, Arifah AK, Waters C. Ketoprofen in the cat:
      pharmacodynamics and chiral pharmacokinetics. Vet J 2003;165(1):21–35.
[79] Lascelles B, Henderson A, Hackett I. Evaluation of the clinical efficacy of meloxicam in cats
      with painful locomotor disorders. J Small Anim Pract 2001;42(12):587–93.
[80] Dodam J, Boedeker B, Gross M, Branson K, Carroll G. Phospholipid-encapsulated
      bupivacaine and analgesia after onychectomy in cats. In: Abstracts from the 26th Annual
      Meeting of the American College of Veterinary Anesthesiologists, New Orleans. American
      College of Veterinary Anesthesiologists; 2001. p. 49.
[81] Fransson BA, Peck KE, Smith JK, Anthony JA, Mealey KL. Transdermal absorption of
      a liposome-encapsulated formulation of lidocaine following topical administration in cats.
      Am J Vet Res 2002;63(9):1309–12.
[82] Bidwell LA, Wilson DV, Caron JP. Systemic lidocaine absorption after placement of
      Lidoderm patches on horses: preliminary findings. In: Abstracts from the Veterinary
      Midwest Anesthesia and Analgesia Conference, Indianapolis. Midwest Veterinary
      Anesthesia and Analgesic Conference; 2004. p. 15.
[83] Ansah OB, Vainio O, Hellsten C, Raekallio M. Postoperative pain control in cats: clinical
      trials with medetomidine and butorphanol. Vet Surg 2002;31(2):99–103.
[84] Ansah O, Raekallio M, Vainio O. Comparing oral and intramuscular administration of
      medetomidine in cats. J Vet Anaesth 1998;25(1):41–6.
[85] Petrenko AB, Yamakura T, Baba H, Shimoji K. The role of N-methyl-D-aspartate
      (NMDA) receptors in pain: a review. Anesth Analg 2003;97(4):1108–16.
[86] Sawyer D, Rech R, Durham RA. Does ketamine provide adequate visceral analgesia when
      used alone or in combination with acepromazine, diazepam, or butorphanol in cats. J Am
      Anim Hospl Assoc 1993;29:257–63.
[87] Slingsby LS, Lane EC, Mears ER, Shanson MC, Waterman-Pearson AE. Postoperative pain
      after ovariohysterectomy in the cat: a comparison of two anaesthetic regimens. Vet Rec 1998;
      143(21):589–90.
[88] Robertson S, Lascelles BD, Taylor P. Effect of low dose ketamine on thermal thresholds in
      cats. Vet Anaesth Analg 2003;30(2):110.
[89] Gaynor JS. Other drugs used to treat pain. In: Gaynor JS, Muir WW, editors. Handbook of
      veterinary pain management. 1st edition. St. Louis: Mosby; 2002. p. 251–60.
[90] Chew DJ, Buffington CA, Kendall MS, DiBartola SP, Woodworth BE. Amitriptyline
      treatment for severe recurrent idiopathic cystitis in cats. J Am Vet Med Assoc 1998;213(9):
      1282–6.
[91] Morello CM, Leckband SG, Stoner CP, Moorhouse DF, Sahagian GA. Randomized
      double-blind study comparing the efficacy of gabapentin with amitriptyline on diabetic
      peripheral neuropathy pain. Arch Intern Med 1999;159(16):1931–7.
[92] Lamont LA, Tranquilli WJ, Mathews KA. Adjunctive analgesic therapy. Vet Clin North Am
      Small Anim Pract 2000;30(4):805–13.

ELSEVIER
SAUNDERS

Vet Clin Small Anim
35 (2005) 147–170

VETERINARY
CLINICS
Small Animal Practice

Recent Concepts in Feline Lower Urinary Tract Disease

Roger A. Hostutler, DVM, MS*,
Dennis J. Chew, DVM, Stephen P. DiBartola, DVM

*Department of Clinical Sciences, The Ohio State University, College of Veterinary Medicine,
Columbus, OH 43210, USA*

A clinical description of lower urinary tract disease (LUTD) in cats in 1925 [1] accurately described the clinical signs and the disease, and reported it to be commonplace. The terms *feline urologic syndrome* (FUS) and *feline lower urinary tract disease* (FLUTD) have since been used to describe the constellation of clinical signs related to irritative voiding but do not identify the underlying etiology. Most cats with LUTD have feline idiopathic or interstitial cystitis (FIC), but urolithiasis, bacterial urinary tract infection (UTI), anatomic malformations, neoplasia, behavioral disorders, and neurologic problems (eg, reflex dysnergia) may also occur, although more uncommonly than FIC. Regardless of the underlying etiology, the resultant clinical signs are similar and include dysuria, stranguria, hematuria (macroscopic and microscopic), pollakiuria, and periuria (a word used to refer to urination in inappropriate places).

Obstructive and nonobstructive uropathy are broader concepts that may also be used to classify LUTD by the presence or absence of urethral obstruction, respectively. Obstructive uropathy is rare in female cats and is primarily seen in male cats. The diameter of the urethra and frequency of obstructive uropathy do not differ between castrated and intact male cats, but urethral obstruction occurs with higher frequency in castrated male cats [2].

Diseases of the lower urinary tract are becoming more apparent clinically as indoor cats and multicat households are becoming more common. Inappropriate elimination results in the relinquishment of approximately 4 million cats annually to animal shelters because of behavior that is unacceptable to owners [3]. The estimated prevalence of LUTD in primary care practice in the United States has been reported to be approximately

---

* Corresponding author.
E-mail address: Hostutler.4@osu.edu (R.A. Hostutler).

0195-5616/05/$ - see front matter © 2005 Elsevier Inc. All rights reserved.
doi:10.1016/j.cvsm.2004.08.006
vetsmall.theclinics.com

1.5% [4]. Based on referral institution studies of cats presented with nonobstructive urinary tract disease, the two most common causes have been found to be FIC (55%–69%) and urolithiasis (13%–28%) [5,6]. A diagnosis of FIC is made after routine diagnostic tests, including urinalysis, urine culture and sensitivity, radiography, ultrasonography, and contrast radiography, fail to identify an etiology. If uroendoscopy is performed and submucosal petechial hemorrhages (ie, glomerulations) are seen, a diagnosis of FIC is made. This nomenclature is used based on similarities of clinical signs seen in human beings with interstitial cystitis.

Recently, many studies have evaluated the effects of dietary and environmental factors on development of LUTD in cats. The influence of behavioral disturbances and interactions with other cats in development of lower urinary tract signs cannot be overemphasized. Most cats with lower urinary tract signs are presented between 2 and 6 years of age, and the disorder is uncommon in cats less than 1 year of age or greater than 10 years of age. When looking solely at nonobstructive disease, LUTD occurs with equal frequency in male and female cats. The risk is higher for castrated or spayed cats when adjusted for age, but the age of neutering does not seem to be clinically relevant [2].

Body weight and diet have been reported to be risk factors when compared with nonaffected cats. Cats that are obese and sedentary have been shown to have a higher incidence of LUTD, as do cats that are fed solely dry food or fed intermittently throughout the day [2].

Another study found an association with indoor elimination, confinement, and sleeping; recent moves; and decreased water intake with the development of LUTD [7]. Environmental factors, such as interactions with owners, multicat households, and changes in routine, have been associated with LUTD and are discussed in detail later. Regardless of the ultimate manifestations of LUTD, changes in environment, husbandry, and feeding may decrease the recurrence rate. Recurrence rates have been reported to be as high as 45% within 6 months in male cats with obstructive uropathy [8] and 39% within 1 year in cats with nonobstructive uropathy [9].

Diagnostic workup

No clinical sign or combination of clinical signs is diagnostic of a particular LUTD in cats. Making a diagnosis involves integrating findings from the signalment, history, physical examination, clinical signs, time course of the disease, urinalysis with sediment evaluation, urine culture and sensitivity testing, and urinary tract imaging. The modality of imaging chosen may include a combination of plain abdominal radiography, ultrasonography of the urogenital system (which affords minimal urethral evaluation), contrast radiography, and uroendoscopy (including urethroscopy and cystoscopy).

Consideration of the signalment may be helpful in developing a list of differential diagnoses. It would be uncommon (<5%) for a cat older than 10 years of age to develop idiopathic cystitis. Bacterial UTIs are diagnosed in more than 50% of cats older than 10 years of age presented with lower urinary tract signs [10]. Likewise, it would be unusual for a young cat to develop a bacterial UTI. Laboratory evaluation of blood work generally is unremarkable unless other diseases, such as chronic renal failure, are present. If concomitant disease is suspected, a complete blood cell count and serum biochemistry profile should be evaluated.

Periuria is a word that has been coined to describe the tendency of cats with irritative voiding to urinate in places other than the litter box (inappropriate urination). Periuria is the most common clinical sign reported by owners of cats with LUTD, and these cats often are suspected by veterinarians to have a behavioral disorder. Approximately half of cats with inappropriate urination as the only client-reported clinical sign have been reported to have interstitial cystitis diagnosed by uroendoscopy [6]. The time course of the clinical signs also may be helpful in arriving at a diagnosis. Initial bouts of interstitial cystitis generally resolve within 7 days with or without treatment. Other diseases, such as urolithiasis and bacterial UTI, often result in clinical signs that are present for longer periods and may be progressive in severity unless adequate therapy is instituted.

Urinalysis with sediment evaluation should be performed if there is recurrence of clinical signs, evidence of underlying chronic renal failure, or previous urinary catheterization or if a perineal urethrostomy is present. Urine dipstick pads that detect white blood cell (WBC) esterase often are positive in the absence of pyuria in cats (ie, they frequently yield false-positive results). When evaluating feline urine sediment, care must be taken not to overinterpret the presence of bacteria. Cellular debris may exhibit Brownian motion and be misinterpreted as bacteria. Dilute urine in the face of pyuria or significant pyuria (>5 WBCs per high-power field [hpf]) regardless of urine specific gravity (USG) warrants urine culture and sensitivity testing on urine collected by cystocentesis. The presence of crystals in urine sediment may have no clinical importance in cats without a stone or urethral plug, because crystals do not damage healthy urothelium. Urine that has been refrigerated or stored for hours often contains crystals in the urinary sediment, and this phenomenon is exaggerated in urine that is highly concentrated [11].

Plain abdominal radiographs that include the pelvic and penile urethra can be helpful in identifying radiopaque calculi (eg, struvite, oxalate) more than 3 mm in diameter. Contrast radiography, including cystography, urethrography, and urethrocystography, is indicated in cats with recurrent or lingering clinical signs. Contrast cystography often is normal in FIC, but the technique may be helpful in detecting small calculi, radiolucent calculi, urachal diverticula and neoplasia as well as in determining bladder wall thickness. Occasionally, contrast material may be seen permeating through the bladder wall in severe cystitis. Contrast evaluation of the urethra generally is normal but may be helpful in diagnosing urethral strictures in male cats and stones in the urethra [12,13]. Generally, these procedures are performed simultaneously as a contrast urethrocystogram in male cats, thus maximizing the information the clinician obtains from one procedure.

Abdominal ultrasonography is useful to evaluate the bladder but is unrewarding for evaluation of the entire length of the urethra. Abdominal ultrasonography may detect small calculi, radiolucent calculi, and bladder masses like polyps and neoplasia and may aid in assessing bladder wall thickness if the bladder is sufficiently distended.

Uroendoscopy is a valuable tool in evaluation of cats that have recurrent or persistent clinical signs associated with the lower urinary tract. Uroendoscopy allows visualization of the urethral and bladder mucosa, detection of small calculi not seen on abdominal ultrasonography, evaluation for urachal remnants, and direct visualization of masses that may be present. Uroendoscopy of female cats is performed using a rigid pediatric cystoscope, which affords much greater detail and manipulation than can be obtained with the flexible fiberoptic ureteroscope that is used in male cats. The rigid cystoscope may be used in male cats that have had a perineal urethrostomy performed and allows the clinician to obtain biopsies. The 1.1-mm flexible urethroscope used in male cats is not as optimal for evaluation of the bladder as the 3.0-mm rigid cystoscope, but it is adequate for evaluation of the urethra for the presence of strictures, plugs, spasms, and stones.

Most cases of LUTD in the cat can be managed successfully in primary care practice. Generally, clinical signs resolve within 7 days. If clinical signs persist or recur repeatedly, further diagnostics and referral to an internist or behaviorist may be indicated. If a cat has two or three episodes of lower urinary tract signs within a short period, further imaging and diagnostics, such as uroendoscopy, may be indicated. Veterinary behaviorists can play an important role in evaluation and management of behavioral and environmental factors. Strategies to enrich the environment of the cat and lessen stresses associated with multicat households and indoor living should become a routine part of husbandry of cats (discussed in detail later in section on treatment of interstitial cystitis).

Feline interstitial/idiopathic cystitis

Pathophysiology

Multiple abnormalities of the bladder, central nervous system, and hypothalamic-pituitary-adrenal axis may lead to the clinical manifestations of FIC. The pelvic and hypogastric nerves and their central connections in the dorsal horn of the sacral and lumbar spinal cord provide sensory innervation to the bladder [14]. Normal bladder urothelium is lined by a specific glycosaminoglycan (GAG) called GP-51 that is believed to inhibit bacterial adherence and protect the urothelium from noxious urine constituents. People and animals with interstitial cystitis excrete decreased amounts of urine GAG [15] and GP-51 [16]. If the GAG layer or urothelium is compromised, constituents of the urine can contact the sensory nerves and result in neurogenic bladder inflammation. The sensory neurons are located in the submucosa and are composed primarily of unmyelinated pain fibers (C-fibers). Once these sensory fibers are stimulated, action potentials are transmitted to the spinal cord and are perceived as pelvic pain. In addition to transmitting the sensation of pain to the brain, local axon reflexes that lead to the release of substance P (SP), a neurotransmitter that results in local potentiation of the inflammation, are released. Local SP release results in increased vascular permeability by means of direct action on vessel walls and through SP-mediated release of inflammatory mediators, such as histamine from mast cells. Receptors for SP also are present on smooth muscle and cause contraction when stimulated. Figs. 1 and 2 illustrate the normal bladder and the described changes that lead to the clinical signs seen with FIC.

Histologic findings in the bladders of FIC-affected cats are typical but not pathognomonic. Changes include edema, hemorrhage, and dilatation of blood vessels in the submucosa. Increased mast cell density has been reported in some cats with FIC when toluidine blue stain is applied [17]. Routine hematoxylin and eosin staining of specimens may reveal an intact or partially denuded urothelium. Electron microscopy, however, has shown areas that lack urothelium and distortion of gap junctions [18]. These findings support the role of local neurogenic inflammation potentially mediated by SP and the findings of other studies on increased bladder permeability in cats with FIC [19].

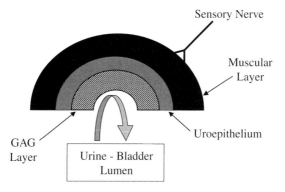

Fig. 1. Normal bladder with intact urothelium and glycosaminoglycan (GAG) layer. The urothelium and GAG act as a natural barrier to protect the underlying layers and sensory nerves from the noxious urine.

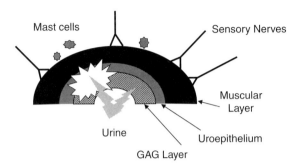

Fig. 2. Schematic of bladder of cat affected with feline interstitial cystitis (FIC). This demonstrates loss of integrity of the glycosaminoglycan layer and urothelium. Loss of integrity of these layers leads to recruitment of sensory nerves, recruitment and activation of mast cells, and changes in the central nervous system that lead to the clinical signs seen with FIC.

The overall clinical manifestations and high recurrence rates in cats with FIC also seem to involve intimate changes in the neurochemistry of the brain. The locus coeruleus (LC) [20] and paraventricular nucleus [21] recently have been reported to be involved in the pathogenesis of FIC. The LC is responsible for excitatory stimulation to the bladder and is activated on bladder distention [22]. These areas in cats with FIC recently have been reported to possess increased tyrosine hydroxylase immunoreactivity, suggesting increased catecholamine synthesis [20,21]. Affected animals also have increased concentrations of circulating catecholamines [23] at rest and during stressful situations. α_2-Adrenoceptors also seem to play a role in the development of FIC in cats. Centrally, α_2-adrenoceptors are found in the LC and spinal cord, where they inhibit catecholamine release and pain input to the brain, respectively [24,25]. Peripherally, α_2-adrenoceptors are found in the bladder mucosa, where they are believed to regulate blood flow. Desensitization of the central α_2-receptors as a result of chronic stimulation and enhanced catecholamine release from the bladder of cats with FIC has been reported [26] and may result in potentiation of the inflammatory response. Finally, cats with FIC have been shown to have a suboptimal response to exogenous corticotropin stimulation when compared with control cats [27], decreased adrenal volume when evaluated by CT [28], and a histologically greater adrenal medulla area than normal cats. These findings suggest that FIC results in overactivation of the sympathetic nervous system with suboptimal activation of the hypothalamic-pituitary-adrenal axis.

Diagnosis

The terms *idiopathic cystitis* and *interstitial cystitis* often are used interchangeably. Idiopathic cystitis is the most common diagnosis in cats with lower urinary tract signs. The term *idiopathic cystitis* is used if all diagnostics fail to confirm the presence of another disease, such as urolithiasis or a bacterial UTI. Idiopathic cystitis generally is seen in middle-aged cats and is rarely diagnosed in cats older than 10 years of age, and no gender predisposition has been reported in cats with nonobstructive FIC [7]. No clinical signs are specific for FIC, but owners of affected cats most commonly report periuria. Cats may exhibit solely periuria, or they may also show signs of pollakiuria, stranguria, and hematuria.

Results of radiography and urinalysis often are nonspecific in cats with FIC. Abdominal radiography may be performed to aid in the elimination of urolithiasis as a differential diagnosis in cats with multiple recurrences of clinical signs. Double-contrast cystography and positive-contrast urethrography are recommended for cats with recurrent lower urinary tract signs in which no cause has been found on urinalysis, urine culture, and plain abdominal radiographs. Results from cats with FIC are normal in approximately 85% of the cases. Focal or diffuse thickening of the bladder wall is seen in some, and contrast agent may be observed dissecting through the bladder wall in a few cases [13]. Ultrasonography is less invasive than urethrocystography but is less sensitive in the detection of small lesions and provides little information about the urethra.

Urinalysis may identify hematuria and proteinuria, the severity of which can vary substantially throughout the day or over the course of several days. The absence of hematuria does not exclude a diagnosis of FIC. A paucity of WBCs is found in the urine sediment. Crystalluria is variable and of no pathologic significance in cats with FIC. Often, crystalluria is an artifact of refrigeration and time of storage. Many times, bacteria are reported from the laboratory when, in fact, they are not present. This problem is common in the cat and is caused by particulate material (eg, small crystals, cellular debris, lipid droplets) that exhibit Brownian motion and may be misidentified as bacteria. The results of urine cultures in cats with FIC are negative (ie, no growth or <1000 colony-forming units/mL on urine collected by cystocentesis). USG should be greater than 1.025 in cats eating canned foods and greater than 1.035 in cats eating dry foods. Urinalysis findings, however, are not specific for any one LUTD. Fig. 3 shows typical urine sediment found in cats affected with FIC.

If clinical signs are continuous or frequently recur or if the episodes become more severe, direct visualization of the lower urinary tract using uroendoscopy may be indicated to eliminate other differential diagnoses and to confirm the diagnosis of FIC. If uroendoscopy is performed and submucosal petechial hemorrhages (ie, glomerulations) are seen, the term *interstitial cystitis* is appropriate (Fig. 4). Glomerulations are not seen in all cats with FIC and may be seen in some sensitive asymptomatic cats that have undergone recent stress [29]. Other findings on cystoscopy in cats with FIC include edema, debris in the lumen of the bladder, and increased vascularity. The severity of cystoscopic lesions does not seem to correlate with the severity of clinical signs observed by the owner; therefore,

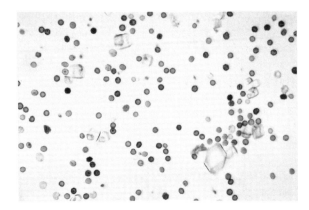

Fig. 3. Urine sediment of cat affected with feline interstitial cystitis. Notice the presence of red blood cells, with a paucity of white blood cells. The presence of crystalluria does not indicate that they are the cause of the clinical signs. A normal urothelium should not be adversely affected by their presence.

cystoscopic re-evaluation of the bladder is not routinely performed once a diagnosis of FIC is made.

FIC is a diagnosis of exclusion, and diagnostic tests must be chosen with the signalment, history, and clinical signs in mind. A young cat with clinical signs lasting 5 to 7 days most likely has FIC. With increasing frequency or severity of episodes, more invasive diagnostics are warranted, however.

Treatment

Treatment of FIC may include environmental enrichment, dietary alterations, pheromone therapy, and pharmacologic intervention in refractory cases. In treating FIC, the owner must be made aware that his or her cat has

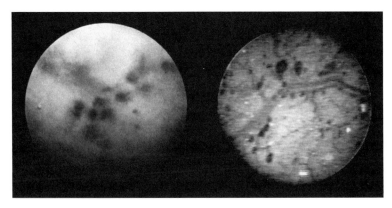

Fig. 4. Cystoscopic evaluation of the urinary bladder in cats affected with feline interstitial cystitis. The figure on the left depicts a cat with multiple large glomerulations. The figure on the right depicts multiple smaller glomerulations with increased vascularity.

a disease with an unknown cause and with no known cure and that the goal of therapy is to decrease the severity and recurrence rate of episodes. Successfully managing affected cats takes a dedicated and understanding owner and equally dedicated veterinary staff.

Environmental enrichment and modification can reduce stress and decrease the severity and intervals of FIC episodes. These changes often are used as initial treatments before other modalities are attempted. Environmental modification includes changes in management of litter boxes, food dishes, and water bowls. To be optimally appealing to the cat, the litter box should be viewed as its own "plastic palace." The litter boxes of cats with FIC should be cleaned frequently. Nonclumping unscented litter is preferred by most cats, but a variety of litter types and depths may be offered in separate boxes [30]. Litter boxes should be totally emptied and cleaned weekly to avoid buildup of odors, such as ammonia. The litter boxes also should be placed in an area that is free of intrusion by other pets and children and should not be placed in high-traffic areas or next to an appliance that may suddenly make noise and disturb the cat. Some cats prefer boxes of different sizes and may not prefer boxes that are covered [31]. An adequate number of litter boxes also is important. The "1 + 1" rule states that there should be one more litter box in the house than there are cats. Perhaps just as important as litter box management is adequate cleaning of areas where inappropriate urination has occurred. Inadequate cleaning may attract affected and nonaffected cats to the area despite adequate litter box management.

Environmental modification also may extend to the manner in which food and water are provided to the cat. To ensure adequate water intake, the cat's water bowl preferences should be determined. Depth of water, type of bowl, flavoring, and the use of fountains all may need to be adjusted until the individual cat's preferences are determined. The type of food that is fed also should be evaluated. Affected cats should be fed moist food exclusively if accepted by the cat. Some cats accustomed to dry food may refuse moist food, however. If a change in diet is attempted, the new food should be introduced alongside the current diet in a separate dish. As with litter boxes, food and water bowls should be cleaned with a mild detergent regularly. The 1 + 1 rule used for litter boxes may be extended to food and water bowls, especially in multicat households. This practice may decrease competition for food and water and decrease stress, which may exacerbate FIC.

Environmental enrichment is designed to simulate activities that are natural and enjoyable to the cat. The environment should afford the cat opportunities to climb, scratch, hide, and rest undisturbed. Providing cats with raised walkways, climbing trees (Fig. 5), window seats, and tents can simulate these activities [32]. Simulating natural hunting behavior by the use of laser pointers, hiding food throughout the house, providing a variety of toys, and using containers or toys that intermittently release food during play serves this purpose well [33].

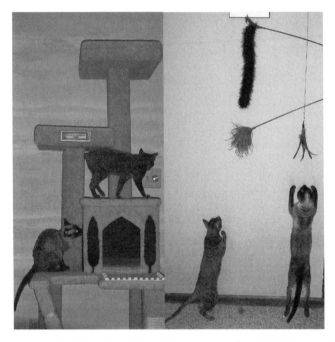

Fig. 5. Environmental enrichment and play with owners are often helpful in cats affected with feline interstitial cystitis. Interactions and enrichment that simulate natural behavior, such as climbing, hunting, and jumping, seem to be helpful.

Interactions of the affected cat with the owners also may aid in reducing stress unless the owner is the source of perceived stress. Some cats enjoy being petted and groomed, whereas others enjoy play interactions with the owner [34]. Especially sensitive cats may perceive any change in routine, feeding schedule, owner work schedule, addition or removal of people or pets from the household, and the owner's emotions as stressful. Therefore, changes in the environment of a sensitive cat should be kept to a minimum.

Dietary modification also may be instituted for animals during their first or second episode of FIC. Attempts to acidify urine and minimize struvite crystalluria often are misguided. No available evidence supports the notion that struvite crystalluria damages normal urothelium or worsens existing cystitis. Perhaps more important is maintaining the constancy, consistency, and composition of the diet that is being fed.

Constancy refers to minimizing changes in the diet that is being fed. If a change in diet is deemed advisable, it should be the cat's choice to switch to the new diet. For example, if a change is made from dry to moist food, both diets should be made available during feedings. If the cat chooses the moist diet, the dry food can be slowly removed as a choice. Consistency refers to the water content of the food. In one report, cats fed a canned formulation of a food had only an 11% recurrence of signs over a 1-year period, whereas cats fed the dry formulation of the same food had a 39% recurrence rate over the same period [35]. Feeding a canned formulation increases the amount of water the animal is consuming and decreases USG. As a result, the concentration of potentially noxious substances in urine is reduced. Composition refers to the nutrient content of the diet being fed. Feeding of certain diets may result in excretion of noxious substances in the urine. Highly acidic urine may activate sensory nerve fibers in the urothelium. The optimal diet for cats with FIC has yet to be determined, and no commercially available cat foods are specifically designed for the treatment of FIC.

Recently, a synthetic formulation of feline facial pheromone (Feliway; Abbott Laboratories, Abbott Park, IL) has been developed to decrease anxiety-related behavior in cats, including urine marking and destructive scratching. This product also may have salutary benefits for cats with FIC, but such effects have not been reported. One report suggested different behavior in hospitalized cats exposed to Feliway compared with placebo-treated cats [36]. Other reports show reduced urine marking during Feliway treatment, which may be a consequence of reduced vigilance of the cats, because perception of their environment has been favorably altered [37,38]. Although not specifically studied, reduced vigilance likely is related to reduction in activation of the sympathetic nervous system. The use of Feliway may be justified in cats with FIC to reduce the impact of an activated sympathetic nervous system on the disease process. Feline facial pheromone often is used in combination with environmental enrichment to decrease stress in cats with FIC. Feliway is available as a spray form and, more recently, as a room diffuser. The diffuser form is reported to cover approximately 650 sq ft and lasts for approximately 30 days. The spray form is formulated in an ethanol vehicle and may be sprayed in carriers approximately 15 minutes before transport, sprayed in cages in a veterinary hospital, or sprayed on areas of inappropriate elimination in the house.

Drug therapy may be indicated if environmental enrichment and modification in combination with dietary modification, enhanced water turnover, and feline facial pheromone use do not control clinical signs. Long-term drug use is reserved for the most severely affected cats that have persistent clinical signs or those that have multiple episodes of FIC. Cats suffering from a current bout of FIC usually are treated with systemic analgesics. Nonsteroidal anti-inflammatory drugs, such as carprofen and ketoprofen, and potent analgesics, such as opioids, including butorphanol, buprenorphine, and fentanyl, seem to be beneficial in short-term pain relief. Scientific evidence to support their routine use in cats with FIC is lacking, however.

Amitriptyline is a tricyclic antidepressant that has been reported to have benefit in the outcome of cats with FIC that is chronic and has failed other more routine treatments [29]. Unfortunately, this study was not blinded, and no placebo group was included Amitriptyline has many effects. It provides analgesia by decreasing C-fiber sensory nerve fiber transmission in the bladder, inhibits norepinephrine reuptake in the LC with subsequent downregulation of norepinephrine outflow, potentially inhibits nociceptive neurons in the spinal trigeminal nucleus, inhibits serotonin reuptake, stabilizes mast cells, blocks glutamate receptors and sodium channels [39], and may have anticholinergic effects. Amitriptyline was not effective in short-term treatment of acute FIC in two recent studies [40,41]. In one study, clinical signs of FIC were worse in cats treated with amitriptyline, possibly as a result of abrupt withdrawal of treatment after 7 days [40]. Extending the duration of therapy may have beneficial effects, however. The severity of clinical signs in severely affected cats treated with amitriptyline at a dose of 10 mg daily was dramatically reduced in 60% of affected cats 1 year after starting therapy. Because of the potential for hepatotoxicity in people, serum biochemistry should be evaluated before and 1 month, 2 months, and 6 months after starting amitriptyline. Other adverse effects include urine retention as a result of anticholinergic effects. In the authors' experience, low doses of amitriptyline often are used with promising results. The dosage range is 2.5 to 12.5 mg given orally once daily. A typical starting dose is 5 mg daily, which is effective in many cats. The dosage may be slowly increased until a calming effect is seen in addition to resolution of clinical signs. If no favorable results are seen after approximately 4 months, the drug should be gradually tapered and discontinued. Other medications that have been used for FIC in cats include clomipramine, fluoxetine, and buspirone. Oral diazepam is not recommended because of its potential to cause hepatic necrosis after oral administration in cats [42]. Glucocorticoids have not been shown to lessen clinical signs or hasten recovery in cats with FIC.

Oral GAG replacement has been used in people with interstitial cystitis with minimally favorable results. Theoretically, orally administered GAG is excreted in the urine and attaches to the defective urothelium, leading to decreased bladder permeability and less neurogenic inflammation. Elmiron (pentosan polysulfate, 100-mg capsules) has been used in human patients with IC. No evidence is available in veterinary medicine to indicate that such replacement decreases the severity or recurrence rate of FIC. GAG replacements, however, can be considered for treatment of cats with severe cystitis in conjunction with other treatments. Adverse effects have not been observed with pentosan polysulfate when given to cats at a dose of 50 mg twice a day. Overdosage theoretically could result in coagulation abnormalities because of the anticoagulant effects of glycosaminoglycans. Adequan (polysulfated glycosaminoglycan) and Cosequin (chondroitin sulfate) are used by some practitioners for treatment of FIC in cats, but such use is off label and no reports document the effectiveness of these treatments. Fig. 6 depicts an approach to diagnosing and treating cats that have recurrent episodes of LUTD.

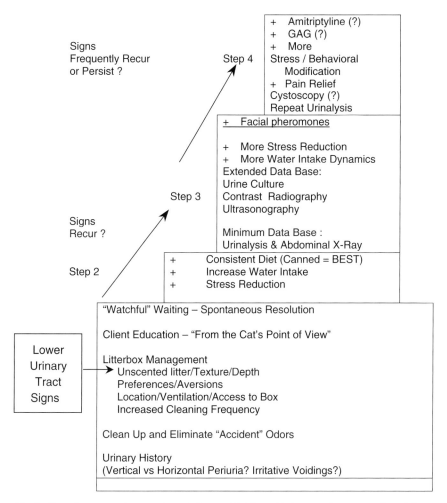

Fig. 6. Stepwise approach to treatment of cats with idiopathic lower urinary tract signs. More diagnostics should be performed when cats fail to clear their initial lower urinary tract signs spontaneously and when signs recur to ensure that the diagnosis is really idiopathic lower urinary tract disease. Properly controlled clinical trials may provide better approaches to treatment in the future, but this is what we do in the interim.

Urinary tract infections

Bacterial UTIs are relatively rare in cats. In younger cats, bacterial UTIs affect less than 2% of cats presented for evaluation of LUTD [6]. In cats older than 10 years of age presented for evaluation of lower urinary tract signs, the probability of bacterial UTIs increases to greater than 50%. Cats that have recurrent UTIs were initially suspected to have reinfection based on results of susceptibility antibiotograms. More recently, it seems that cats with recurrent UTIs and chronic renal failure suspected of having reinfections actually have relapsing infection based on genetic analysis of the bacteria [43]. Cats that have a concurrent disease, such as diabetes mellitus or chronic renal failure [10,44], are at increased risk for developing a bacterial UTI. Cats that have recently had a urinary catheter placed for obstructive uropathy or other reasons and cats that have had a perineal urethrostomy performed also are at increased risk of developing a UTI. In such cases, culture and sensitivity of urine obtained by cystocentesis is a more important diagnostic consideration at first presentation.

Urinalysis with sediment evaluation may be helpful but should not be used alone to definitively diagnose UTI. As mentioned previously, identification of "bacteria" in feline urine sediment is problematic, because cellular debris commonly found in the urine sediment exhibits Brownian motion and can easily misinterpreted as bacteria. The presence of dilute urine (USG <1.030) increases the index of suspicion that a UTI may be present. Also, the presence of WBCs is not diagnostic of a UTI, but it increases the index of suspicion. Pyuria may be present with many LUTDs, including FIC, without a concomitant bacterial UTI. Some cats with a confirmed UTI do not have obvious pyuria, especially when the UTI occurs in association with dilute urine.

If a cat is definitively diagnosed with a UTI based on quantitative urine culture and sensitivity testing, antibacterial therapy should be based on sensitivity results. Treatment with the appropriate antibacterials generally is performed for 2 to 3 weeks or for 4 to 6 weeks if pyelonephritis is suspected based on the physical examination, complete blood cell count, biochemistry profile, and abdominal ultrasonography. Routine monitoring of cats predisposed to UTIs by use of urine culture is recommended. As many as 33% of cats with chronic renal failure can be expected to have or develop a UTI during the next 6 months to 1 year.

Special caution is warranted with the use of fluoroquinolones in treatment of cats with a UTI associated with chronic renal failure (CRF). Initial reports of sudden blindness in cats treated with enrofloxacin showed what seemed to be a dose-related effect in some cats treated with higher dosages [45]. Some cats treated with lower dosages also developed blindness, but the affected cats were found to have reduced renal function. After dosage recommendations were reduced to 5 mg/kg every 24 hours, reports of blindness decreased dramatically. Cats with renal dysfunction develop higher plasma concentrations of fluoroquinolones and their metabolites. Retinal toxicity of fluoroquinolones may be related to peak concentrations of drug, which favor enhanced tissue distribution. All fluoroquinolones demonstrate dose-dependent retinal toxicity at higher dosages. In cats with CRF and a UTI, a dosage of 3 mg/kg every 24 hours or 2.5 mg/kg every 12 hours is recommended to reduce the potential for retinal toxicity. In normal cats, the concentration of fluoroquinolones in urine is high and well above the minimum inhibitory concentration for most pathogens. In CRF, the concentration of fluoroquinolones in urine is decreased, but the concentration achieved is still above the minimum inhibitory concentration for most uropathogens. Whether the reduced dosage regimen achieves tissue concentrations above the minimum inhibitory concentration for offending organisms in the kidney of cats with upper UTI is not known.

Urolithiasis

The formation of uroliths depends on supersaturation of the urine with calculogenic minerals. If supersaturation is sufficient and sustained, a nidus may form on which subsequent calculus may develop. The type of calculus formed is dependent on many factors, including renal excretion of minerals, pH of the urine, presence of promoters, absence of inhibitors, concomitant bacterial infections, and possibly underlying inflammation. Clinical signs associated with urolithiasis generally are similar to those of other LUTDs, but obstruction may occur if the stone becomes lodged in the urethra. This complication may occur in male and female cats but is much more common in male cats.

The diagnosis of urolithiasis includes a combination of abdominal palpation and urinary tract imaging. Routine abdominal radiography is helpful if the uroliths are large enough (>3 mm) and radiodense. Abdominal ultrasonography and double-contrast cystography are beneficial for the detection of stones that are small (<3 mm) or radiolucent. Care must be taken not to assume that urolithiasis is present based on occurrence of crystals in the urine sediment. Likewise, crystals in the urine typically are not the cause of lower urinary tract signs, and one should not equate the type of crystals seen with the type of urolith that may be present. Crystals may be present without disease, calculi may be present without crystals, and crystals of a different type may be present in cats with calculi of a specific type. Quantitative stone analysis is the only way to ascertain definitively the type of urolith present. If uroliths are present, however, the index of suspicion for a particular type is greatly increased when taking into account the urine pH, presence or absence of UTI, and crystal type. Definitive long-term treatment of urolithiasis depends on the type of calculus present. Medical dissolution may be attempted for urate and struvite calculi, but no protocol is available to dissolve calcium oxalate calculi. For large calculi or those that do not respond to dissolution protocols, surgical intervention often is required. Voiding urohydropulsion may be attempted for stones up to 5 mm in female cats and 1 to 2 mm in male cats. Using this technique in male cats may result in obstruction if the size of the uroliths is underestimated; thus, it should only be performed by clinicians familiar with the technique.

All calculi that are removed from a cat should be analyzed by a diagnostic laboratory using quantitative analysis to determine the specific type of urolith present. Quantitative analysis is especially useful if a mixed urolith (more than one mineral) is present. Qualitative analysis should not be performed, because frequent false-positive and false-negative results occur and the relative contribution of the different crystalloids present is not determined.

Urate urolithiasis

Urate urolithiasis accounted for approximately 6% of 20,343 calculi evaluated by the University of Minnesota [46]. Portosystemic vascular anomalies can contribute to urate urolithiasis in cats, but the exact pathogenesis in most affected cats remains unknown [47]. Several risk factors, such as UTI leading to increased urine ammonia, excessive dietary protein, and metabolic acidosis, have been noted. It is not possible to predict which cats ultimately will develop urate urolithiasis, however. The bladder is the most common site for urate calculi, but they also are found in the urethra and kidneys.

Urate calculi generally are radiolucent and are not detected on survey radiographs unless other mineral constituents are present. Double-contrast cystography and ultrasonography may be used to facilitate detection of these calculi. Prevention of urolith formation and dissolution of calculi may be attempted by combining diets that are low in nucleoproteins (containing purines) and by the addition of allopurinol. Allopurinol acts by inhibiting the enzyme xanthine oxidase, which is required for uric acid production. Use of allopurinol may increase the risk of xanthine urolithiasis in the cat, however. The recommended dosage for allopurinol in cats is 9 mg/kg/d [48]. If medical dissolution is unsuccessful, as is generally the case in urate urolithiasis secondary to portosystemic shunts, surgical removal or urohydropulsion may be necessary. Correction of the portosystemic shunt, if present, should prevent recurrence.

Struvite urolithiasis

Struvite calculi analyzed at two major laboratories performing quantitative analysis far outnumbered oxalate uroliths before the late 1980s. Since that time, possibly as a result of a shift by the pet food industry to magnesium-restricted acidifying diets, struvite calculi have declined to approximately 42%, whereas oxalates have increased to approximately 46% of the calculi analyzed [47]. The urine is sterile in approximately 95% of cases of struvite urolithiasis in cats, which is in sharp contrast to the situation in dogs, in which struvite urolithiasis is almost always associated with a bacterial UTI. Consequently, struvite urolithiasis in the cat is thought to be metabolic in origin. Struvite urolithiasis associated with a UTI generally is caused by the presence of urease-producing bacteria. Urease production results in an increase in urine pH that favors struvite crystallization in supersaturated urine. Struvite urolithiasis not associated with a bacterial UTI often is associated with concentrated urine and possibly with excess consumption and excretion of calculogenic minerals (especially magnesium) and alkaline urine.

A diagnosis of struvite urolithiasis is definitively made by quantitative stone analysis. Urinalysis and urine culture and sensitivity testing are indicated in cats with suspected struvite urolithiasis to determine the underlying etiology. Struvite uroliths usually are identified on plain abdominal radiographs because they are radiopaque and generally easily seen. If the calculi are extremely small, ultrasonography and double-contrast cystography may be required to identify them.

Treatment of struvite urolithiasis can include surgical removal of calculi, voiding urohydropulsion, or medical calculolysis depending on the individual situation. Increasing water intake is imperative in medical management of urolithiasis to promote formation of urine that is not supersaturated with calculogenic minerals. One commercially available calculolytic diet (Hills s/d, Science Diet, Topeka, KS) specifically designed for cats is acidifying, magnesium restricted, and supplemented with salt and has been reported to be effective in cats fed the canned preparation. Unlike the similar calculolytic diet for dogs, the formulation devised for cats is not restricted in protein. While feeding a calculolytic diet, it is important to emphasize to the owner that no other foods, including treats, should be given. The goal is to achieve a urine pH less than 6.3 and USG less than 1.030. During therapy, abdominal radiographs should be re-evaluated at 3-week intervals to ensure that therapy is working. In cats in which concomitant bacterial UTI is present, appropriate antibiotics should be given during dissolution and for 2 weeks after uroliths are no longer apparent radiographically. The average time for dissolution of struvite calculi in cats without infection was 36 days (range: 14–141 days), and in those with UTI, it was 44 days (range: 14–92 days) [49]. If uroliths persist or increase in size despite adequate dissolution therapy, the initial diagnosis must be questioned or the possibility of a mixed urolith should be considered. Occasionally, medical dissolution can be used to decrease the size of calculi so that voiding urohydropulsion can be employed.

After clinical signs have abated and dissolution is complete, routine monitoring by urinalysis and abdominal radiography may be indicated. In cats predisposed to bacterial UTIs (ie, those with chronic renal failure, diabetes mellitus, or perineal urethrostomy), periodic urine cultures are warranted. In all cats that repeatedly form uroliths, regardless of type, decreasing USG by feeding canned cat foods is indicated if the cat can be successfully transitioned to a moist diet. Many commercial diets have been designed to prevent formation of new struvite stones, but no reports confirm the effectiveness of any of these diets.

Oxalate urolithiasis

Calcium oxalate uroliths have become the most frequent type of urolith in cats based on calculi submitted to laboratories for quantitative analyses. The percentage of uroliths from cats analyzed at the University of

Minnesota Urolith Center that were oxalates increased from approximately 2% to more than 40% over an 11-year period [50]. This shift may have been associated with a change in diet formulation by the pet food industry in an attempt to decrease the formation of sterile struvite uroliths by decreasing the magnesium and increasing the acid content of the diets. This strategy could have uncovered a group of cats predisposed to calcium oxalate stone formation not previously identified because they had not been exposed to a provocative environment. Calcium oxalate urolithiasis generally occurs in older cats (7–10 years of age) [51], frequently recurs, and generally is not associated with a bacterial UTI. Breeds that have been reported to be at an increased risk for calcium oxalate uroliths include the Ragdoll, British Shorthair, Foreign Shorthair, Himalayan, Havana Brown, Scottish Fold, Persian, and Exotic Shorthair. Birman, mixed-breed, Abyssinian, and Siamese cats have been reported to have a lower risk for developing calcium oxalate uroliths [51]. Indoor housing also has been reported as a risk factor for calcium oxalate urolithiasis [52]. This risk factor may be a consequence of decreased voiding and water intake.

Other than the previously mentioned dietary factors, the etiology of calcium oxalate urolith formation generally is unknown. Systemic metabolic derangements, such as acidosis and hypercalcemia, seem to increase the risk, however. Systemic acidosis results in release of calcium carbonate from bone (a normal buffering response) and secondary calciuresis. Acidosis also may decrease the urinary excretion of citrate, an inhibitor of calcium oxalate urolith formation. All cats that are presented with calcium oxalate urolithiasis should have their serum calcium concentration evaluated. Systemic hypercalcemia results in increased calciuresis and may increase the risk of urolith formation. As many as 35% of calcium oxalate stone-forming cats evaluated at the University of Minnesota Urolith Center have been noted to have hypercalcemia [50]; many of these cats likely had idiopathic hypercalcemia. If the hypercalcemia is not corrected, it is likely that calcium oxalate urolithiasis will recur.

Currently, no medical dissolution protocol is available for calcium oxalate calculi. If the uroliths are not voided and clinical signs are present, voiding urohydropulsion or surgical intervention is indicated. After surgical removal, a nonacidifying diet that is low in calcium and oxalate should be fed. Phosphorus should not be restricted because of the potential for increased gut absorption of calcium and secondary calciuresis arising as a result of low serum phosphorus concentration, and magnesium should not be restricted because of its inhibitory effect on oxalate urolith formation. Excessive supplementation with sodium to stimulate water consumption is not indicated because of potential augmentation of calciuresis. Potassium citrate (100–150 mg/kg/d) may be helpful in decreasing recurrence because of the inhibitory effects of citrate on calcium oxalate stone formation and its alkalinizing effect. This effect assumes that some of the administered citrate will be excreted unmetabolized into the urine. Reports documenting the effectiveness of this treatment are lacking, however. Increasing water consumption by feeding canned food if possible is paramount in the management of urolithiasis.

Several commercially available diets have been developed that are designed to prevent recurrence of calcium oxalate calculi. No evidence-based outcome studies have been reported showing the effectiveness of any of these diets to prevent recurrent urolith formation. These diets have been developed based on the assumption that less urinary acidification is beneficial. Some companies have data indicating that dietary changes alter the relative supersaturation or activity product ratio of urine from normal cats fed these diets. Relative supersaturation and activity product ratio data provide surrogate information about the possibility of decreasing recurrence of urolithiasis in clinically affected cats.

Urethral obstruction

The most common cause of urethral obstruction in male cats was urethral plugs in one study [5] and idiopathic disease in a more recent report [53]. When evaluated with fiberoptic urethroscopy, plugs were identified in approximately 30% of obstructed cats in a preliminary study at The Ohio State University (K.L. Cannizzo, DVM, MS; D.J. Chew, DVM, un-published observations). Other potential causes include urolithiasis with or without a bacterial UTI, urethral spasm, and, rarely, stricture or neoplasia. Male cats are greatly predisposed to urethral obstruction compared with female cats because of their extremely narrow penile urethra (Fig. 7). Large (>5 mm) uroliths cause obstruction of the female urethra, however.

The exact pathogenesis of urethral plugs has not been definitively proven. One theory is that the occurrence of UTI or inflammation with crystalluria leads to the aggregation of protein, crystals, WBCs, and red blood cells, which, in turn, are surrounded by amorphous material, leading to plug formation. Another theory suggests that chronic bladder inflammation leads to a decrease in vascular integrity. Loss of vascular integrity then leads to an increase in urine protein concentration, increased urine pH, crystalluria, and, ultimately, plug formation. Urethritis without plug formation is severe in some cats with urethral obstruction examined by urethroscopy. It is not known what role, if any, calicivirus-like particles seen by electron microscopy of urethral plugs play in the pathogenesis of urethral plug development. Any plug that is obtained after re-establishment of patency should be evaluated for composition by quantitative analysis. Urethral plugs generally are composed of struvite crystals. This observation continues to be true, despite the increased frequency of calcium oxalate calculi and, presumably, calcium oxalate crystalluria.

At presentation, an obstructed cat should be treated on an emergency basis. Cats that have been obstructed for more than 48 hours are most likely to be severely ill and require uremic crisis management. Placement of an

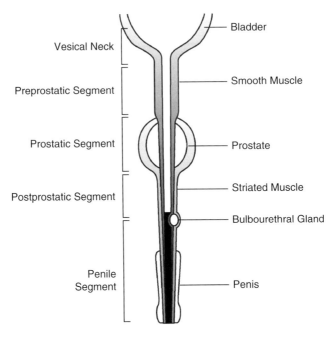

Fig. 7. Diagram of the lower urinary tract of a male cat. Notice the thin circumference of the urethra as it leaves the bladder. This narrow urethra can easily be obstructed secondary to inflammation, calculi, and urethrospasm.

intravenous catheter and administration of analgesic medication should be performed at presentation. Decompressive cystocentesis may be advisable before re-establishing urethral patency. Cystocentesis can be performed with a single puncture into the bladder using a 22- or 23-gauge butterfly needle or a 22-gauge needle attached to an extension set, stopcock, and syringe. The needle is inserted halfway between the apex and neck of the bladder, and all the urine that can be obtained is removed. More complete removal of urine is accomplished when digital compression is maintained on the bladder wall. Some leakage of urine into the abdomen accompanies this procedure but is minimized by more complete evacuation of urine from the bladder.

Laboratory evaluation, including a complete blood cell count, serum biochemistry, urinalysis, and urine culture, should be performed in all obstructed cats. Obstructed cats may have life-threatening dehydration, hyperkalemia, acidosis, or hypocalcemia that may need to be corrected. Hyperkalemia and acidosis generally resolve adequately with volume expansion using a balanced electrolyte solution. The use of calcium salts, glucose, or glucose and insulin may be required to correct hyperkalemia in some instances. In a recent study of 223 obstructed cats, serum potassium concentration was evaluated in 199. Twelve percent of these 199 cats had mildly increased serum potassium concentrations (≥ 6.0 mEq/L and < 8.0

mEq/L), 11.6% had potassium concentrations greater than or equal to 8.0 mEq/L and less than 10.0 mEq/L, and 0.5% had serum potassium concentrations greater than 10.0 mEq/L [54]. One study reported a 75% frequency of ionized hypocalcemia in cats with urethral obstruction [55]. The presence of severe metabolic acidosis as determined by blood gas analysis (pH <7.1) may necessitate sodium bicarbonate administration.

Establishment of urethral patency is obtained after the patient is stabilized and properly sedated or anesthetized based on its clinical condition and overall stability. During establishment of patency, the penis should be handled gently to avoid aggravating inflammation. After sedation and gentle penile manipulation or massage, a urethral plug or extremely small calculi contributing to the obstruction may be expelled. All cats that are presented with urethral obstruction may not need placement of an indwelling urinary catheter depending on the quality of the urethral stream and presence or absence of systemic illness. If the animal is moribund, has a severely large bladder, or has severe azotemia or other metabolic derangements, catheter placement is essential for adequate patient management.

Marked postobstructive diuresis may occur in cats that were obstructed for several days or are severely azotemic. The degree of postobstructive diuresis is often proportional to the degree of azotemia. A balanced electrolyte solution, such as lactated Ringer's solution or Plasmalyte, often is adequate for rehydration and stabilization. Urine output should be monitored to ensure that dehydration does not occur because of the magnitude of diuresis. Management of postobstructive diuresis by monitoring the patient's input and output ("ins and outs") may be needed. This procedure is accomplished by providing sensible and insensible fluid needs. Insensible losses cannot be measured and are generally considered to be 10 mL/lb/d. Sensible losses are losses, such as urine, that can be easily measured. The insensible loss replacement is kept constant, and the sensible losses generally are measured for a given period (eg, 2–4 hours) and then replaced over the following time interval. Fluids may be gradually tapered after azotemia resolves. After the cat is stabilized and while the catheter is still in place, acepromazine (0.02–0.05 mg/kg every 4–6 hours) and buprenorphine (5–20 µg/kg) or butorphanol (0.2–0.4 mg/kg every 6–8 hours) can be administered in cats with urethral obstruction. These medications aid in relaxing the urethral sphincter and provide pain relief. α_1-Antagonists, such as phenoxybenzamine (2.5–7.5 mg every 12–24 hours) and prazosin (0.5 mg every 8 hours), may be added to decrease urethral tone as an alternative to acepromazine. In animals that have bladder atony secondary to severe prolonged distention of the bladder, parasympathomimetic drugs, such as bethanecol (1.25–5.0 mg every 12 hours) may be added once urethral patency has been established. After successful medical management, owner counseling about long-term medical treatment of FIC is necessary if it is suspected as the underlying cause. Fig. 8 depicts an approach to treatment of a severely obstructed cat on initial presentation.

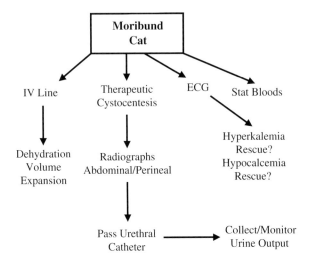

Fig. 8. Algorithm approach to an obstructed cat. Decompressive cystocentesis, fluid therapy, and baseline blood work (including blood gas analysis with electrolytes) should be performed at presentation. Obtaining patency of the urethra should be performed after other life-saving measures and diagnostics are completed.

If medical management fails despite exhaustive treatment or in recurrent severe episodes of urethral obstruction, perineal urethrostomy may be indicated. This surgery is used only in severely affected animals and only after extensive owner education about the potential complications, such as urinary incontinence and stricture formation (both of which are unlikely) and increased risk of ascending UTIs [56].

References

[1] Kirk H. Urinary deposits and retention. In: The diseases of the cat and it general management. London: Bailliere, Tindall and Cox; 1925. p. 261–7.

[2] Willeberg P. Epidemiology of naturally-occurring feline urologic syndrome. Vet Clin N Am Small Anim Prac 1984;14:455–69.

[3] Patronek GJ, Glickman LT, Beck AM, et al. Risk factors for relinquishment of cats to an animal shelter. J Am Vet Med Assoc 1996;209:582–8.

[4] Lund EM, Armstrong PJ, Kirk CA, et al. Health status and population characteristics of dogs and cats examined at private veterinary practices in the United States. J Am Vet Med Assoc 1999;214:1336–41.

[5] Kruger JM, Osborne CA, Goyal SM, et al. Clinical evaluation of cats with lower urinary tract disease. J Am Vet Med Assoc 1991;199:211–6.

[6] Buffington CA, Chew DJ, Kendall MS, et al. Clinical evaluation of cats with nonobstructive lower urinary tract diseases. J Am Vet Med Assoc 1997;210:46–50.

[7] Jones B, Sanson RL, Morris RS. Elucidating the risk factors of feline urologic syndrome. NZ Vet J 1997;45:100–8.

[8] Bovee KC, Reif JS, Maguire TG, et al. Recurrence of feline urethral obstruction. J Am Vet Med Assoc 1979;174:93–6.

[9] Barker J, Povey RC. The feline urolithiasis syndrome: a review and an inquiry into the alleged role of dry cat food in its aetiology. J Small Anim Pract 1973;14:445–57.

[10] Bartges JW. Lower urinary tract disease in geriatric cats. In: Proceedings of the 15th American College of Veterinary Internal Medicine Forum; 1997. p. 322–4.

[11] Sturgess CP, Hesford A, Owen H, et al. An investigation into the effects of storage on the diagnosis of crystalluria in cats. J Feline Med Surg 2001;3:81–5.

[12] Scrivani PV, Chew DJ, Buffington CA, et al. Results of double-contrast cystography in cats with idiopathic cystitis: 45 cases (1993–1995). J Am Vet Med Assoc 1998;212:1907–9.

[13] Scrivani PV, Chew DJ, Buffington CA, et al. Results of retrograde urethrography in cats with idiopathic, nonobstructive lower urinary tract disease and their association with pathogenesis. J Am Vet Med Assoc 1997;211:741–8.

[14] de Groat WC, Yoshimura N. Pharmacology of the lower urinary tract. Annu Rev Pharmacol Toxicol 2001;41:691–721.

[15] Buffington CA, Blaisdell JL, Binns SP Jr, et al. Decreased urine glycosaminoglycan excretion in cats with interstitial cystitis. J Urol 1996;155:1801–4.

[16] Byrne DS, Sedor JF, Estojak J, et al. The urinary glycoprotein GP51 as a clinical marker for interstitial cystitis. J Urol 1999;161:1786–90.

[17] Buffington CA, Chew DJ, Woodworth BE. Animal model of human disease—feline interstitial cystitis. Comp Pathol Bull 1997;29:3, 6.

[18] Lavelle JP, Meyers SA, Ruiz WG, et al. Urothelial pathophysiological changes in feline interstitial cystitis: a human model. Am J Physiol Renal Physiol 2000;278(Suppl):F540–53.

[19] Gao X, Buffington CA, Au JL. Effect of interstitial cystitis on drug absorption from the urinary bladder. J Pharmacol Exp Ther 1994;271:818–23.

[20] Reche AJ, Buffington CA. Increased tyrosine hydroxylase immunoreactivity in the locus coeruleus of cats with interstitial cystitis. J Urol 1998;159:1045–8.

[21] Welk K, Buffington CA. Effects of interstitial cystitis on central neuropeptide and receptor immunoreactivity in cats. Columbus: The Ohio State University; 2003. p. 31.

[22] de Groat WC, Booth AM, Yoshimura N. Neurophysiology of micturition and its modification in animal models of human disease. In: Maggi CA, Hill CE, editors. Nervous control of the urogenital system. The autonomic nervous system. Chur: Harwood; 1993. p. 227–90.

[23] Buffington CA, Pacak K. Increased plasma norepinephrine concentration in cats with interstitial cystitis. J Urol 2001;165:2051–4.

[24] Stevens CW, Brenner GM. Spinal administration of adrenergic agents produces analgesia in amphibians. Eur J Pharmacol 1996;316:205–10.

[25] Sabbe MB, Penning JP, Ozaki GT, et al. Spinal and systemic action of the alpha 2 receptor agonist dexmedetomidine in dogs. Antinociception and carbon dioxide response. Anesthesiology 1994;80:1057–72.

[26] Petrovaara A, Kauppila T, Jyvasjarvi E, et al. Involvement of supraspinal and spinal segmental alpha-2-adrenergic mechanisms in the medetomidine-induced antinociception. Neuroscience 1991;44:705–14.

[27] Westropp JL, Buffington CA. Evaluation of the hypothalamic-pituitary-adrenal axis in cats with FIC. Presented at 15th Annual American College of Veterinary Internal Medicine Forum. American College of Veterinary Internal Medicine; 2003.

[28] Westropp JL, Welk K, Buffington CA. Small adrenal glands in cats with feline interstitial cystitis. J Urol 2002;170:2492–7.

[29] Chew DJ, Buffington CA, Kendall MS, et al. Amitriptyline treatment for severe recurrent idiopathic cystitis in cats. J Am Vet Med Assoc 1998;213:1282–6.

[30] Neilson JC. Feline house soiling: elimination and marking behaviors. Vet Clin N Am Small Anim Pract 2003;33:287–301.

[31] Overall KL. Feline elimination disorders. In: Overall KL, editor. Clinical behavioral medicine for small animals. St. Louis: Mosby; 1997. p. 160–94.

[32] Delzio S, Ribarich C. Felinestein. New York: Harper Perennial; 1999.

[33] McCune S. Environmental enrichment for cats—a review. Second International Conference on Environmental Enrichment, 1997.

[34] Turner DC. The human-cat relationship. In: Bateson P, editor. The domestic cat—the biology of its behavior. 2nd edition. Cambridge: Cambridge University Press; 2000. p. 194–206.

[35] Markwell PJ, Buffington CA, Chew DJ, et al. Clinical evaluation of commercially available urinary acidification diets in the management of idiopathic cystitis in cats. J Am Vet Med Assoc 1999;214:361–5.

[36] Griffith CA, Steigerwald ES, Buffington CA. Effects of a synthetic facial pheromone on behavior of cats. J Am Vet Med Assoc 2000;217:1154–6.

[37] Mills DS, White JC. Long-term follow up of the effect of a pheromone therapy on feline spraying behaviour. Vet Rec 2000;147:746–7.

[38] Hunthausen W. Evaluating a feline facial pheromone analogue to control urine spraying. Vet Med 1998;143:151–6.

[39] Pena F, Neaga E, Amuzescu B, et al. Amitriptyline has a dual effect on the conductive properties of the epithelial Na channel. J Pharm Pharmacol 2002;54:1393–8.

[40] Kruger JM, Conway TS, Kaneene JB, et al. Randomized controlled trial of the efficacy of short-term amitriptyline administration for treatment of acute, nonobstructive, idiopathic lower urinary tract disease in cats. J Am Vet Med Assoc 2003;222:749–58.

[41] Kraijer M, Fink-Grimmels J, Nickel RF. The short-term clinical efficacy of amitriptyline in the management of idiopathic feline lower urinary tract disease: a controlled clinical study. J Feline Med Surg 2003;5(3):191–6.

[42] Center SA, Elston TH, Rowland PH, et al. Fulminant hepatic failure associated with oral administration of diazepam in 11 cats. J Am Vet Med Assoc 1996;209:618–25.

[43] Freitag T, Squires RA, Schmid J, et al. Antibiotic sensitivity profiles underestimate the proportion of relapsing infections in cats with chronic renal failure and urinary tract infection [abstract 10]. Presented at the American College of Veterinary Medicine Forum. Minneapolis, June 9–12, 2004.

[44] Lulich JP, Osborne CA, O'Brien TD, et al. Feline renal failure: questions, answers, questions. Compend Contin Educ Pract Vet 1992;14:127–53.

[45] Gelatt KN, van der Woerdt A, Ketring KL, et al. Enrofloxacin-associated retinal degeneration in cats. Vet Ophthalmol 2001;4(2):99–106.

[46] Osborne CA, Kruger JM, Lulich J, et al. Feline lower urinary tract diseases. In: Ettinger SJ, Feldman E, editors. Textbook of veterinary internal medicine. Philadelphia: WB Saunders; 2000. p. 1710–47.

[47] Duval D, Barsanti JA, Cornelius LM, et al. Ammonium acid urate urolithiasis in a cat. Feline Pract 1995;23:18–22.

[48] Plumb DC. Allopurinol. In: Plumb veterinary drug handbook. 4th edition. Ames: Iowa State University Press; 2002. p. 20.

[49] Osborne CA, Lulich JP, Kruger JM, et al. Medical dissolution of feline struvite urocystoliths. J Am Vet Med Assoc 1990;196:1053–63.

[50] Osborne CA, Lulich JP, Thumachi R, et al. Feline urolithiasis. Etiology and pathophysiology. Vet Clin N Am Small Anim Pract 1996;26:217–32.

[51] Lekcharoensuk C, Lulich JP, Osborne CA, et al. Association between patient-related factors and risk of calcium oxalate and magnesium ammonium phosphate urolithiasis in cats. J Am Vet Med Assoc 2000;217:520–5.

[52] Kirk CA, Ling GV, Franti CE, et al. Evaluation of factors associated with development of calcium oxalate urolithiasis in cats. J Am Vet Med Assoc 1995;207:1429–34.

[53] Gerber B. Short-term followup of cats with obstructive lower urinary tract disease. In: Proceedings of the 13th European Congress of Veterinary Internal Medicine. Uppsala; 2003.

[54] Lee JA, Drobatz KJ. Characterization of the clinical characteristics, electrolytes, acid-base, and renal parameters in male cats with urethral obstruction. J Vet Emerg Crit Care 2003; 13:227–33.

[55] Drobatz KJ, Hughes D. Concentration of ionized calcium in plasma from cats with urethral obstruction. J Am Vet Med Assoc 1997;211:1392–5.

[56] Smith CW. Perineal urethrostomy. Vet Clin N Am Small Anim Pract 2002;32(4):917–25.

ELSEVIER
SAUNDERS

Vet Clin Small Anim
35 (2005) 171–210

VETERINARY
CLINICS
Small Animal Practice

Feline Endocrinopathies

Danièlle Gunn-Moore, BVM&S, PhD, ILTM, MACVSc, MRCVS, RCVS

*Feline Clinic, University of Edinburgh Hospital for Small Animals,
Easter Bush Veterinary Clinics, Midlothian, Scotland EH25 9RG*

Hyperthyroidism

Pathogenesis

Hyperthyroidism is one of the most common feline endocrinopathies [1–9], affecting approximately 1 in 300 cats [10]. Ninety-nine percent of cases result from benign nodular hyperplasia, adenomatous hyperplasia, or adenoma [4,11,12]. The autonomous secretion of thyroxine (T_4) and triiodothyronine (T_3) produces a negative feedback effect on the pituitary gland, suppressing the release of thyroid-stimulating hormone (TSH) such that any normal thyroid tissue atrophies. In 70% to 75% of the cats with hyperthyroidism, both thyroid glands are affected [4,11,12]. Only 1% to 3% of cases are caused by mild to moderately malignant thyroid carcinoma [13].

Although the incidence of feline hyperthyroidism has increased steadily since the early 1980s, the cause is still unknown [14]. A number of theories have been proposed, however, involving factors related to diet (possibly including the presence of goitrogens, eating canned cat food, iodine content, or frequent changes) [14–17], environmental causes (possibly associated with cat litter, toxins, pollution, or exposure to allergens) [16,18], a genetic mutation [19], abnormal immune responses [20], or altered hormonal responses [4].

Clinical signs

Hyperthyroidism is seen mainly in middle-aged to older cats, with the age at presentation ranging from 4 to 23 years (mean = 13 years) [11,21]. It has occasionally been seen in younger cats (including one 8-month-old kitten),

The author received funding support for her lectureship from Nestlé Purina Petcare.
E-mail address: Danielle.Gunn-Moore@ed.ac.uk

however [22]. There is no sex or breed predisposition [11,17,21], although Siamese and Himalayan (Color-point Persian) cats seem to be underrepresented in some studies [16,18].

Increasing levels of thyroid hormones affect nearly all organ systems, and in most cases, clinical signs are insidious and progressive. Most affected cats have a history of weight loss (90%) and polyphagia (61%), usually occurring over several months [4,21,23]. They are frequently restless (40%) and have a matted, ill-kempt, or greasy coat (36%). They have often been vomiting (38%) or had diarrhea, usually with bulky feces (39%). Some become polyuric or polydipsic (47%) [11,21,23]. Polyphagia results from increased energy expenditure secondary to the increase in metabolic rate. Diarrhea may result from malabsorption or intestinal hypermotility. Vomiting may result from overrapid eating or be the direct effect of T_4 on the chemoreceptor trigger zone within the brain. Polyuria or polydipsia may result from the diuretic effects of T_4, increased renal blood flow, associated renal insufficiency, or compulsive polydipsia. Less common clinical signs include respiratory signs (23%, including dyspnea, coughing, and sneezing), aggression (8%), seizures (7%), or severe muscle weakness (<1%, caused by hyperthyroidism-associated hypokalemic myopathy or thiamine deficiency) [4,23,24].

Associated cardiac hypertrophy may eventually result in congestive heart failure, with dyspnea, apathy, hind limb weakness caused by aortic thromboemboli, or collapse [25]. Cardiac effects result from a high-output state, induced, in part, by a demand for increased tissue perfusion to meet the needs of increased tissue metabolism. In addition, thyroid hormones can have a direct effect on cardiac muscle. Cardiovascular changes include left ventricular hypertrophy, left atrial and ventricular dilation, increased myocardial contractility, and decreased peripheral vascular resistance [25].

Between 20% and 85% of cats with hyperthyroidism develop systemic hypertension [26–29]. In addition, the risk may actually increase after successful thyroidectomy [29]. The presence of systemic hypertension may be detected as hypertensive retinopathy, including ocular hemorrhage [30], or may cause clinical signs associated with cerebrovascular accidents, dementia, or renal failure [4].

Approximately 10% of cats with hyperthyroidism present with signs of inappetence rather than polyphagia and are often depressed and weak ("apathetic hyperthyroidism") [11]. In contrast, there are also many hyperthyroid cats that are brought in for their routine vaccination in apparent good health, because their owners presume that the clinical signs are the normal result of aging [23].

Diagnosis

Hyperthyroidism should be suspected when any older cat presents with weight loss, especially when the weight loss is associated with a good appetite.

Inappetence should not rule out hyperthyroidism, however. Physical examination usually reveals a rather poor body condition, an ill-kempt coat, and a palpable thyroid nodule on either or both sides of the trachea (80%–90% of cases) [11,21,23]. Affected cats often have tachycardia (48%), a systolic murmur (41%), a gallop rhythm (12%), or ectopic beats. Hyperthyroid cats are often agitated, difficult to examine, and become easily stressed [4,11,23].

Clinical pathologic examination almost always reveals raised liver enzymes (serum alanine transferase [ALT, 85%], or alkaline phosphatase [ALP, 62%]) [4,11,21,23]. This hepatopathy may be secondary to a direct toxic effect of the thyroid hormones, hepatic lipidosis, malnutrition, or hepatic hypoxia resulting from cardiac failure [21]. The ALP may also be raised because of increased bone metabolism [31,32]. In some cases, the serum glucose concentration may be increased (5%), or azotemia may be present (26%) [11]. The latter may result from increased protein catabolism, reduced renal perfusion caused by associated cardiac insufficiency, or renal damage induced by associated systemic hypertension, or it may be related to concomitant but unrelated chronic renal insufficiency. Hyperphosphatemia (18%), hypocalcemia, and secondary hyperparathyroidism (77%) may also be detected, irrespective of the presence of renal insufficiency, possibly resulting from T_4-mediated alterations in bone metabolism and increased phosphate absorption [11,33]. Hypokalemia may be present or may develop in response to the stress of the diagnostic investigations. When this occurs, the resulting hypokalemic myopathy may be seen as severe muscle weakness and neck ventroflexion, and the serum creatinine kinase (CK) concentration increases [24].

Hematologic testing may reveal erythrocytosis (39%), macrocytosis (20%), or, in severe disease, mild anemia. Leukocyte changes may include a mature neutrophilia, lymphopenia, lymphocytosis, eosinopenia, or eosinophilia [11,21]. Unless there is concurrent renal insufficiency, the urine is usually concentrated [21,23,34], and microalbuminuria may be present [35].

When investigating a cat for possible hyperthyroidism, it is important to consider all possible differential diagnoses and to look for evidence of multiple interacting diseases. This is because hyperthyroidism is seen most commonly in older cats and this group of patients is often affected by more than one disorder. Diabetes mellitus, renal disease, malassimilation syndromes (including inflammatory bowel disease, early intestinal lympho-sarcoma, pancreatitis, and exocrine pancreatic insufficiency), acromegaly, and hyperadrenocorticism are perhaps the most important differential diagnoses.

A full cardiac investigation is recommended before considering treatment options for hyperthyroidism. Thoracic radiography may reveal cardiome-galy, pulmonary edema, or pleural effusion [11]. Electrocardiography (ECG) and echocardiography commonly reveal abnormalities. ECG changes include sinus tachycardia, increased R-wave amplitude, prolonged QRS duration, atrial and ventricular arrhythmias, and intraventricular conduction disturbances [11,23,36,37]. Echocardiographic abnormalities include concentric hypertrophy of the left ventricular free wall and, less frequently, of the interventricular septum, increased left atrial diameter at end diastole, and hyperdynamic wall motion [37,38].

A definitive diagnosis of hyperthyroidism is based on detecting elevated serum concentrations of total T_4 (and sometimes T_3) [11,21,39]. Measurement of T_3 alone is not usually recommended because it is less sensitive than measuring T_4 [23,39,40]. Unfortunately, some cats with hyperthyroidism have a T_4 concentration that is within the normal range. This may be a result of early or mild hyperthyroidism, daily variations in T_4 concentrations, or the concurrent presence of severe systemic illness causing a reduction in T_4 (euthyroid sick syndrome) [21,39,41–44].

If hyperthyroidism is suspected despite a high normal T_4 concentration, there are a number of possible investigative options.

Retest the cat

The simplest and most appropriate way to deal with a cat that is suspected of having hyperthyroidism but has a T_4 level within the normal range is to retest its total T_4 concentration immediately or in a few weeks [41]. Assessing free T_4 (by equilibrium dialysis) [39,43] as well as total T_4 may help in confirming the presence of hyperthyroidism [39,45]. Although the methods described below are other possible approaches, they all have limitations.

Triiodothyronine suppression test

The protocol is to collect a blood sample, give T_3 orally at a rate of 25 mg every 8 hours for seven doses, and then collect a blood sample 2 to 4 hours after the seventh dose (ie, on day 3). An increase in T_3 concentration confirms successful medication. Suppression of the total T_4 concentration to below 50% of baseline, or less than 1.5 µg/dL (<20 nmol/L), does not occur in hyperthyroid cats [46,47]. This is a useful test for ruling out hyperthyroidism, but it cannot reliably confirm the presence of the disease [46,47]. In addition, unless the cat is hospitalized, this test relies on the owner being able to administer the T_3.

Thyrotropin-releasing hormone stimulation test

The protocol is to collect a blood sample, give thyrotropin-releasing hormone (TRH) intravenously at a dose of 0.1 mg/kg, and then collect a second blood sample 4 hours later. Assess both samples for serum total T_4 concentration. Stimulation to greater than 50% does not occur in hyperthyroid cats. Side effects of TRH include transient salivation, vomiting, tachypnea, and defecation [48,49]. Although this test is good at detecting mild or early hyperthyroidism [49], it is not so good at detecting hyperthyroidism in a cat with severe concurrent disease (euthyroid sick syndrome) [50].

Thyroid-stimulating hormone response test
This test is not recommended in the diagnosis of hyperthyroidism because it cannot reliably differentiate between normal cats and cats with mild hyperthyroidism [12,45,46]. In addition, TSH is difficult to obtain.

Nuclear isotope scanning
Scintigraphy can be used to detect hyperactive thyroid tissue and to determine whether one or both thyroid glands are overactive [11]. The procedure is relatively safe and simple to perform but requires that the cat be anesthetized (or heavily sedated) and can only be performed in a licensed facility.

Trial course of antithyroid therapy
Administering a trial course of antithyroid therapy for approximately 30 days and observing for improvements in clinical signs can help in trying to decide whether or not a cat has clinical hyperthyroidism. It is important to monitor hematology and serum biochemistry, however, and there is a potential risk of side effects [4].

Treatment

Hyperthyroidism can be treated medically, surgically, or with radioiodine (I^{131}). Before deciding which treatment to use, the cat should be assessed for concurrent disease, especially renal disease, systemic hypertension, and heart disease, all of which occur commonly in association with hyperthyroidism. It is particularly important to assess the cat's renal function (check blood urea nitrogen [BUN], creatinine concentrations, and urine specific gravity). This is because resolution of the hyperthyroid state often is associated with an increase in BUN and creatinine concentrations and a decrease in glomerular filtration rate (GFR) and effective renal blood flow. Because of this, some cats without prior evidence of renal insufficiency or with only mild renal impairment develop signs of uremia after treatment for hyperthyroidism [34,51]. To determine what effect resolving the hyperthyroid state may have on renal function, a short course of medical therapy is recommended before considering radiotherapy or surgery [34,51,52]. Cats that show significant uremia or develop renal failure should then be maintained on a lower dose of medical therapy and should not be considered as suitable candidates for radiotherapy or surgery. Similarly, cats that develop significant uremia or renal failure after radiotherapy or surgery should be given L-thyroxine to maintain a euthyroid or mild hyperthyroid state [34,51].

Medical therapy
Medical therapy tends to be given to stabilize the patient before surgical treatment, to help determine whether or not masked renal disease may be

present before thyroidectomy or I^{131} treatment, or when neither I^{131} treatment nor surgery is possible.

Methimazole and carbimazole are antithyroid drugs that block T_3 and T_4 synthesis. They share the same mechanism of action; carbimazole is almost entirely broken down to methimazole in vivo (carbimazole, 5 mg, is broken down to methimazole, 3 mg). It usually takes 1 to 3 weeks of treatment to achieve a significant decrease in T_4 concentration [53,54]. The dose for both drugs is 2.5 to 5.0 mg per cat administered orally every 12 to 24 hours initially, increasing to every 8 to 12 hours as necessary, adjusted to maintain a euthyroid state, and given for the rest of the cat's life. (An algorithm is available for the treatment and monitoring of hyperthyroid cats during methimazole therapy [4]. The drugs are most effective given twice or three times daily [55]. The dose should start low (especially when renal insufficiency is suspected), and the renal values should be monitored as the dose is gradually increased. When cat and owner compliance is good, the successful response rate is approximately 85% [53,54]. Difficulty in administration causes many treatment failures, however. In an attempt to make medicating simpler, many clinicians are now using topical transdermal applications of methimazole, and initial studies seem to show promise [56].

Poor compliance results from the need for frequent medication and the requirement for regular blood sampling to look for side effects and to monitor T_4 concentration. Up to approximately 20% of treated cats develop side effects, which are usually seen within the first 3 months of treatment. They commonly include anorexia, vomiting, lethargy, hepatopathy, jaundice, cutaneous reactions (typically pruritus of the head and neck), bleeding tendencies, or, occasionally, myasthenia gravis or immune-mediated hemolytic anemia (IMHA). Blood dyscrasias occur in 2% to 10% of treated cats and include eosinophilia, lymphocytosis, leukopenia, thrombocytopenia, agranulocytosis, prolonged clotting times, and IMHA. Although mild side effects may resolve despite continued treatment, it is usually recommended that treatment be stopped. Side effects are seen more commonly with methimazole than with carbimazole at standard prescribed doses [53,54].

Other medical therapies

β-adrenoceptor blocking agents may be administered to reduce the effect of the enhanced catecholamine activity of hyperthyroidism and thus reduce the incidence of tachycardia, arrhythmia, and hypertension (eg, propranolol at a dose of 2.5–5.0 mg per cat administered orally every 8–12 hours) [57].

Calcium or sodium ipodate is an oral cholecystographic iodine-based contrast agent. Ipodate has been shown to inhibit the conversion of T_4 to the more active T_3. It can successfully reduce T_3 concentrations and resolve clinical signs of hyperthyroidism in most cats treated (8 of 12 cats in the study by Murray and Peterson [58]). Although the effect may be transient in some cases, in others, cats have been maintained for up to 6 months. The recommended dosage is 15 mg/kg administered orally every 12 hours (maximum of 100 mg/d per cat). Ipodate may be difficult to obtain and needs to be reformulated into smaller capsules (which adds to the cost).

Stable iodine (eg, potassium iodate) can help to decrease T_3 and T_4 synthesis and reduce thyroid gland vascularity before thyroid surgery. The effect can be transient and inconsistent, however. The suggested dose of potassium iodate is 30 to 100 mg/d per cat administered orally for 10 to 14 days before surgery using potassium iodate at a rate of approximately 20 mg per cat administered orally every 12 hours (using 100 g of potassium iodide per 100-mL of water solution). Side effects include variable anorexia, salivation, depression, and, occasionally, cardiovascular collapse and death [57].

Surgical thyroidectomy

The success of surgery depends on the stability of the patient, the expertise of the surgeon, and the expertise of the anesthetist (eg, do not give atropine). To reduce the risks of anesthesia, the cat should be made euthyroid before surgery (see section on medical therapy). For the same reasons, some clinicians also like to administer β-blockers to cats with severe tachycardia (eg, propranolol at a rate of 2.5–5.0 mg per cat orally three times daily 1–2 weeks before surgery). A bilateral thyroidectomy is usually performed, because 70% to 75% of cases have bilateral hyperplasia. Some clinicians prefer a staged procedure, however, removing one thyroid gland at a time. Although there are a number of different techniques available, most clinicians perform a modified extracapsular approach, because the risk of recurrence is reduced, whereas the risk of postoperative hypocalcemia is only slightly increased [59–61]. Preoperative considerations, anesthetic options, and surgical techniques are reviewed elsewhere [4,62]. The successful response rate is generally greater than 95%. Some cats have ectopic overactive thyroid tissue that is not easily accessible at surgery, however, and this can result in treatment failure. Surgical risks include the usual anesthetic risks of older patients (which often have concurrent renal or cardiac disease), iatrogenic damage to parathyroid tissue leading to transient or permanent hypocalcemia, damage to the local nerves leading to laryngeal paralysis or Horner's syndrome, and, rarely, clinical hypo-thyroidism.

If a bilateral thyroidectomy is performed, the cat should be monitored for possible hypocalcemia for 3 to 7 days after surgery and observed for associated clinical signs, including restlessness, weakness, twitching, tetany, and seizures [4,60]. If acute hypocalcemia occurs, it should be treated by slow intravenous administration of 1 to 1.5 mL/kg of 10% calcium gluconate, followed by 2.0 mL/kg of 10% calcium gluconate in 100 mL of saline every 12 hours. Once oral medication is possible, vitamin D (eg, dihydrotachysterol at a dose of 0.03 mg/kg administered orally daily or calcitriol at a dose of 2.5–10 ng/kg daily) and calcium (eg, calcium lactate or carbonate at a dose of 0.5–3.0 g per cat daily in divided doses) should be given. The doses should be adjusted so that the serum calcium level stays at the low end of the reference range; whenever possible, the dihydrotachys-terol should be weaned down by approximately 0.01 mg/kg every other day.

Radioiodine

I^{131} is taken up by and destroys overactive thyroid tissue while sparing normal tissue. Where facilities are available, this therapy is considered by many to be the treatment of choice for cases uncomplicated by renal insufficiency. It is also the only treatment option for cats with thyroid carcinoma that is not amenable to surgery [63]. The technique is simple, safe, and effective. It is noninvasive, carries no anesthetic risk, and poses no risk to the parathyroid glands or to the bone marrow [13]. The procedure is of particular use in those cats that are considered poor candidates for surgery or when the thyroid glands are not readily accessible. The disadvantages of I^{131} treatment are the lack of availability of facilities, the hospitalization period required for radioactive decay of the isotope (from 2 days to 4 weeks depending on the country and state), and the special requirements for handling radioactive substances.

A success rate of greater than 80% has been reported in most studies; where approximately 80% of patients become euthyroid after treatment, 10% fail to respond and 10% become hypothyroid [13,64–71]. Few of the resulting hypothyroid cats are presented with clinical problems, and the normal thyroid tissue usually recovers function, although it may take a few weeks or, occasionally, months. Side effects are few but include unmasking occult renal failure, transient dysphagia or dysphonia, or permanent hypothyroidism [64–73]. Enhanced thyroid uptake of I^{131} can occur immediately after the withdrawal of methimazole [74,75]. Because this may carry a risk of greater local tissue damage, some authors recommend that methimazole treatment be stopped 2 weeks before I^{131} is given [75]. Other studies do not support the assumption that stopping treatment early gives any benefit [76], however, and doing so incurs the possibility that a medically stable cat may become unstable in the interim period.

Other procedures

Percutaneous intrathyroid ethanol injections have been used to treat hyperplastic thyroid nodules in a small number of cats. Using ultrasound guidance, the injections have been administered to cats under general anesthesia. Bilateral treatment cannot be recommended because it carries a significant risk of side effects (Horner's syndrome, dysphonia, and laryngeal paralysis) [77]. Unilateral treatment could be considered in cats that are unable to undergo conventional treatment; however, there is still a risk of dysphonia, and advanced ultrasonographic equipment and skills are essential [78].

Percutaneous ultrasound-guided radiofrequency heat ablation has resulted in transient remission of hyperthyroidism in a small number of cats. It should only be administered unilaterally, however, and side effects include transient Horner's syndrome and laryngeal paralysis. In addition, advanced ultrasonographic equipment and skills are required [79].

Prognosis

Without treatment, cats with hyperthyroidism usually die of concurrent renal disease, heart disease, liver disease, or systemic hypertension. With treatment, the prognosis varies from extremely good to guarded, dependent on the presence of heart disease, renal disease, and systemic hypertension; whether or not any systemic damage has become permanent before treatment of the hyperthyroidism; and which treatment options are available. On average, the mean life expectancy of treated cats is approximately 2 years [71,73].

Hypothyroidism

Pathogenesis

Hypothyroidism is a relatively rare condition of cats. Most cases are iatrogenic and occur after treatment for hyperthyroidism by bilateral thyroidectomy, I^{131} treatment, or an overdose of antithyroid drugs [3,71]. Although there is only one well-described case of adult-onset primary hypothyroidism [80], congenital hypothyroidism has been recognized more frequently [81–84]. It has resulted from a number of different causes, including defective thyroid hormone synthesis (presumably related to abnormal peroxidase activity) [83,84], thyroid dysgenesis [82], an inability of the thyroid gland to respond to TSH [85], and juvenile-onset immune-mediated thyroiditis [86]. In most affected cats, hypothyroidism seems to be inherited as an autosomal recessive trait [83–85]. In addition, feeding kittens on an all-meat diet occasionally may result in hypothyroidism [3].

Clinical signs

Many iatrogenic cases remain subclinical [71]. When they do have clinical signs, affected cats tend to show marked weight gain, lethargy, inappetence, and, occasionally, hypothermia and bradycardia. Skin changes may include a dull, dry, ill-kempt hair coat with matting and seborrhea. In addition, affected cats may develop alopecia of the pinnae, which also affects the pressure points, tail base, and caudal flanks in some cases [71]. A cat with adult-onset hypothyroidism was presented with extreme lethargy, hypo-thermia, poor hair growth, seborrhea, and puffy facial features, presumably resulting from myxedema [80].

Congenital hypothyroidism has been seen in domestic shorthair cats and Abyssinian cats, with no sex predisposition [83,84,86]. The clinical signs depend on the type and severity of the underlying defect. Affected kittens typically appear normal at birth, but by 4 to 8 weeks of age, their growth rate slows down. Signs of disproportionate dwarfism develop by the time the kittens are 6 to 9 months old. This is characterized by short limbs, a round body, and an enlarged broad head. Affected kittens are generally mentally dull and lethargic, become hypothermic and bradycardic, and may suffer recurrent episodes of severe constipation. Deciduous teeth are usually retained until 12 to 18 months of age, and the coat may have only a few guard hairs and retain its undercoat [84] or become shaggy [86]. In cats with thyroid peroxidase defects, goiter is evident from 6 months of age [82,83]. Kittens with immune-mediated thyroiditis die within 1 to 2 weeks of developing clinical signs at 1 to 2 months of age [85]; kittens with TSH resistance usually die by 16 weeks of age [85], whereas in kittens with thyroid peroxidase defects, the clinical signs become less pronounced with time [84].

Diagnosis

Routine hematologic testing may demonstrate mild anemia, whereas serum biochemistry may show hypercholesterolemia (particularly in iatrogenic cases). In affected kittens, radiographic changes may include delayed closure of ossification centers of the long bones [83,84].

The circulating T_4 concentration is low or low normal in all cases. Care is required with interpretation, however, because low T_4 concentrations are commonly associated with nonthyroidal illness [39,41,43]. In addition, although the thyroid-suppressive effects of certain drugs (eg, glucocorticoids, anticonvulsants, sulfonamide antibiotics, and some nonsteroidal anti-inflammatory agents) are well known in dogs, their effects in cats have generally been less well understood [3].

Confirmation usually relies on results from TSH or TRH response tests [84,85]. The TSH test is performed by collecting a blood sample for a basal total T_4 determination, giving TSH intravenously at a rate of 0.1 IU per kilogram of body weight and then collecting a second blood sample for repeat total T_4 assessment after 6 hours. In a hypothyroid cat, there should be no stimulation. Unfortunately, TSH is now difficult to obtain. The TRH test is performed in the same manner as described in the section on hyperthyroidism. The total T_4 increase is less than that seen after TSH administration, however, and is more prone to being complicated by severe nonthyroidal illness [3].

Other tests can also be considered. These include assessing a baseline TSH level. Although feline-specific reagents are not currently available, preliminary studies using canine reagents look promising [87]. Cats with hypothyroidism should have an increased TSH concentration. Once feline-specific tests are available for detecting the presence of circulating thyroglobulin and thyroid hormone antibodies, these may help in confirming the presence of lymphocytic thyroiditis. A diagnosis of lymphocytic thyroiditis has previously been confirmed by thyroid biopsy in an adult cat [80] and some kittens [86]. Diagnosis of the specific underlying defects requires specific investigations [3].

The major differential diagnoses for congenital hypothyroidism include a number of lysosomal storage diseases (eg, mucopolysaccharidosis) and, possibly, chondrodysplasia.

Treatment and prognosis

Treatment requires giving oral L-thyroxine (0.05–0.1 mg per cat daily) and then adjusting the dose based on the clinical response after 4 to 6 weeks. In iatrogenic and adult-onset hypothyroidism, the response to treatment is usually excellent and the prognosis is extremely good [71,80]. In kittens, the response can be variable, often with incomplete resolution of clinical signs. Without treatment, kittens with TSH resistance usually die by 16 weeks of age. Giving prophylactic L-thyroxine to kittens genetically at risk of developing immune-mediated thyroiditis reduces the severity of the disease [86].

Acromegaly

Pathogenesis

In cats, acromegaly (hypersomatotropism with associated enlargement of the cranial features and internal organs) is caused by the presence of a growth hormone (GH)–secreting tumor within the anterior lobe of the pituitary gland [2,46,88–96] and is a relatively rare disease (approximately 30 published cases). Unlike the situation in dogs, increased levels of circulating progestogens or progesterone do not stimulate GH secretion in cats [97,98].

Clinical signs

Clinical findings result from the catabolic and diabetogenic effects of GH, the anabolic actions of insulin-like growth factor-1 (IGF-1), and the growth of the pituitary macroadenoma [2]. The disease is typically seen in older (range: 4–19 years, mean 10 years), male, mixed-breed cats (Table 1) [2,46,88–96]. Affected cats are usually presented with clinical signs related to poorly controlled diabetes mellitus, including polyuria, polydipsia, and polyphagia. More chronically affected cats may have "dropped hocks," resulting from peripheral diabetic neuropathy. Although the diabetes mellitus is resistant to insulin [46,92,94] in most cases, some cats have variable insulin requirements (see Table 1) [96]; some cats may even stop requiring insulin, presumably because they suffer an infarct within their pituitary tumor (see Table 1). GH causes peripheral resistance to insulin by antagonizing its action at a postreceptor level [99].

Cats with acromegaly are typically rather large, and they may initially show weight gain or weight loss [46,94,95]. In the long term, however, they tend to increase in weight and size slowly, with somewhat disproportionate

Table 1
Cats with acromegaly that the author has treated in the last 10 years

Age[a] (years)	Sex	Breed	Presenting complaint	IGF-1 (µg/mL)	Insulin	Weight (kg)	Concurrent findings	Outcome
12	MN	DSH	Resistant DM for 2 months	>1000	5–30 IU lente q12h	5.9 → 9.1	HCM, organomegaly	After 2 years with DM → acute neurologic episode → non-DM for 1 year; 3 months → died from hepatic rupture PME → macro-adenoma in pituitary
10	MN	DSH	Resistant DM for 4 months	Initially 843; 1 year later >1000	20–25 IU PZI q12h	6 → 9	HCM, organomegaly	Died after 4 years of CHF PME → macro-adenoma in pituitary
19	MN	DSH	DM for 6 years, now unstable	>1000	6 IU PZI q12h	6	Organomegaly	Lost to follow-up after ~1 year
15	MN	DSH	Unstable DM for 2 months	>1000	5–10 IU lente q12h	4.5	HCM + CHF, CRF, organomegaly	Died 1 month later of CHF No PME
14	MN	DSH	Unstable DM for 6 weeks	987	3 IU lente q12h	6.3	HCM + CRF	Euthanised after 2 weeks No PME
13	FN	DSH	Resistant DM for 1 month	>1000	9 IU PZI q12h	6.2	Hepatomegaly + hepatic neoplasia	Euthanised after 8 months No PME

10	MN	DSH	Resistant DM for 2 months	>1000	6–12 IU lente q12h	4.4 → 5.8	HCM, CHF, CRF, organomegaly + severe pancreatic pathologic findings on ultrasound examination	Died after 3 years of CHF / No PME
10	MN	DSH	Resistant DM for 1 month	>1000	10 IU lente q12h	5.7	HCM	Still alive after 2 years
13	MN	DSH	Resistant DM for 4 months	>2000	7 IU lente q12h	5.0	None	Still alive after 6 months
14	FN	DSH	Unstable DM for 2 weeks	1802	2 IU PZI q12h	3.6	Hyperthyroid, pancreatic pathologic findings, neurologic signs	Still alive after 2 months

Abbreviations: CHF, congestive heart failure; CRF, chronic renal failure; DM, diabetes mellitus; DSH, domestic shorthair; FN, female neutered; h, hour; HCM, cardiac hypertrophy; IGF-1, insulin-like growth factor 1; MN, male neutered; PME, postmortem examination; q, every; PZI, protamine zinc insulin.
[a] Age at presentation.

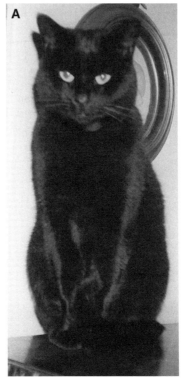

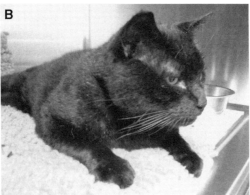

Fig. 1. (*A*) Photograph of a cat with acromegaly before onset of signs attributable to acromegaly. (*B*) Photograph taken 5 years after the first photograph. Note the disproportionate enlargement of the facial features.

enlargement and thickening of the head and feet and marked abdominal distention (Figs. 1 and 2) [2,46,96]. Weight gain may result from direct anabolic effects of IGF-1 or arise secondary to chronic insulin overdose [2,46].

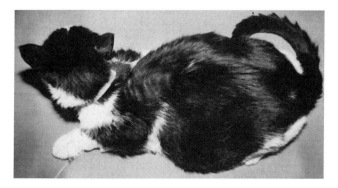

Fig. 2. Acromegalic cat with a pot-bellied appearance resulting from enlargement of intra-abdominal organs. (Courtesy of John Randolph, DVM, Cornell University Hospital for Animals, Ithaca, NY.)

Other changes may also been detected. These include growth of the jawbones, which may result in obvious interdental spaces and prognathism of the lower jaw [2,46,93,94,96,100]. The latter can result in separation of the upper and lower canine teeth, and this altered dental spacing may cause malocclusion or secondary labial ulceration. Distortion of the joints can lead to destructive arthritis [100]. Abdominal distention and a pot-bellied appearance result from ongoing enlargement of the abdominal organs, with hepatomegaly and renomegaly being the easiest to detect on palpation [92,94,96,100]. A mild increase in respiratory noise may result from increased soft tissue thickness around the airways [97]. Organ enlargement may eventually lead to organ dysfunction and eventual failure, with clinical signs reflecting the particular organ systems that have been affected. Cardiac hypertrophy seems to be present in most cases and often leads to congestive heart failure [2,92,95,100]. Chronic renal failure is also seen in many cases, whereas fewer cats develop liver failure (see Table 1) [94,96,100]. Concurrent hypertension has been documented in some cats and may result in ocular hemorrhages, sudden blindness, or neurologic signs [2]. Only rarely do neurologic signs result from the pituitary tumor compressing and invading the hypothalamus [2,93,95,100].

Diagnosis

Although acromegaly is not a common disease in cats, it should be considered in any large-sized cat that develops insulin-resistant or poorly controlled diabetes mellitus. Clinical pathologic examination typically reveals hyperglycemia and glycosuria, but ketosis is rare. Affected cats may also show azotemia, hypercholesterolemia, hyperphosphatemia, hyperpro-teinemia, mildly raised liver enzymes, erythrocytosis, and persistent pro-teinuria [95,100]. Although clinical pathologic examination often reveals a number of different changes, none are diagnostic of acromegaly. It is important to rule out other causes of insulin resistance, particularly hyperadrenocorticism. Comparing the cat with a previous photograph of itself can be helpful in confirming the disproportionate enlargement and thickening of its head (see Fig. 1).

Other tests can be used to gain supportive evidence. Because almost all cases are caused by the presence of a macroadenoma within the pituitary gland, CT or MRI may be useful for detecting these tumors and determining their size [2,93,94,96,100]. CT and MRI may also be useful in detecting organomegaly, as can radiography, which can also be used to detect increased interdental spaces, hyperostosis of the skull, or degenerative arthritis [2,100].

A diagnosis can usually be made by measuring GH levels (where available) [92,94,100] or IGF-1 concentrations (see Table 1) [96], which tend to give similar results [89,93,96]. Unfortunately, the degree of elevation does not always correlate with the clinical signs [95], and although IGF-1 levels greater than 100 nmol/L (>1000 µg/mL) are usually present in cats with acromegaly, care should be taken when assessing cats that have been diabetic for a prolonged period because they may also have raised IGF-1 levels [101,102]. In human beings, it is known that there are a large number of other diseases that can also lead to increased IGF-1 levels, including renal failure, some forms of cancer, and altered T_4 levels [2]. Unfortunately, the effects of these variables are not yet known in cats; thus, care should be taken when interpreting a raised IGF-1 concentration. In theory, the presence of acromegaly can be confirmed by evaluating the GH response to a glucose suppression test; however, because normal cats do not necessarily suppress, this test is of questionable use in cats with suspected acromegaly [96,100,103]. Perhaps the most reliable diagnosis is based on the presence of typically clinical findings; a raised IGF-1 level; and CT, MRI, or postmortem confirmation of a pituitary mass.

Treatment

Acromegaly can be treated in three ways: external beam radiotherapy, surgical removal of the pituitary gland, or medical therapy. In people with acromegaly, external beam radiotherapy is often effective, although clinical improvement may be slow to develop. The few cats that have been treated with cobalt[60] irradiation have shown variable results, ranging from no response to dramatic resolution of hypersomatotropism and hyperglycemia [2,46,94,100,104]. Overall, in cats, this form of treatment probably offers the best chance for control of acromegaly; however, treatment requires repeated anesthetics, and suitable facilities are limited. Surgical excision of the tumor provides another treatment possibility, and in human patients, this usually results in rapid and effective treatment. Hypophysectomy has rarely been performed in cats [93,100].

Medical treatment options include the use of somatostatin analogues (eg, octreotide), dopamine agonists (eg, bromocriptine), and GH-receptor antagonists (eg, pegvisomant). Although they all require frequent administration and often cause side effects, they are sometimes used in the treatment of people with acromegaly. Unfortunately, limited trials with octreotide in acromegalic cats have not been promising [92,95,100], and dopamine agonists and GH-receptor antagonists have not yet been evaluated in this species [2].

Temporary management consists of trying to stabilize the diabetes mellitus and control any other concurrent or related disorders (eg, hypertension, heart failure, renal disease). Control of the diabetes mellitus can usually be achieved by giving high doses of exogenous insulin (20–130 IU/d), sometimes in various combinations of short-, intermediate-, or long-acting insulin [100]. Because the severity of the insulin resistance can fluctuate, it has been suggested that doses should not exceed 12 to 15 IU per injection so that the risk of iatrogenic hypoglycemia is reduced [95]. Rarely, spontaneous necrosis of the tumor can result in temporary or permanent remission of clinical signs (see Table 1).

Prognosis

The long-term prognosis is poor. Because the tumors grow slowly, however, the short-term prognosis may be good to guarded, with survival times ranging from 2 weeks to 4 years reported (median survival time 20 months) (see Table 1) [96,100]. Longer durations have been reported when the pituitary tumor has been successfully treated [2,94].

Hyposomatotropism

Pathogenesis

Hyposomatotropism can result from a congenital defect in the structure or function of the pituitary gland or be idiopathic or acquired in adults secondary to destruction of the pituitary gland (by inflammatory, traumatic, vascular, or neoplastic processes) or suppression by concurrent disorders. In cats, clinical signs have never been reported associated with acquired disease. Congenital hyposomatotropism (pituitary dwarfism) has been seen only rarely, where it results from a congenital deficiency of GH [2]. In some cases, it may also be associated with deficiencies in other hormones produced by the anterior lobe of the pituitary gland (TSH, corticotropin, prolactin, follicle-stimulating hormone, and luteinizing hormone).

Clinical signs

Kittens affected with pituitary dwarfism are born normal, but by 1 to 2 months of age, their growth slows down and they never achieve adult proportions. In addition, their coat tends to appear ill-kempt, with a retained kitten coat and a lack of guard hairs. Dwarfs, which are only deficient in

GH, retain normal body proportions, whereas cats those with concurrent deficiencies (particularly in TSH) develop a rather chunky and dispropor-tionate appearance.

Diagnosis

The results of routine hematology and serum biochemistry are usually unaltered, and diagnosis relies on demonstrating subnormal levels of GH or IGF-1. Because the basal GH concentration of some affected animals attains a normal range, stimulation tests may be needed. Unfortunately, these have not been well investigated in cats [2].

Treatment and prognosis

In theory, the early administration of exogenous recombinant GH to a kitten with pituitary dwarfism may allow it to grow to reach adult proportions. This treatment option has not yet been reported in cats, however. The prognosis for affected kittens therefore remains guarded, because they tend to develop infectious or degenerative disease or neuro-logic dysfunction.

Diabetes insipidus

Pathogenesis

Diabetes insipidus (DI) is a disorder of water metabolism characterized by polyuria, with dilute urine, and a compensatory polydipsia. DI can result from a deficiency in the production of antidiuretic hormone (ADH), called central DI (CDI), or from a failure of the kidneys to respond to ADH, called nephrogenic DI (NDI). Congenital CDI can result from defective synthesis or secretion of ADH and can be partial or complete. CDI can also be acquired as a result of inflammatory, traumatic, vascular, neoplastic, or idiopathic processes affecting ADH production or regulation by the hypothalamic-pituitary axis. CDI is a rare diagnosis in cats (approximately eight published cases) [1,105–111], resulting from congenital defects [110], pituitary neoplasia [109], or trauma [106] or being idiopathic [108,111].

NDI can result from a congenital lack of ADH receptors or be caused by defects in postreceptor binding and can also be partial or complete. Congenital NDI has not yet been documented in the cat; thus, most cases of NDI are secondary to renal or metabolic disorders, such as pyelonephritis, interstitial nephritis, hypokalemia, hypocalcemia, hyperthyroidism, or liver disease.

Clinical signs

Most cats with CDI have been young adults [1,108,109,111], although there have also been two kittens that were believed to have congenital defects [110]. The clinical signs of CDI are marked polyuria and polydipsia, usually with water consumption greater than 100 mL/kg/d [1,105–111] (normal is approximately 40–70 mL/kg/d) [112].

Diagnosis

The results of routine hematology and serum biochemistry may be unremarkable or may reveal changes consistent with dehydration, and plasma osmolality may be increased. Urinalysis is usually unremarkable other than the urine being quite dilute (<1.012, typically 1.003–1.007) [1,105–111]. A diagnosis of DI can only be made after ruling out all other causes of polyuria and polydipsia and demonstrating a lack of ability to concentrate urine in a water deprivation test. Patients with CDI can concentrate their urine after the administration of exogenous ADH or ADH analogue (eg, the synthetic ADH analogue 1 deamino (8 D-arginine) vasopressin [DDAVP]), whereas patients with NDI are nonresponsive. The urine specific gravity of cats reported with CDI did not rise above 1.014 after a water deprivation test but concentrated to greater than 1.020 after the administration of ADH or an ADH analogue [1,105–111].

Treatment

Treatment for CDI is the daily administration of DDAVP by subcutaneous injection or intranasal or conjunctival instillation. DDAVP is expensive, however, and some owners find it simpler to have the cat live outside, where its regular need to urinate is less problematic. Other potential therapies include chlorpropamide for partial CDI and thiazide diuretics for CDI and NDI [1,105–111].

Prognosis

The prognosis for uncomplicated CDI is good if the clinical signs can be controlled or the cat can live outside.

Hyperadrenocorticism

Pathogenesis

In cats, naturally occurring hyperadrenocorticism, more correctly termed *hypercortisolism*, is a relatively rare disease (approximately 70 cases reported). It is most frequently caused by the presence of a corticotropin-secreting pituitary tumor (approximately 80% of cases), most of which are adenomas [5,113–119]. The high circulating levels of corticotropin result in bilateral adrenal hyperplasia (ie, pituitary-dependent hyperadrenocorticism [PDH]). Approximately 20% of cases are caused by functional adrenal tumors that autonomously secrete cortisol; approximately 50% of these tumors are benign adenomas, and approximately 50% are malignant adenocarcinomas [5,114–117,120].

Iatrogenic hyperadrenocorticism has only been seen occasionally in cats, probably because cats seem to be relatively resistant to the deleterious effects of exogenous corticosteroids [5]. When it has occasionally been seen, it has usually been caused by the administration of long courses of exogenous corticosteroids (parenteral, oral, or topical) or megestrol acetate [97,121–125].

Clinical signs

Hyperadrenocorticism is typically seen in middle-aged to older cats (range: 4–16 years, mean approximately 10 years) [5,113–120]. There seems to be no breed predisposition, and although female cats seemed to be overrepresented in some initial studies [95,115], it is now clear that there is no sex predisposition [5].

History and clinical signs are often vague; however, they usually include polyuria, polydipsia, polyphagia, weight loss, generalized muscle loss, and lethargy and may include a history of recurrent infections or abscesses. Affected cats typically have a coat that is in poor condition, with spontaneous alopecia, and fragile thin inelastic skin that bruises easily (ie, fragile skin syndrome). Occasionally, they develop seborrhea or bacterial dermatitis [113–117,120]. Affected cats usually have a pot-bellied appearance resulting from weakened abdominal muscles, obesity, and, in some cases, hepatomegaly, which may be palpable [113–117,120,126]. Less frequently seen clinical signs include generalized muscle weakness; dropped hocks (resulting from diabetic neuropathy); diarrhea; constipation; dyspnea or panting; cystitis (caused by bacterial or fungal urinary tract infections); or signs related to congestive heart failure, renal failure, or acute pancreatitis [5,114,117,118,120,127].

Because cortisol antagonizes insulin, approximately 80% of affected cats develop diabetes mellitus, which may or may not be insulin resistant [5,114–117,119].

Diagnosis

Hyperadrenocorticism should be suspected in any cat with the clinical signs described previously, particularly if it has unstable diabetes mellitus or a history of exogenous corticosteroid administration.

Clinical pathologic changes are variable. Because hyperadrenocorticism is frequently associated with diabetes mellitus, serum biochemistry and urinalysis often reveal persistent hyperglycemia and glucosuria but rarely show ketonuria [5,113,114,117,120]. Increased liver enzymes and hypercholesterolemia may be seen regardless of whether or not the cat has diabetes; however, the increases are much less dramatic than those seen in dogs with hyperadrenocorticism. Other less common findings include hypokalemia, hyperglobulinemia, azotemia, and hypothyroxinemia [5,114,117,120]. Hematologic examination may reveal a stress leukogram (neutrophilia or lymphopenia) or, occasionally, a mild variably regenerative anemia [5,113,114,117,120].

Radiographic changes may include hepatomegaly, osteopenia, abdominal enlargement, distention of the urinary bladder, or dystrophic mineralization [5,128]. Occasionally, adrenal neoplasia may be large enough to see radiographically. The presence of adrenal mineralization should not be overinterpreted, however, because it occurs in approximately 30% of normal cats [126].

Making a diagnosis of hyperadrenocorticism can be difficult. This is because the clinical signs are often less dramatic in cats than in dogs, the results of the specific tests are often inconsistent, and few of the tests have well-established specificity and sensitivity in cats [5,117]. It is usually necessary to use a combination of tests.

In cats, screening tests include the urine cortisol-to-creatinine ratio (UC/CR), low-dose dexamethasone suppression (screening) test (LDDST), and corticotropin stimulation test.

Urine cortisol-to-creatinine ratio

The protocol is to collect a urine sample, centrifuge it, and submit the supernatant. The test is quite sensitive, such that a normal ratio almost always rules out hyperadrenocorticism ($<3.6 \times 10^{-5}$) [129]. Unfortunately, the test is not extremely specific, because an increased ratio can also be associated with nonadrenal illness, especially diabetes mellitus and hyperthyroidism [130,131]. The test is more reliable if the sample is collected at home, because the cat is less likely to be stressed [5,132].

Low-dose dexamethasone suppression (screening) test

The protocol is to collect a baseline blood sample, give dexamethasone intravenously at a dose of 0.1 mg/kg, and then collect further blood samples after 4 to 8 hours.

In normal cats, the serum cortisol concentration should be less than 1.4 μg/dL (<30 nmol/L), or less than 50% of the predexamethasone level 4 to 8 hours after administration of dexamethasone. Most cats with hyperadrenocorticism (80%–95%) fail to suppress at 8 hours (suppression at 4 hours but not at 8 hours is consistent with PDH). Although false-negative results may occur in mild cases of hyperadrenocorticism, this test is sensitive and therefore a good screening test for hyperadrenocorticism [5,115].

This dose of dexamethasone is higher than the 0.01 mg/kg used in dogs. This is because the lower dose was found to be less sensitive in cats [133] in studies in which 10% to 15% of normal cats and some cats with nonadrenal illness failed to suppress [134,135].

Corticotropin stimulation test

The protocol is to collect a baseline blood sample, give synthetic corti-cotropin intravenously at a dose of 0.125 to 0.25 mg, and then collect further blood samples after 1 to 2 hours.

The normal basal serum cortisol concentration should be 0 to 5 µg/dL (10–110 nmol/L). One or 2 hours after administration of corticotropin, the cortisol concentration in a normal cat should be 5 to 15 µg/dL (210–330 nmol/L) but is greater than 19 µg/dL (>500 nmol/L) in most cats with hyperadrenocorticism [136–139].

Although intravenous and intramuscular routes of administration have been investigated [114,116,134,136–138], the intravenous route is generally preferred because it gives a more marked and prolonged elevation in cortisol, with the peak occurring between 60 and 240 minutes after the dexamethasone injection [117,136,138].

Unfortunately, false-negative results may be seen in a significant per-centage (30%–40%) of cats with hyperadrenocorticism, and false-positive results can also occur [114,117,135,139]. For this reason, the UC/CR and LDDST are the preferred screening tests in cats [5].

Additional tests are used to try to differentiate PDH from adrenal neoplasia. These include the high-dose dexamethasone suppression test (HDDST), measurement of endogenous (basal) corticotropin, the combi-nation test, ultrasonography, and, when available, CT or MRI.

High-dose dexamethasone suppression test

This test is performed like the LDDST, with the exception that the cat is given dexamethasone at a dose of 1.0 mg/kg. It has been suggested that the 8-hour sample can be omitted because it adds little information [5]. Cats with PDH may or may not suppress, whereas cats with adrenal-dependent hyperadrenocorticism do not suppress [5,140].

An alternative "at home" protocol has gained favor because it is easy to perform and interpret, gives more consistent results than the standard HDDST, reduces the stress to the cat, and reduces the risk of bruising post venipuncture [5]. The owner collects a urine sample from the cat on the morning of day 1 and day 2; gives three oral doses of dexamethasone (0.1 mg/kg) at 8-hour intervals at 8:00 AM, 4:00 PM, and 12:00 PM [129] or two doses at 4:00 PM and 12:00 PM [141]; and then collects a third urine sample on the morning of day 3. All three samples are then delivered to the veterinarian for UC/CR assessment.

The mean of the first two UC/CRs gives the "basal value" and acts as a screening test, confirming the presence of hyperadrenocorticism. The cat is then described as having suppressed if the UC/CR on day 3 is less than 50% of the basal value. Cats with PDH may or may not suppress, whereas cats with adrenal-dependent hyperadrenocorticism do not suppress [5].

Measurement of endogenous (basal) corticotropin

The protocol is to collect a blood sample in EDTA, spin it immediately, transfer the plasma into a plastic tube, and then ship it overnight on ice or freeze it for storage. In cats with PDH, the plasma corticotropin concentration is usually high normal or greater (>15 pg/mL) compared with being low (<10 pg/mL) in those cats with adrenal tumors [5]. This test is an effective method of differentiating PDH from adrenal-dependent hyperadrenocorticism [115]. Because normal cats may also have low corticotropin levels, they cannot be differentiated from cats with adrenal-dependent hyperadrenocorticism using this test, which is why this test should not be used as a screening test for hyperadrenocorticism [134].

Combination test

The protocol is to collect a blood sample, give dexamethasone intravenously at a dose of 1.0 mg/kg, collect a further blood sample after 4 hours, and then immediately perform a corticotropin stimulation test as previously described.

The interpretation is the same as for a corticotropin stimulation test and HDDST (taking the HDDST result as the result at 4 hours). Because the corticotropin stimulation test is no longer recommended as a screening test for cats with hyperadrenocorticism, however, this combined test has also fallen out of favor.

Ultrasonography and CT or MRI

Each of these imaging modalities can be used to determine the shape and size of the adrenal glands [114,116,117,128]. Ultrasonography is a relatively useful method of determining adrenal size [142,143]; unilateral adrenal enlargement is typical of an adrenal tumor; bilateral enlargement usually indicates PDH, although it can occasionally result from bilateral adrenal tumors. CT and MRI can be used to image the pituitary gland as well as the adrenal glands; approximately 50% of the pituitary tumors are large enough to be visualized using these techniques [5,141,144].

A number of other diseases may need to be excluded because they can cause clinical signs similar to those seen in hyperadrenocorticism. One of these conditions is acromegaly (because it also causes insulin-resistant diabetes mellitus); for more information, the reader is referred to the previous section on this disease. Acromegaly can usually be diagnosed by assessing the IGF-1 concentration, however [2]. Another condition that may need to be considered is the presence of a progesterone-secreting adrenal tumor. Although these tumors have been seen only rarely in cats, they can cause cutaneous changes indistinguishable from those seen with hyperadrenocorticism and may also result in diabetes mellitus [145,146]. Although, by definition, they do cause a form of hyperadrenocorticism, they do not cause hypercortisolism and can usually be diagnosed via evaluation of the sex hormones.

Treatment

There are a number of possible treatment options for cats with hyperadrenocorticism. There have been few large-scale studies on their use in this species, however.

Initial studies on a number of different medical therapies have generally given poor results. It has therefore been suggested that medical therapy is perhaps best reserved for presurgical stabilization rather than for long-term control [5]. Although mitotane has been shown to be well tolerated in healthy cats [133,137], it has been used to treat few cats with hyperadrenocorticism. Although it gave poor results in one cat at a dose of 25 mg/kg/d for 25 days [114], longer courses or higher doses have been more effective in a small number of cases [126,147]. Treatment with ketoconazole has given mixed results and has caused considerable toxicity in some cats [120,148–151]. Metyrapone has shown potential positive effects in a small number of cats; however, it is difficult to obtain [150–154]. There is little information available on the use of L-deprenyl in cats, and it has no proven efficacy in the treatment of feline hyperadrenocorticism.

Of all of the medical approaches, the use of trilostane has given the most promising results, albeit in a small number of cats, and certainly warrants further investigation [118,119]. Trilostane inhibits 3β-17-hydroxysteroid dehydrogenase; in doing so, it blocks the synthesis of adrenal and gonadal steroid hormones. It has been used for the treatment of PDH and adrenal-dependent hyperadrenocorticism in dogs with good results [155,156]. In the small number of cats with PDH that have been treated, trilostane reduced their clinical signs and improved their endocrine test results. Although they still required exogenous insulin, they survived for many months on treatment [118,119]. Trilostane has also been used to treat a single feline case of bilateral adrenal enlargement with excessive sex hormone production (but no hypercortisolemia), in which it induced moderate clinical improvement [157]. Trilostane has typically been given at a dose of 30 mg/cat orally once or twice daily (ranging from 15 mg per cat once daily to 60 mg per cat twice daily) long-term [118,119]. Although side effects seem to be few, the administration of trilostane is not recommended in patients with renal insufficiency [119], and it has caused adrenal necrosis in a dog [158]. It should only be used with caution in cats, and close monitoring is essential (repeated serum biochemistry, hematology, and assessment of the pituitary-adrenal axis).

Cobalt irradiation for the treatment of PDH by ablation of the pituitary tumor has been used in a small number of cats [5,104,114]. It has given mixed results and requires specialist facilities.

There are a number of surgical options for the treatment of hyperadrenocorticism, including uni- or bilateral adrenalectomy and hypophysectomy. Because of the difficulties with medical therapy, adrenalectomy has been considered the treatment of choice in cats with hyperadrenocorticism [114,116,117,133]. This may be changing, however, with the apparent success of trilostane treatment. When a single adrenal tumor is present, the removal of the affected adrenal gland is recommended. With PDH or bilateral adrenal tumors, bilateral adrenalectomy is recommended [114,116,117]. Early diagnosis helps to reduce postoperative complications [114]. Although surgery can provide successful treatment, the risk of a fatal perioperative hypoadrenal crisis, cardiac or renal failure, sepsis, or surgical complications is great [114,116,117,126]. The procedure should only be performed by an experienced surgeon. Consideration of the diabetic state must be given, and perioperative treatment with glucocorticoids and mineralocorticoids is essential [5,114,117]. Short-term postoperative glucocorticoid administration is needed after unilateral adrenalectomy, because the contralateral gland is temporarily atrophied. Long-term treatment is needed after bilateral adrenalectomy, however, and should also include mineralocorticoids [114,116,117].

Transsphenoidal hypophysectomy is the treatment of choice in people with PDH and has been successfully performed in a small number of cats with the PDH. It requires specialist surgical facilities and the same type of perioperative management as with bilateral adrenalectomy, and it carries many potential complications [141,159].

When attempting to treat the cause of the hyperadrenocorticism, exogenous insulin may still be required. Stabilization of the diabetes can usually be achieved using high doses of exogenous insulin, sometimes in various combinations of short-, intermediate-, or long-acting insulin [100]. Because the severity of the insulin resistance can fluctuate, it is recommended that doses do not exceed 2.2 IU/kg per dose [5].

Prognosis

Without successful treatment, the prognosis is poor, with most untreated cats dying or being euthanized within a month of diagnosis [5,114,117]. When PDH is present, successful bilateral adrenalectomy can reduce the signs of hyperadrenocorticism, but the risk of a hypoadrenal crisis or other perioperative complications is high. In addition, tumor expansion may eventually lead to neurologic signs [117]. If adrenal tumors are successfully removed, the hyperadrenocorticism should resolve and the diabetic state may become less insulin resistant or even resolve [5,114,116,117]. Because early studies of trilostane seem to show that although it may ameliorate the signs of hyperadrenocorticism, it may not alter the need for exogenous insulin, diabetic cats are still susceptible to diabetic complications [119].

Primary sex hormone–secreting adrenal tumors

Pathogenesis and clinical signs

There have been a small number of cats that have been found to have sex hormone–secreting adrenal tumors. The four cases in the literature have occurred in older (7–14 years) neutered cats; three were male and found to have progesterone-secreting tumors, and one was female with an estradiol- and testosterone-producing tumor [5,145,146,157]. The three male cats were presented with cutaneous changes indistinguishable from those seen with classic hyperadrenocorticism; an unkempt greasy hair coat, nonpruritic symmetric alopecia, and fragile easily bruised and damaged skin. In addition, one had demodicosis [146]. Two of the cats were diabetic, whereas the third was periodically hyperglycemic and glucosuric [5,145,146]. The female cat was presented because it had become aggressive, its urine had developed a strong "tom-cat" odor, and it had vulval hyperplasia [157]. Although the cat's coat was unkempt, there was no alopecia or skin thinning.

Diagnosis

The only significant findings on clinical pathologic examination were persistent hyperglycemic and glucosuric in the two diabetic male cats. Unilateral adrenal enlargement was found on ultrasound examination in the male cats, whereas both adrenals were enlarged in the female cat [5,145,146,157].

Extensive endocrine testing was performed in each case. In all four cats, corticotropin stimulation tests revealed low-normal basal plasma cortisol concentrations, and poststimulation results were consistent with iatrogenic hyperadrenocorticism (despite no exogenous steroid having been given). None of the cats had hypercortisolemia. In the male cats, the LDDST produced results variably consistent with hyperadrenocorticism, and one of the cats had an undetectable endogenous corticotropin level. Each of the male cats had a high basal progesterone level (reference range <0.35 ng/mL, 3.6–13.2 ng/mL in affected cats) [5,145,146]. The female cat had markedly elevated basal estradiol and testosterone levels [157].

Treatment

Before adrenalectomy, two of the male cats were successfully treated with aminoglutethimide (AGT) (approximately 6 mg/kg administered orally twice daily) [5,146]. AGT inhibits the enzyme responsible for converting cholesterol to pregnenolone during the synthesis of adrenocortical steroids. The female cat responded temporarily to treatment with a different steroid hormone inhibitor, trilostane [157].

Primary hyperaldosteronism

Pathogenesis

Primary hyperaldosteronism is a rare disease in the cat (five published cases) and 11 cases presented in abstract. Hyperaldosteronism is caused by the presence of an aldosterone-secreting adrenal tumor, typically unilateral adrenal adenomas or carcinomas, but also occasional bilateral adenomas [5,154,160–163,192]. Aldosterone is the primary hormone responsible for maintaining normal sodium, potassium, chloride, and acid-base homeostasis. Excessive aldosterone secretion results in hypokalemia (because of increased urinary excretion of potassium), metabolic alkalosis (because of increased renal tubular bicarbonate transport), and systemic hypertension (secondary to sodium and water retention). The cats in the cases that have been reported have all been older (6–20 years of age) neutered cats, and there has been no sex predisposition [5,154,160–163,192].

Clinical signs and diagnosis

The cats were presented with muscle weakness (13 cats), cervical ventroflexion, polyuria or polydipsia, weight loss, reduced appetite, ataxia, blindness caused by hypertensive retinopathy, nocturia, and/or abdominal enlargement. All were hypokalemic, eight were moderately to severely hypertensive, and two had concurrent diabetes mellitus. Serum CK levels were elevated because of the hypokalemic myopathy, and urine was dilute (two cats). All had markedly increased concentrations of serum aldosterone, with low or normal concentrations of renin. Abdominal ultrasound (or MRI) detected an adrenal mass in most cases.

Treatment

Short-term treatment was achieved by giving high doses of oral potassium supplementation. This can usually be administered in the form of potassium gluconate solution, tablets, or powder (4–10 Eq [mmol] administered orally every 24 hours in divided doses). In severe cases, intravenous potassium supplementation may be necessary. This should be administered carefully, with cardiac monitoring. Although it is not usually recommended to exceed administered potassium at a rate of 0.5 Eq (mmol)/kg/h, this may occasionally be necessary in severe cases to prevent death from paralysis of the respiratory muscles. Cats with significant systemic hypertension may also require amlodipine (0.625–1.25 mg/d per cat orally) to reduce their blood pressure. The addition of spironolactone, a potassium-sparing diuretic (which is a synthetic homologue and competitive antagonist of aldosterone), can help in maintaining serum potassium levels. The recommended dose is 2 to 4 mg/kg/d administered orally, although some clinicians have used considerably higher doses (up to 50 mg/kg/d). Surgical removal of the adrenal tumor has successfully achieved in some cases [5,154,160–163,192].

Pheochromocytoma

Pathogenesis

Pheochromocytomas are endocrine tumors arising from the chromaffin cells of the adrenal gland. They are usually solitary and can occasionally arise outside the adrenal gland (extra-adrenal pheochromocytoma, also termed *paraganglioma*). They are rarely reported in cats. Functional adrenal pheochromocytomas have been reported in an 11-year-old female domestic shorthair cat [164] and seen in a 20-year-old neutered Burmese cat (seen by the author). They have more typically been detected as incidental antemortem findings [165,166] or postmortem findings [7,167]. Functional pheochromocytoma may produce epinephrine (adrenalin), norepinephrine (noradrenalin), and, occasionally, dopamine and other hormones [168].

Clinical signs

In cats, an antemortem diagnosis of a pheochromocytoma is rare. This reflects the low incidence of the tumor but may also result from a low index of suspicion, the vague and often episodic nature of the clinical signs, and the lack of easy diagnostic tests. Clinical signs may result from the direct presence of the tumor and its space-occupying nature or be secondary to the excessive secretion of large amounts of catecholamines. The clinical signs in three cats consisted of polyuria and polydipsia [164,167], whereas in another cat, they were caused by severe systemic hypertension, and included congestive heart failure, pleural effusion, and hypertensive retinopathy (seen by the author). In other species, clinical signs often include acute collapse, cardiovascular shock, pulmonary edema, cardiac arrhythmia, epistaxis, cerebral hemorrhage, and seizures [168].

Diagnosis

Diagnosis is difficult. The investigation should include routine hematologic testing, serum biochemistry, serum total T_4 concentration, dynamic tests to exclude hyperadrenocorticism, evaluation of the systemic blood pressure, chest and abdominal radiography, abdominal ultrasound examination, and a full cardiac investigation. The presence of an adrenal mass in a cat with systemic hypertension should alert the clinician to the possibility of a pheochromocytoma. Other potentially useful diagnostic investigations include abdominal CT or MRI, vena cava venography, ultrasound-guided needle biopsy of the mass, and measurement of plasma or urine catecholamines [7,168].

Treatment

Surgical removal of the tumor remains the only definitive treatment but requires considerable perioperative care and should only be performed by an experienced surgeon [7]. Medical treatment may achieve temporary control of the clinical signs. It entails the use of α-blockers (eg, phenoxybenzamine) and, if needed, β-blockers (eg, propranolol or atenolol). Currently, there are too few cases of pheochromocytoma in cats to determine an accurate prognosis; however, it is likely that in cats, as in other species, the prognosis is determined by the size and activity of the tumor and the extent of its invasion.

Hypoadrenocorticism

Pathogenesis

Primary hypoadrenocorticism is a rare condition in cats (approximately 40 reported cases). Most cases are believed to have resulted from the immune-mediated destruction of the adrenal gland, resulting in glucocorticoid and mineralocorticoid deficiency [169]. There are also occasional cases with other causes, including two cases that resulted from trauma (the author has also treated a similar case) [170,171] and two cases that resulted from bilateral adrenal infiltration with lymphoma [172]. Naturally occurring secondary hypoadrenocorticism has not been reported in the cat, except iatrogenically, where it has followed the rapid withdrawal of exogenous corticosteroids [121,124,173].

Clinical signs

Although a wide age range of cats have been affected (range: 1.5–14 years, typically early middle age), there seems to be no breed or sex predisposition [7,170,172–177,191]. There is usually a history of lethargy, depression, anorexia, and weight loss. Less common signs include collapse, muscle weakness, vomiting, polydipsia, polyuria, and dysphagia [172,175,177,191]. Clinical examination typically reveals dehydration, weakness, and hypothermia, although weak pulses, bradycardia, and abdominal pain are seen less frequently. Clinical signs typically wax and wane and often respond partially to symptomatic treatment with intravenous fluids and glucocorticoid therapy [170,172–175,177,191].

Diagnosis

Typical clinical pathologic findings include hyperkalemia (5.4–7.6 mEq [mmol]/L), hyponatremia, hypochloremia, azotemia, hyperphosphatemia, and urine specific gravity of less than 1.030. Less common findings include anemia, lymphocytosis, and eosinophilia [170,172–175,177]. The corticotropin stimulation test is considered a reliable test for the diagnosis of hypoadrenocorticism in cats (see section on hyperadrenocorticism for the methodology) [140,178]. Diagnosis is based on a lack of stimulation. Measurement of the endogenous corticotropin concentration is useful in confirming that the hypoadrenocorticism is primary (it should be elevated) [170,172–175,177]. Microcardia and pulmonary hypoperfusion may be seen on thoracic radiography [177].

Treatment

Treatment of an acute hypoadrenal crisis involves restoration of the fluid volume, correction of any acid-base imbalance, and provision of glucocorticoid and mineralocorticoid supplementation. In some cases, resolution of the clinical signs may be somewhat slower than typically seen in dogs, taking 3 to 5 days. Long-term management requires the administration of fludrocortisone (approximately 0.1 mg/d per cat) plus or minus a glucocorticoid (typically prednisolone at approximately 1.5 mg/d per cat administered orally or methylprednisolone acetate at 10 mg/month per cat administered intramuscularly). The dosage of the fludrocortisone may need to be adjusted based on serial serum biochemistry analysis; serum biochemistry is measured every 1 to 2 weeks until the cat is stable [170,173–175].

Prognosis

The prognosis for most cats, provided they survive the initial crisis, seems to be good [173–175,177]. The prognosis for cats with hypoadrenocorticism caused by infiltrating neoplasia is dependent on the amenability of the tumor to treatment, however [172]. Depending on the severity of the damage, cases that result from trauma may be transient (the author's case resolved within 2 months) [170].

Hyperparathyroidism

Pathogenesis

Hypercalcemia is seen less commonly in cats than in dogs. Although primary hyperparathyroidism can cause hypercalcemia in cats, it is seen only rarely (approximately 6% of cases of hypercalcemia, approximately 20 published cases) [8,179–184]. In cats, hypercalcemia is most commonly associated with neoplasia (30%, most commonly, lymphoma and squamous cell carcinoma caused by production of parathyroid hormone–related protein [PTHrP], increased vitamin D_3 production by lymphoma cells, or increased bone lysis surrounding the tumor); renal failure (25%, caused by secondary renal hyperparathyroidism); calcium oxalate urolithiasis (15%, where the hypercalcemia is usually idiopathic); granulomatous infections (6%, typically mycobacterial or deep fungal infections, where macrophage activation results in increased vitamin D_3 production), and, occasionally, hypoadrenocorticism or vitamin D toxicosis [125,182,185]. Most cases of primary hyperparathyroidism have been caused by a solitary parathyroid adenoma. Occasional cases have resulted from solitary or bilateral carcinoma, bilateral cystadenoma, and parathyroid hyperplasia, however [8,179–184].

Clinical signs

Although the mean age of cats with hypercalcemia is approximately 9 years (range: 1–19 years) [182], the mean age for cats with primary hyperparathyroidism is older, at approximately 13 years (range: 8–20 years) [8,179–184]. There is no sex predisposition, but Siamese cats may be overrepresented with primary hyperparathyroidism [179].

Clinical signs associated with hypercalcemia include anorexia and lethargy (50%), gastrointestinal signs (27%, including vomiting, diarrhea, and constipation), polyuria or polydipsia (24%), lower urinary tract signs (23%), and neuromuscular signs (14%, including weakness and muscle tremors). Although the clinical signs seem to be similar regardless of the underlying cause, cats with primary hyperparathyroidism are less likely to show signs relating to the lower urinary tract and the nervous system. In addition, a parathyroid mass is usually palpable in cats with primary hyperparathyroidism (11 of 19 cats) [8,179–184].

Diagnosis

In cats with primary hyperparathyroidism, the only consistent abnormal finding on hematology and serum biochemistry is hypercalcemia, with total and ionized calcium concentrations being increased. Many affected cats eventually develop raised BUN and creatinine concentrations. Serum parathyroid hormone levels range from within the normal range to increased, but these are still abnormal because, physiologically, they should be reduced in the face of hypercalcemia. Ideally, the diagnostic investigation should also include assessment of PTHrP and vitamin D metabolites, both of which should be low in cats with primary hyperparathyroidism. (An algorithm is available to explain the use of these different assays in diagnosing the underlying cause of hypercalcemia [8]). Cervical ultrasound examination may detect one or more enlarged parathyroid glands.

Treatment

Most cats with primary hyperparathyroidism have been treated surgically. Once the overactive parathyroid gland(s) has been removed, the cats have generally recovered well, although in the case of malignant neoplasia, it may recur. Vitamin D and calcium have usually been given after surgery to reduce the risk of clinical hypocalcemia (see section on the surgical treatment of hyperthyroidism). Clinical signs relating to hypocalcemia have been few, however [8,179,181,184].

Hypoparathyroidism

Pathogenesis

In cats, hypocalcemia is seen reasonably commonly and may be associated with hypoalbuminemia, renal failure, administration of phosphate-containing enemas, intestinal malabsorption, acute pancreatitis, puerperal tetany, or ethylene glycol toxicity; as a complication of bilateral thyroidectomy; and resulting from primary hypoparathyroidism [9]. Noniatrogenic primary hypoparathyroidism has been seen rarely (approximately 14 cases reported) [31,186–190] and is believed to result from an immune-mediated attack on the parathyroid glands [186,188].

Clinical signs

The age at presentation for cats with primary hypoparathyroidism has ranged from 5 months to 7 years (mean = approximately 2 years). Male cats have been seen slightly more frequently than female cats, but there does not seem to be a breed predisposition [9,186–190].

The clinical course has been acute or insidious in onset, and affected cats are usually lethargic and anorexic and have intermittent neurologic or neuromuscular disturbances. The latter may include focal or generalized muscle tremors, ataxia, stilted gait, disorientation, weakness, tetanic spasms, and seizures. In addition, some cats may show panting, protrusion of the nictitating membranes, mydriasis, dysphagia, pruritus, or ptyalism. Physical findings may include depression, weakness, fever or hypothermia, bradycardia, dehydration, and the presence of lenticular cataracts [9,186–190].

Diagnosis

Routine serum biochemistry reveals profound hypocalcemia, with severe hyperphosphatemia and, occasionally, an elevated ALT concentration. ECG may show bradycardia or a prolonged QT interval. A diagnosis of primary hypoparathyroidism relies on demonstrating a lack of parathyroid hormone and, where possible, the histological evaluation of a parathyroid gland biopsy [9,186–188].

Treatment and prognosis

Treatment is the same as for iatrogenic hypoparathyroidism, for example, when it occurs after bilateral thyroidectomy, and entails the initial intravenous administration of 10% calcium gluconate, followed by oral calcium and vitamin D supplementation. Because lifelong treatment is needed, however, it is important to monitor response to therapy so that the lowest possible doses are given. Once the doses have been adjusted, the long-term prognosis seems to be good [9,186–188].

References

[1] Feldman EC, Nelson RW. Water metabolism and diabetes insipidus. In: Feldman EC, Nelson RW, editors. Canine and feline endocrinology and reproduction. 3rd edition. Philadelphia: WB Saunders; 2004. p. 2–44.

[2] Feldman EC, Nelson RW. Disorders of growth hormone. In: Feldman EC, Nelson RW, editors. Canine and feline endocrinology and reproduction. 3rd edition. Philadelphia: WB Saunders; 2004. p. 45–84.

[3] Feldman EC, Nelson RW. Hypothyroidism. In: Feldman EC, Nelson RW, editors. Canine and feline endocrinology and reproduction. 3rd edition. Philadelphia: WB Saunders; 2004. p. 86–151.

[4] Feldman EC, Nelson RW. Feline hyperthyroidism (thyrotoxicosis). In: Feldman EC, Nelson RW, editors. Canine and feline endocrinology and reproduction. 3rd edition. Philadelphia: WB Saunders; 2004. p. 152–218.

[5] Feldman EC, Nelson RW. Hyperadrenocorticism in cats (Cushing's syndrome). In: Feldman EC, Nelson RW, editors. Canine and feline endocrinology and reproduction. 3rd edition. Philadelphia: WB Saunders; 2004. p. 358–93.

[6] Feldman EC, Nelson RW. Hypoadrenocorticism in cats. In: Feldman EC, Nelson RW, editors. Canine and feline endocrinology and reproduction. 3rd edition. Philadelphia: WB Saunders; 2004. p. 425–37.

[7] Feldman EC, Nelson RW. Pheochromocytoma and multiple endocrine neoplasia. In: Feldman EC, Nelson RW, editors. Canine and feline endocrinology and reproduction. 3rd edition. Philadelphia: WB Saunders; 2004. p. 440–63.

[8] Feldman EC, Nelson RW. Hypercalcemia and primary hyperparathyroidism. In: Feldman EC, Nelson RW, editors. Canine and feline endocrinology and reproduction. 3rd edition. Philadelphia: WB Saunders; 2004. p. 660–715.

[9] Feldman EC, Nelson RW. Hypocalcemia and primary hypoparathyroidism. In: Feldman EC, Nelson RW, editors. Canine and feline endocrinology and reproduction. 3rd edition. Philadelphia: WB Saunders; 2004. p. 716–42.

[10] Gerber H, Gerber H, Peter H, et al. Etiopathology of feline toxic nodular goiter. Vet Clin N Am Small Anim Pract 1994;24:541–65.

[11] Peterson ME, Kintzer PP, Cavanagh PG, et al. Feline hyperthyroidism: pretreatment clinical and laboratory evaluation of 131 cases. J Am Vet Med Assoc 1983;183(1):103–10.

[12] Peterson ME, Ferguson DC. Thyroid disease. In: Ettinger SJ, editor. Textbook of veterinary internal medicine. Philadelphia: WB Saunders; 1989. p. 1654–67.

[13] Turrel JM, Feldman EC, Nelson RW, et al. Thyroid carcinoma causing hyperthyroidism in cats: 14 cases (1981–1986). J Am Vet Med Assoc 1988;193(3):359–64.

[14] Edinboro CH, Scott-Moncrieff JC, Janovitz E, et al. Epidemiologic study of the relationships between consumption of commercial canned food and risk of hyperthyroidism in cats. J Am Vet Med Assoc 2004;224(6):879–86.

[15] Tarttelin MF, Johnson LA, Cooke RR, et al. Serum free thyroxine levels respond inversely to changes in levels of dietary iodine in the domestic cat. NZ Vet J 1992;40:66–8.

[16] Kass PH, Paterson ME, Levy J, et al. Evaluation of environmental, nutritional, and host factors in cats with hyperthyroidism. J Vet Intern Med 1999;13:323–9.

[17] Martin KM, Rossing MA, Ryland LM, et al. Evaluation of dietary and environmental risk factors for hyperthyroidism in cats. J Am Vet Med Assoc 2000;217:853–6.

[18] Scarlett JM, Moise NS, Rayl J. Feline hyperthyroidism: a descriptive and case-control study. Prev Vet Med 1988;6:295–309.

[19] Merryman JI, Buckles EL, Bowers G, et al. Overexpression of c-Ras in hyperplasia and adenomas of the feline thyroid gland: an immunohistopathological analysis of 34 cases. Vet Pathol 1999;36:117–24.

[20] Nguyen LQ, Arseven OK, Gerber H, et al. Cloning of the cat TSH receptor and evidence against an autoimmune etiology of feline hyperthyroidism. Endocrinology 2002;143(2):395–402.

[21] Thoday KL, Mooney CT. Historical, clinical and laboratory features of 126 hyperthyroid cats. Vet Rec 1992;131:257–64.

[22] Gordon JM, Ehrart EJ, Sisson DD. Juvenile hyperthyroidism in a cat. J Am Anim Hosp Assoc 2003;39(1):67–71.

[23] Broussard JD, Peterson ME, Fox PR. Changes in clinical and laboratory findings in cats with hyperthyroidism from 1983 to 1993. J Am Vet Med Assoc 1995;206:302–5.

[24] Nemzek JA, Kruger JM, Walshaw R, et al. Acute onset of hypokalemia and muscular weakness in four hyperthyroid cats. J Am Vet Med Assoc 1994;205:65–8.

[25] Liu S, Peterson ME, Fox PR. Hypertrophic cardiomyopathy and hyperthyroidism in the cat. J Am Vet Med Assoc 1984;185(1):52–7.

[26] Kobayashi DL, Peterson ME, Graves TK, et al. Hypertension in cats with chronic renal failure and hyperthyroidism. J Vet Intern Med 1990;4:58–62.

[27] Littman MP. Spontaneous systemic hypertension in 24 cats. J Vet Intern Med 1994;8: 79–86.

[28] Bodey AR, Samson J. Epidemiological study of blood pressure in domestic cats. J Soc Adm Pharm 1998;39:567–73.

[29] Syme HM. Hypertension and the endocrine system. In: Proceedings of 22nd American College of Veterinary Internal Medicine Forum, Minneapolis, 2004. Lakewood (CO): American College of Veterinary Internal Medicine; 2004. p. 603.

[30] Stiles J, Polzin DJ, Bistner SI. The prevalence of retinopathy in cats with systemic hypertension and chronic renal failure or hyperthyroidism. J Am Anim Hosp Assoc 1994; 30:564–72.

[31] Horney BS, Farmer AJ, Honor DJ, et al. Agarose gel electrophoresis of alkaline phosphatase isoenzyme in the serum of hyperthyroid cats. Vet Clin Pathol 1994;23: 98–102.

[32] Foster DJ, Thoday KL. Tissue sources of serum alkaline phosphatase in 34 hyperthyroid cats: a qualitative and quantitative study. Res Vet Sci 2000;68:89–94.

[33] Barber PJ, Elliott J. Study of calcium homeostasis in feline hyperthyroidism. J Soc Adm Pharm 1996;37:575–82.

[34] Graves TK, Olivier NB, Nachreiner RF, et al. Changes in renal function associated with treatment of hyperthyroidism in cats. Am J Vet Res 1994;55(12):1745–9.

[35] Syme HM, Elliott J. Prevalence and significance of proteinuria in cats with hyperthyroidism. In: BSAVA Congress Proceedings, 2003. Gloucester, UK: BSAVA; 2003. p. 533.

[36] Peterson ME, Keene B, Ferguson DC, et al. Electrocardiographic findings in 45 cats with hyperthyroidism. J Am Vet Med Assoc 1982;180(8):934–7.

[37] Moise NS, Dietze AE. Echocardiographic, electrocardiographic, and radiographic detection of cardiomegaly in hyperthyroid cats. Am J Vet Res 1986;47(7):1487–94.

[38] Bond BR, Fox PR, Peterson ME, et al. Echocardiographic findings in 103 cats with hyperthyroidism. J Am Vet Med Assoc 1988;192(11):1546–9.

[39] Peterson ME, Melian C, Nichols R. Measurement of serum concentrations of free thyroxine, total thyroxine and total triiodothyronine in cats with hyperthyroidism and cats with nonthyroidal disease. J Am Vet Med Assoc 2001;218(4):529–36.

[40] Peterson ME, Graves TK, Cavanagh I. Serum thyroid hormone concentrations fluctuate in cats with hyperthyroidism. J Vet Intern Med 1987;1(3):142–6.

[41] Peterson ME, Gamble DA. Effect of nonthyroidal illness on serum thyroxine concentrations in cats: 494 cases (1988). J Am Vet Med Assoc 1990;197:1203–8.

[42] McLoughlin MA, DiBartola SP, Birchard SJ, et al. Influence of systemic nonthyroidal illness on serum concentration of thyroxine in hyperthyroid cats. J Am Anim Hosp Assoc 1993;29:227–34.

[43] Mooney CT, Little CJL, Macrae AW. Effects of illness not associated with the thyroid gland on serum total and free thyroxine concentration in cats. J Am Vet Med Assoc 1996; 208:2004–8.

[44] Paradis M, Page N. Serum free thyroxine concentrations measured by chemiluminescence in hyperthyroid and euthyroid cats. J Am Anim Hosp Assoc 1996;32:489–94.

[45] Mooney CT, Thoday KL, Doxey DL. Serum thyroxine and triiodothyronine responses of hyperthyroid cats to thyrotropin. Am J Vet Res 1996;57(7):987–91.

[46] Peterson ME, Graves TK, Gamble DA. Triiodothyronine (T3) suppression test: an aid in the diagnosis of mild hyperthyroidism in cats. J Vet Intern Med 1990;4(5):233–8.

[47] Refsal KR, Nachreiner RF, Stein BE, et al. Use of the triiodothyronine suppression test for diagnosis of hyperthyroidism in ill cats that have serum concentration of iodothyronines within normal range. J Am Vet Med Assoc 1991;199:1594–601.

[48] Sparkes AH, Jones BR, Gruffydd-Jones TJ, et al. Thyroid function in the cat: assessment by the TRH response test and the thyrotrophin stimulation test. J Soc Adm Pharm 1991;32: 59–63.

[49] Peterson ME, Broussard JD, Gamble DA. Use of the thyrotropin releasing hormone stimulation test to diagnose mild hyperthyroidism in cats. J Vet Intern Med 1994;8(4): 279–86.

[50] Tomsa K, Glaus TM, Kacl GM, et al. Thyrotropin-releasing hormone stimulation test to assess thyroid function in severely sick cats. J Vet Intern Med 2001;15:89–93.

[51] Adams WH, Daniel GB, Legendre AM. Investigation of the effects of hyperthyroidism on renal function in the cat. Can J Vet Res 1997;61:53–6.

[52] Becker TJ, Graves TK, Kruger JM, et al. Effects of methimazole on renal function in cats with hyperthyroidism. J Am Anim Hosp Assoc 2000;36:215–23.

[53] Peterson ME, Kintzer PP, Lewis SI. Methimazole treatment of 262 cats with hyperthyroidism. J Vet Intern Med 1988;2:150–7.

[54] Mooney CT, Thoday KL, Doxey DL. Carbimazole therapy for feline hyperthyroidism. J Soc Adm Pharm 1992;33:228–35.

[55] Trepanier LA, Hoffman SB, Kroll M, et al. Efficacy and safety of once versus twice daily administration of methimazole in cats with hyperthyroidism. J Am Vet Med Assoc 2003; 222:954–8.

[56] Hoffmann G, Marks SL, Taboada J, et al. Transdermal methimazole treatment in cats with hyperthyroidism. J Feline Med Surg 2003;5(2):77–82.

[57] Foster DJ, Thoday KL. Use of propranolol and potassium iodate in the presurgical management of hyperthyroid cats. J Soc Adm Pharm 1999;40:307–15.

[58] Murray LAS, Peterson ME. Ipodate treatment of hyperthyroidism in cats. J Am Vet Med Assoc 1997;211:63–7.

[59] Birchard SJ, Peterson ME, Jacobson A. Surgical treatment of feline hyperthyroidism: results from 85 cases. J Am Anim Hosp Assoc 1984;20(5):705–9.

[60] Flanders JA, Harvey HJ, Erb HN. Feline thyroidectomy: a comparison of postoperative hypocalcemia associated with three different surgical techniques. Vet Surg 1987;16(5): 362–6.

[61] Welches CD, Scavelli TD, Matthieson DT, et al. Occurrence of problems after three techniques of bilateral thyroidectomy in cats. Vet Surg 1989;18(5):392–6.

[62] Flanders JA. Surgical options for the treatment of hyperthyroidism in the cat. J Feline Med Surg 1999;1(3):127–34.

[63] Guptill L, Scott-Moncrieff CR, Janovitz EB, et al. Response to high-dose radioactive iodine administration in cats with thyroid carcinoma that had previously undergone surgery. J Am Vet Med Assoc 1995;207(8):1055–8.

[64] Meric SM, Hawkins EC, Washabau RJ, et al. Serum thyroxine concentrations after radioactive iodine therapy in cats with hyperthyroidism. J Am Vet Med Assoc 1986;188(9): 1038–40.

[65] Klausner JS, Johnston GR, Feeney DA, et al. Results of radioactive iodine therapy in 23 cats with hyperthyroidism. Minn J Vet Med 1987;27:28–32.

[66] Meric SM, Rubin SI. Serum thyroxine concentrations following fixed-dose radioactive iodine treatment in hyperthyroid cats: 62 cases (1986–1989). J Am Vet Med Assoc 1990; 197(5):621–3.

[67] Malik R, Lamb WA, Church DB. Treatment of feline hyperthyroidism using orally administered radio-iodine: a study of 40 consecutive cases. Aust Vet J 1993;70: 218–9.

[68] Mooney CT. Radioactive iodine therapy for feline hyperthyroidism: efficacy and administration routes. J Soc Adm Pharm 1994;35:289–94.

[69] Slater MR, Komkov A, Robinson LE, et al. Long-term follow-up of hyperthyroid cats treated with iodine-131. Vet Radiol Ultrasound 1994;35(3):204–9.

[70] Theon AP, Van Vechten MK, Feldman EC. Prospective randomised comparison of intravenous versus subcutaneous administration for treatment of hyperthyroidism in cats. Am J Vet Res 1994;55(12):1734–8.

[71] Peterson ME, Becker DV. Radioiodine treatment of 524 cats with hyperthyroidism. J Am Vet Med Assoc 1995;207:1422–8.

[72] Turrel JM, Feldman EC, Hays M, et al. Radioactive iodine therapy in cats with hyperthyroidism. J Am Vet Med Assoc 1984;184(5):554–9.

[73] Slater MR, Geller S, Rogers K. Long-term health and predictors of survival for hyperthyroid cats treated with iodine 131. J Vet Intern Med 2001;15:47–51.

[74] Nieckarz JA, Daniel GB. The effect of methimazole on thyroid uptake of pertechnetate and radioiodine in normal cats. Vet Radiol Ultrasound 2001;42(5):448–57.

[75] Chastain CB, Panciera D. The effect of methimazole on thyroid uptake of pertechnetate and radioiodine in normal cats. Small Anim Clin Endocrinol 2002;12(2):448–57.

[76] Chun R, Garrett LD, Sargeant J, et al. Predictors of response to radioiodine in hyperthyroid cats. Vet Radiol Ultrasound 2002;43(6):587–91.

[77] Wells AL, Long GD, Hornof WJ, et al. Use of percutaneous ethanol injection for treatment of bilateral hyperplastic thyroid nodules in cats. J Am Vet Med Assoc 2001;218(8):1293–7.

[78] Goldstein RE, Long GD, Swift NC, et al. Percutaneous ethanol injection for treatment of unilateral hyperplastic thyroid nodules in cats. J Am Vet Med Assoc 2001;218(8):1298–302.

[79] Mallery KF, Pollard RE, Nelson RW, et al. Percutaneous ultrasound-guided radio-frequency heat ablation for the treatment of hyperthyroidism in cats. J Am Vet Med Assoc 2003;223(11):1602–7.

[80] Rand JS, Levine J, Best SJ, et al. Spontaneous adult-onset hypothyroidism in a cat. J Vet Intern Med 1993;7(5):272–6.

[81] Arnold U, Opitz M, Grosser I, et al. Goitrous hypothyroidism and dwarfism in a kitten. J Am Anim Hosp Assoc 1984;20:753–8.

[82] Peterson ME. Feline hypothyroidism. In: Kirk RW, editor. Current veterinary therapy X. Philadelphia: WB Saunders; 1989. p. 1000–1.

[83] Sjollema BE, den Hartog MT, de Vijlder JJ, et al. Congenital hypothyroidism in two cats due to defective organification: data suggesting loosely anchored thyroperoxidase. Acta Endocrinol 1991;125(4):435–40.

[84] Jones BR, Gruffydd-Jones TJ, Sparkes AH, et al. Preliminary studies on congenital hypothyroidism in a family of Abyssinian cats. Vet Rec 1992;131:145–8.

[85] Tanase H, Kudo K, Horikoshi H, et al. Inherited hypothyroidism with thyrotropin resistance in Japanese cats. J Endocrinol 1991;129(2):245–51.

[86] Schumm-Draeger PM, Fortmeyer HP. Autoimmune thyroiditis: spontaneous disease models—cat. Exp Clin Endocrinol Diabetes 1996;104:12–3.

[87] Graham PA, Refsal KR, Nachreiner RF, et al. The measurement of feline thyrotropin (TSH) using a commercial canine immunoradiometric assay [abstract]. J Vet Intern Med 2000;14:342.

[88] Eigenmann JE, Wortman JA, Haskins ME. Elevated growth hormone levels and diabetes mellitus in a cat with acromegalic features. J Am Anim Hosp Assoc 1984;20:747–52.

[89] Middleton DJ, Culvenor JA, Vasak E, et al. Growth hormone-producing adenoma, elevated serum somatomedin C concentration and diabetes mellitus in a cat. Can Vet J 1985;26:169–71.

[90] Lichtensteiger CA, Wortman JA, Eigenmann JE. Functional pituitary acidophil adenoma in a cat with diabetes mellitus and acromegalic features. Vet Pathol 1986;23:518–21.

[91] Kittleson MD, Pion PD, Lothrop CDJ, et al. Hypersomatotropism in a cat presented with hypertrophic cardiomyopathy (HCM) and insulin resistance but without diabetes mellitus (DM) [abstract]. J Vet Intern Med 1989;3:126.

[92] Morrison SA, Randolph J, Lothrop CD. Hypersomatotropism and insulin-resistant diabetes mellitus in a cat. J Am Vet Med Assoc 1989;1:91–4.

[93] Abrams-Ogg ACG, Holmberg DL, Stewart WA, et al. Acromegaly in a cat: diagnosis by magnetic resonance imaging and treatment by cryohypophysectomy. Can Vet J 1993;34:682–5.

[94] Goossens MM, Feldman EC, Nelson RW, et al. Cobalt 60 irradiation of pituitary gland tumors in three cats with acromegaly. J Am Vet Med Assoc 1998;3(1):374–6.

[95] Feldman EC, Nelson RW. Acromegaly and hyperadrenocorticism in cats: a clinical perspective. J Feline Med Surg 2000;2:153–8.

[96] Norman EJ, Mooney CT. Diagnosis and management of diabetes mellitus in five cats with somatotrophic abnormalities. J Feline Med Surg 2000;1:183–90.

[97] Peterson ME. Effects of megestrol acetate on glucose tolerance and growth hormone secretion in the cat. Res Vet Sci 1987;42:354–7.

[98] Church DB, Watson ADJ, Emslie DR, et al. Effects of proligestone and megestrol on plasma adrenocorticotrophic hormone, insulin and insulin-like growth factor-1 concentrations in cats. Res Vet Sci 1994;56:175–8.

[99] Rosenfeld RG, Wilson DM, Dollar LA, et al. Both human pituitary growth hormone and recombinant DNA-derived human growth hormone cause insulin resistance at a post-receptor site. J Clin Endocrinol Metab 1982;54:1033–8.

[100] Peterson ME, Taylor RS, Greco DS, et al. Acromegaly in 14 cats. J Vet Intern Med 1990;4: 192–201.

[101] Lewitt MS, Hazel SJ, Church DB, et al. Regulation of insulin-like growth factor binding protein-3 ternary complex in feline diabetes mellitus. J Endocrinol 2000;166:21–7.

[102] Starkey SR, Tan K, Church DB. Investigation of serum IGF-1 levels amongst diabetic and non-diabetic cats. J Feline Med Surg 2004;6:149–55.

[103] Kokka N, Garcia JF, Morgan M, et al. Immunoassay of plasma growth hormone in cats following fasting and administration of insulin, arginine, 2-deoxyglucose and hypothalamic extract. Endocrinology 1971;88:359–66.

[104] Kaser-Hotz B, Rohrer CR, Stankeova S, et al. Radiotherapy of pituitary tumours in five cats. J Soc Adm Pharm 2002;43:303–7.

[105] Green RA, Farrow CS. Diabetes insipidus in a cat. J Am Vet Med Assoc 1974;164: 524–6.

[106] Rogers WA, Valdez H, Anderson BC, et al. Partial deficiency in antidiuretic hormone in a cat. J Am Vet Med Assoc 1977;170(5):545–7.

[107] Burnie AG, Dunn JK. A case of central diabetes insipidus in the cat: diagnosis and treatment. J Soc Adm Pharm 1982;23:237–41.

[108] Court MH, Watson AD. Idiopathic neurogenic diabetes insipidus in a cat. Aust Vet J 1983; 60(8):245–7.

[109] Feldman EC, Nelson RW. Polydipsia and polyuria. In: Pedersen D, editor. Canine and feline endocrinology and reproduction. Philadelphia: WB Saunders; 1987. p. 1–26.

[110] Kraus KH. The use of desmopressin in diagnosis and treatment of diabetes insipidus in cats. Compend Contin Educ Pract Vet 1987;9:752–8.

[111] Pittari JM. Central diabetes insipidus in a cat. Feline Pract 1996;24(4):18–21.

[112] Peterson ME, Randolf JH. Endocrine diseases. In: Sherding RG, editor. The cat: diseases and clinical management. New York: Churchill Livingston; 1989. p. 1101–3.

[113] Peterson ME, Steele P. Pituitary-dependent hyperadrenocorticism in a cat. J Am Vet Med Assoc 1986;189(6):680–3.

[114] Nelson RW, Feldman EC, Smith MC. Hyperadrenocorticism in cats: seven cases (1978–1987). J Am Vet Med Assoc 1988;193(2):245–50.

[115] Immink WF, van Toor AJ, Vos JH, et al. Hyperadrenocorticism in four cats. Vet Q 1992;15: 81–5.

[116] Duesberg CA, Nelson RW, Feldman EC, et al. Adrenalectomy for the treatment of hyperadrenocorticism in cats: 10 cases (1988–1992). J Am Vet Med Assoc 1995;207: 1066–70.

[117] Watson PJ, Herrtage ME. Hyperadrenocorticism in six cats. J Soc Adm Pharm 1998;39: 175–84.

[118] Skelly BJ, Petrus D, Nicholls PK. Use of trilostane for the treatment of pituitary-dependent hyperadrenocorticism in a cat. J Soc Adm Pharm 2003;44(6):269–72.

[119] Neiger R, Witt AL, Noble A, et al. Trilostane therapy for treatment of pituitary-dependent hyperadrenocorticism in 5 cats. J Vet Intern Med 2004;18:160–4.

[120] Valentine RW, Silber A. Feline hyperadrenocorticism: a rare case. Feline Pract 1996;24(2): 6–11.

[121] Chastain CB, Graham CL, Nichols CE. Adrenocortical suppression in cats given megestrol acetate. Am J Vet Res 1981;42(12):2029–35.

[122] Greene CE, Carmichael KP, Gratzek A. Iatrogenic hyperadrenocorticism in a cat. Feline Pract 1995;23(5):7–12.

[123] Schaer M, Ginn PE. Iatrogenic Cushing's syndrome and steroid hepatopathy in a cat. J Am Anim Hosp Assoc 1999;35:48–51.

[124] Ferasin L. Iatrogenic hyperadrenocorticism in a cat following a short therapeutic course of methylprednisolone acetate. J Feline Med Surg 2001;3:87–93.

[125] Smith SA, Freeman LC, Bagladi-Swanson M. Hypercalcemia due to iatrogenic secondary hypoadrenocorticism and diabetes mellitus in a cat. J Am Anim Hosp Assoc 2002;38:41–4.

[126] Myers NC, Bruyette DS. Feline adrenocortical diseases: part I—hyperadrenocorticism. Semin Vet Med Surg (Small Anim) 1994;9:137–43.

[127] Toll J, Ashe CM, Trepanier LA. Intravesicular administration of clotrimazole for treatment of candiduria in a cat with diabetes mellitus. J Am Vet Med Assoc 2003;223(8): 1156–8.

[128] Widmer WR, Guptill L. Imaging techniques for facilitating diagnosis of hyperadrenocorticism in dogs and cats. J Am Vet Med Assoc 1995;206(12):1857–64.

[129] Goossens MMC, Meyer HP, Voorhout G, et al. Urinary excretion of glucocorticoids in the diagnosis of hyperadrenocorticism in cats. Dom Anim Endocrinol 1995;12:355–62.

[130] Henry CJ, Clark TP, Young DW, et al. Urine cortisol:creatinine ratio in healthy and sick cats. J Vet Intern Med 1996;10:123–6.

[131] de Lange MS, Galac S, Trip MR, et al. High urinary corticoid/creatinine ratios in cats with hyperthyroidism. J Vet Intern Med 2004;18(2):152–5.

[132] Cauvin AL, Witt AL, Groves E, et al. The urinary corticoid:creatinine ratio (UCCR) in healthy cats undergoing hospitalization. J Feline Med Surg 2003;5:329–33.

[133] Zerbe CA. Feline hyperadrenocorticism. In: Kirk RW, editor. Current veterinary therapy X. Philadelphia: WB Saunders; 1989. p. 1038–42.

[134] Smith MC, Feldman EC. Plasma endogenous ACTH concentration and plasma cortisol response to synthetic ACTH and dexamethasone sodium phosphate in healthy cats. Am J Vet Res 1987;48:1719–24.

[135] Duesberg CA, Peterson ME. Adrenal disorders in cats. Vet Clin N Am Small Anim Pract 1997;27:321–47.

[136] Peterson ME, Kintzer PP, Foodman MS, et al. Adrenal function in the cat: comparison of the effects of cosyntropin (synthetic ACTH) and corticotrophin gel stimulation. Res Vet Sci 1984;37:331–3.

[137] Zerbe CA, Refsal KR, Peterson ME, et al. Effect of non-adrenal illness on adrenal function in the cat. Am J Vet Res 1987;48:451–4.

[138] Sparkes AH, Adams DT, Douthwaite JA, et al. Assessment of adrenal function in cats: response to intravenous synthetic ACTH. J Soc Adm Pharm 1990;31:1–4.

[139] Peterson ME, Kemppainen RJ. Dose-response relation between plasma concentration of corticotrophin and cortisol after administration of incremental doses of cosyntropin for corticotrophin stimulation testing in cats. Am J Vet Res 1993;54:300–4.

[140] Bruyette DS. Adrenal function testing. In: August JR, editor. Consultations in feline internal medicine. 2nd edition. Philadelphia: WB Saunders; 1994. p. 129–32.

[141] Meij BP, Voorhout G, Van Den Ingh TS, et al. Transsphenoidal hypophysectomy for treatment of pituitary-dependent hyperadrenocorticism in 7 cats. Vet Surg 2001;30:72–86.

[142] Cartee RE, Hudson JA, Finn-Bodner S. Ultrasonography. Vet Clin N Am Small Anim Pract 1993;23:345–77.

[143] Zimmer C, Horauf A, Reusch C. Ultrasonographic examination of the adrenal gland and evaluation of the hypophyseal-adrenal axis in 20 cats. J Soc Adm Pharm 2000;41:156–60.

[144] Elliott DA, Feldman EC, Koblik PD, Samii VF, Nelson RW. Prevalence of pituitary tumours among diabetic cats with insulin resistance. J Am Vet Med Assoc 2000;216:1765–8.

[145] Boord M, Griffin C. Progesterone secreting adrenal mass in a cat with clinical signs of hyperadrenocorticism. J Am Vet Med Assoc 1999;214(5):666–9.

[146] Rossmeisl JH, Scott-Moncrieff JCR, Siems J, et al. Hyperadrenocorticism and hyper-progesteronemia in a cat with an adrenocortical adenocarcinoma. J Am Anim Hosp Assoc 2000;36:512–7.

[147] Schwedes CS. Mitotane (o, p'-DDD) treatment in a cat with hyperadrenocorticism. J Soc Adm Pharm 1997;38:520–4.

[148] Willard MD, Nachreiner RF, Howard VC, et al. Effect of long-term administration of ketoconazole in cats. Am J Vet Res 1986;47:2510–3.

[149] Jones CA, Refsal KR, Stevens BJ, et al. Adrenocortical adenocarcinoma in a cat. J Am Anim Hosp Assoc 1992;28:59–62.

[150] Feldman EC, Nelson RW. Hyperadrenocorticism. In: Feldman EC, Nelson RW, editors. Canine and feline endocrinology and reproduction. 2nd edition. Philadelphia: WB Saunders; 1996. p. 187–261.

[151] Feldman EC, Nelson RW. Hypoadrenocorticism in cats. In: Feldman EC, Nelson RW, editors. Canine and feline endocrinology and reproduction. 2nd edition. Philadelphia: WB Saunders; 1996. p. 302–6.

[152] Daley CA, Zerbe CA, Schick RO, et al. Use of metyrapone to treat pituitary-dependent hyperadrenocorticism in a cat with large cutaneous wounds. J Am Vet Med Assoc 1993;202: 956–60.

[153] Moore LE, Biller DS, Olsen DE. Hyperadrenocorticism treated with metyrapone followed by bilateral adrenalectomy. J Am Vet Med Assoc 2000;217:691–4.

[154] Moore LE, Biller DS, Smith TA. Use of abdominal ultrasonography in the diagnosis of primary hyperaldosteronism. J Am Vet Med Assoc 2000;217:213–5.

[155] Neiger R, Ramsey I, O'Connor J, et al. Trilostane treatment of 78 dogs with pituitary-dependent hyperadrenocorticism. Vet Rec 2002;150:799–804.

[156] Eastwood JM, Elwood CM, Hurley KJ. Trilostane treatment of a dog with functional adrenocortical neoplasia. J Soc Adm Pharm 2003;44(3):126–31.

[157] Boag AK, Neiger R, Church DB. Trilostane treatment of bilateral adrenal enlargement and excessive sex steroid hormone production in a cat. J Soc Adm Pharm 2004;45(5):263–6.

[158] Chapman PS, Kelly DF, Archer J, et al. Adrenal necrosis in a dog receiving trilostane for the treatment of hyperadrenocorticism. J Soc Adm Pharm 2004;45(6):307–10.

[159] Meij B, Voorhout G, Rijnberk A. Progress in transsphenoidal hypophysectomy for treatment of pituitary-dependent hyperadrenocorticism in dogs and cats. Mol Cell Endocrinol 2002;197(1–2):89–96.

[160] Eger CE, Robinson WF, Huxtable CR. Primary hyperaldosteronism (Conn's syndrome) in a cat: a case report and review of comparative aspects. J Soc Adm Pharm 1983;24:293–307.

[161] Ahn A. Hyperaldosteronism in cats. Semin Vet Med Surg 1994;9(3):153–7.

[162] Flood SM, Randolph JF, Gelzer ARM, et al. Primary hyperaldosteronism in two cats. J Am Anim Hosp Assoc 1999;35:411–6.

[163] Rijnberk A, Voorhout G, Kooistra HS, et al. Hyperaldosteronism in a cat with metastasized adrenocortical tumour. Vet Q 2001;23:38–43.

[164] Henry CJ, Brewer WG, Montgomery, et al. Clinical vignette: adrenal pheochromocytoma. J Vet Intern Med 1993;7(3):199–201.

[165] Patnaik AK, Erlandson RA, Lieberman PH, et al. Extra-adrenal pheochromocytoma (paraganglioma) in a cat. J Am Vet Med Assoc 1990;197:104–6.

[166] Chun R, Jakovljevic S, Morrison WB, et al. Apocrine gland adenocarcinoma and pheochromocytoma in a cat. J Am Anim Hosp Assoc 1997;33:33–6.

[167] Carpenter JL, Andrews LK, Holzworth J. Tumors and tumor-like lesions. In: Holzworth J, editor. Diseases of the cat: medicine and surgery, vol. 1. Philadelphia: WB Saunders; 1987. p. 541–4.

[168] Maher ER. Pheochromocytoma in the dog and cat: diagnosis and management. Semin Vet Med Surg 1994;9(3):158–66.

[169] Johnessee JS, Peterson ME, Gilbertson SR. Primary hypoadrenocorticism in a cat. J Am Vet Med Assoc 1983;183:881–2.

[170] Berger SL, Reed JR. Traumatically induced hypoadrenocorticism in a cat. J Am Anim Hosp Assoc 1993;29:337–9.

[171] Brain PH. Trauma-induced hypoadrenocorticism in a cat. Aust Vet Pract 1997;27:178–81.

[172] Parnell NK, Powell LL, Hohenhaus AE, et al. Hypoadrenocorticism as the primary manifestation of lymphoma in two cats. J Am Vet Med Assoc 1999;214:1208–11.

[173] Feldman EC. Adrenal gland disease. In: Ettinger S, editor. Textbook of veterinary internal medicine. Philadelphia: WB Saunders; 1989. p. 1771.

[174] Peterson ME, Greco DS. Primary hypoadrenocorticism in the cat. In: American College of Veterinary Internal Medicine Scientific Proceedings, Washington, DC, 1986. Blacksburg (VA): American College of Veterinary Internal Medicine; 1986. p. 42.

[175] Peterson ME, Greco DS, Orth DN. Primary hypoadrenocorticism in 10 cats. J Vet Intern Med 1989;3:55–8.

[176] Hardy RM. Hypoadrenal gland disease. In: Ettinger SJ, Feldman EC, editors. Textbook of veterinary internal medicine. 4th edition. Philadelphia: WB Saunders; 1995. p. 1579–93.

[177] Stonehewer J, Tasker S. Hypoadrenocorticism in a cat. J Soc Adm Pharm 2001;42:186–90.

[178] Myers NC, Bruyette DS. Feline adrenocortical diseases: part I—hypoadrenocorticism. Semin Vet Med Surg (Small Anim) 1994;9:144–7.

[179] Kallet AJ, Richter KP, Feldman EC, et al. Primary hyperparathyroidism in cats: seven cases (1984–1989). J Am Vet Med Assoc 1991;199(12):1767–71.

[180] Marquez GA, Klausner JS, Osborne CA. Calcium oxalate urolithiasis in a cat with a functional parathyroid adenocarcinoma. J Am Vet Med Assoc 1995;206(6):817–9.

[181] Den Hertog E, Goossens MMC, van der Linde-Sipman JS, et al. Primary hyperparathyroidism in two cats. Vet Q 1997;19:81–4.

[182] Savary KCM, Price GS, Vaden SL. Hypercalemia in cats: a retrospective study of 71 cases (1991–1997). J Vet Intern Med 2000;14:184–9.

[183] Sueda MT, Stefanacci JD. Ultrasound examination of the parathyroid glands in two hypercalcemic cats. Vet Radiol Ultrasound 2000;41:448–51.

[184] Kaplan E. Primary hyperparathyroidism and concurrent hyperthyroidism in a cat. Can Vet J 2002;43:117–9.

[185] Mealey KL, Willard MD, Nagode LA, et al. Hypercalcemia associated with granulomatous disease in a cat. J Am Vet Med Assoc 1999;215:959–62.

[186] Forbes S, Nelson RW, Guptill L. Primary hypoparathyroidism in a cat. J Am Vet Med Assoc 1990;196(8):1285–7.

[187] Parker JSL. A probable case of hypoparathyroidism in a cat. J Soc Adm Pharm 1991;32: 470–3.

[188] Peterson ME, James KM, Wallace M, et al. Idiopathic hypoparathyroidism in five cats. J Vet Intern Med 1991;5:47–51.

[189] Bassett JR. Hypocalcemia and hyperphosphatemia due to primary hypoparathyroidism in a six-month-old kitten. J Am Anim Hosp Assoc 1998;34:503–7.

[190] Ruopp JL. Primary hypoparathyroidism in a cat complicated by suspect iatrogenic calcinosis cutis. J Am Anim Hosp Assoc 2001;37:370–3.

[191] Mawhinney AD, Rahaley RS, Belford CJ. Primary hypoadrenocorticism in a cat. Aust Vet Pract 1989;19:46–9.

[192] Ash RA, Harvey AM, Tasker S. Primary hyperaldosteronism in eleven cats [abstract]. J Vet Intern Med 2004;18:793–4.

ELSEVIER
SAUNDERS

Vet Clin Small Anim
35 (2005) 211–224

VETERINARY
CLINICS
Small Animal Practice

Diabetes Mellitus in Cats

Jacquie S. Rand, BVSc, DVSc[a],*,
Rhett D. Marshall, BVSc[a,b]

[a]*Centre for Companion Animal Health, School of Veterinary Science,
The University of Queensland, Brisbane, Queensland 4072, Australia*
[b]*Creek Road Cat Clinic, Brisbane, Australia*

Pathogenesis

Feline diabetes is one of the most common endocrinopathies in cats. The frequency of feline diabetes varies with the population studied, with 1 in 200 cats affected in a first-accession feline practice and higher (1 in 100 cats) and lower (1 in 400 cats) frequencies reported in other populations [1–3]. Burmese cats are predisposed to diabetes in Australia, New Zealand, and the United Kingdom (Gunn-Moore, BVM&S, PhD, unpublished data) [1,4], with 1 in 50 cats affected in Australia [2]. Increasing age is a risk factor for feline diabetes, and most affected cats are older than 8 years, with a peak incidence between 10 and 13 years [2,3]. Increasing age is also important in Burmese cats, with 1 in 10 Burmese cats 8 years of age or older reported to be diabetic [2]. The incidence of diabetes in cats is increasing, as it is in people [5]. The increase is likely because of an increase in obesity in cats, which is a factor recognized to increase the risk for feline diabetes [5,6].

Approximately 80% to 95% of diabetic cats seem to have type 2 diabetes based on islet histology and clinical characteristics of the disease [7]. A relatively small percentage of diabetic cats have other specific types of diabetes characterized by diseases that destroy β cells, such as pancreatitis or neoplasia, or cause marked insulin resistance, such as growth hormone excess (acromegaly) [8,9].

What is type 2 diabetes?

Type 2 diabetes was previously called adult-onset diabetes or non–insulin-dependent diabetes. Type 2 diabetes is characterized by decreased

---

* Corresponding author.
E-mail address: j.rand@uq.edu.au (J.S. Rand).

insulin secretion combined with reduced insulin action, also known as decreased insulin sensitivity or insulin resistance [10]. Diabetic cats are, on average, six times less sensitive to insulin than nondiabetic cats [10].

What causes type 2 diabetes?

Type 2 diabetes results when there is β-cell failure, resulting in insufficient insulin being secreted to maintain normoglycemia [11]. A chronic high demand to secrete insulin is thought to lead to β-cell failure and loss through apoptosis, which is partially mediated by oxidative damage [11]. The major cause of this high demand for insulin secretion is insulin resistance [12]. In an insulin-resistant state, a higher plasma insulin concentration is required to produce the same glucose uptake into tissues compared with when insulin sensitivity is normal. A number of factors contribute to insulin resistance, including genotype, obesity, physical inactivity, diet, and drugs. Some cats have intrinsically low insulin sensitivity and are at risk of developing impaired glucose tolerance with weight gain [13]. Lean cats with insulin sensitivity values below the population median were shown to have three times the risk of developing impaired glucose when body weight increased by 2 kg compared with cats with higher insulin sensitivity values. Impaired glucose tolerance is a state between normal glucose tolerance and diabetes, and these cats are likely at increased risk of diabetes with time. In human beings, the underlying level of insulin sensitivity is genetically determined, but this has not been investigated in cats [11].

Obesity is a major factor decreasing insulin sensitivity, and cats that increased their body weight over 10 months by 2 kg (44%) had a 50% decrease in insulin sensitivity [13]. Insulin resistance from genotype and obesity are the most frequent factors predisposing to type 2 diabetes in people. Physical inactivity in people and dogs also decreases insulin sensitivity independent of body weight [14]. Urban cats, especially cats that are confined indoors and no longer hunt to obtain their food, are physically inactive compared with feral cats and are also likely insulin resistant. High-fat diets produce high fatty acid concentrations and reduce insulin sensitivity. High free fatty acid concentrations also suppress insulin secretion [15].

Drugs like corticosteroids and progestins decrease insulin sensitivity, especially if long-acting forms or repeated administration is used [9]. They also increase appetite, leading to weight gain, further reducing insulin sensitivity. Both drugs increase the risk of diabetes in cats [6].

In addition to β-cell exhaustion from chronic insulin resistance, β cells are lost as a result of amyloid deposition [16,17]. Mature amyloid fibrils surround β cells, isolating them from pancreatic blood vessels, and immature amyloid fibrils that form intracellularly are highly toxic to β cells [18]. On average, 30% of the islet is replaced by amyloid in diabetic cats, although some cats have more profound amyloid deposition [17]. Overt diabetes requires loss of more than 80% of islet cells [10], and although amyloid deposition alone may not cause diabetes in many cats, it contributes to β-cell loss. This loss of β cells increases the susceptibility to diabetes, particularly if there is increased demand for insulin secretion as a result of intrinsic factors and obesity.

Pancreatitis is evident histologically in approximately 50% of diabetic cats [17,19]. In most cats, it is insufficient to cause diabetes by itself, but in many cats, it seems to be a contributor to β-cell loss.

Once blood glucose rises, it causes suppression of insulin secretion, a phenomenon called glucose toxicity. Initially, the suppression of insulin secretion is reversible, but it later causes β-cell loss [20,21]. When first diagnosed, many diabetic cats respond poorly to oral hypoglycemic agents and need insulin for adequate glycemic control. With recovery of β cells from glucose toxicity, however, many cats regain sufficient β-cell function such that they no longer require insulin, which is termed *diabetic remission*.

Diets high in carbohydrates put a large demand on β cells to secrete insulin and likely contribute to β-cell failure when fed long-term in cats predisposed to diabetes because of low insulin sensitivity [22].

Clinical signs and diagnosis

There are no internationally agreed on criteria for the diagnosis of diabetes mellitus in cats [6]. Clinical signs, such as polydipsia/polyuria, weight loss, or polyphagia, are nonspecific, and the diagnosis cannot be confirmed by clinical examination. Diagnosis in cats is often complicated by stress hyperglycemia, which may lead to glycosuria or blood glucose levels in excess of 360 mg/dL (20 mmol/L) in sick nondiabetic cats [23]. Blood glucose in nondiabetic, unstressed, client-owned cats is usually less than 171 mg/dL (9.5 mmol/L) [24]. When sampling blood, it is important to avoid the cat struggling, because this has been shown to be associated with transient hyperglycemia as high as 288 mg/dL (16 mmol/L) in normal cats [25]. Blood glucose should be measured several hours after the first sample to confirm persistent hyperglycemia, especially if the blood glucose level is less than 360 mg/dL (20 mmol/L). Signs of diabetes occur once the blood glucose concentration exceeds the renal threshold, which is approximately 288 mg/dL (16 mmol/L) for normal cats [26].

Fructosamine may be useful in assisting in diagnosis, especially when typical clinical signs of diabetes have not been observed or reported. Some cats that do not have diabetes have elevated fructosamine levels similar to those of diabetic cats (false-positive results), and, occasionally, untreated diabetic cats may have fructosamine levels similar to those of normal cats (false-negative results) [27]. A fructosamine concentration of greater than 400 μmol/L in a cat strongly supports a diagnosis of diabetes [27,28]. In experimentally-induced hyperglycemia in cats, although fructosamine concentration increased significantly from baseline within 3 days when the blood glucose concentration was maintained at 306 or 540 mg/dL (17 or 30 mmol/L), mean fructosamine did not increase higher than 350 µmol/L when glucose was 306 mg/dL (17 mmol/L) for 6 weeks [21].

Elevated glycated hemoglobin demonstrates hyperglycemia over a slightly longer period than fructosamine and can also be used to aid in diagnosis [29,30]. As with fructosamine, glycated hemoglobin is neither fully sensitive nor specific for the diagnosis of feline diabetes mellitus [29]. Reported reference ranges for glycated hemoglobin vary considerably, and values should be interpreted based on the reference range for the laboratory [29,31–33].

Measurement of water intake is inexpensive and useful for confirming polydipsia once the blood glucose concentration is higher than the renal threshold. In normal cats, total water intake, including water in food, ranges from 60 to 100 mL/kg every 24 hours, but water drunk is much less, especially if the cat is consuming canned food, with an average value of approximately 20 mL/kg [34,35]. Measurement of water intake to document polydipsia may only be practical in a cat that is clinically healthy, and the decision to treat can be delayed by a few days.

If there is doubt as to whether the hyperglycemia is transient and associated with stress or is from diabetes, it is prudent to begin insulin therapy and monitor glucose concentrations carefully for the next few days in sick cats. Reducing glucose concentration with exogenous insulin reduces the suppressive effect of glucose toxicity and makes recovery of β cells more likely. Because glucose toxicity can reduce insulin secretion in normal cats to levels of insulin-dependent diabetic cats within 3 to 7 days, do not wait to begin insulin therapy if the blood glucose concentration is 270 mg/dL (15 mmol/L) or higher. Likewise, in cats with iatrogenic or spontaneous hyperadrenocorticism or acromegaly, begin insulin therapy immediately to preserve remaining β cells. Therapy for the underlying disease can then be instituted, and glucose concentrations can be monitored to adjust insulin dose. Do not wait to see if the diabetes resolves once the underlying disease process is treated or the exogenous hormone is eliminated, because this makes permanent diabetes more likely.

Ketoacidosis

Ketoacidosis occurs in approximately 12% to 37% of diabetic cats at the time of diagnosis, and a smaller percentage are ketotic without acidosis [19,27]. Ketoacidosis results in depression, vomiting, and anorexia. Ketoacidosis can be precipitated by concomitant disease, especially infection [36]. It is also important to realize that once cats become markedly insulinopenic, even previously normal cats progress to ketosis within 10 to 30 days, without evidence of precipitating disease [21]. If untreated, acidosis quickly ensues [21]. Small doses of insulin usually correct ketonemia and prevent life-threatening acidosis, even if marked hyperglycemia persists [21]. In experimentally-induced diabetes, ketonemia occurred, on average, 5 days before ketonuria was detected using a urine test strip, and an acetone odor to the breath was also detected before ketonuria [21]. Although ketotic cats usually have low insulin concentrations, with appropriate therapy to overcome glucose toxicity and lipotoxicity, some β-cell function may return.

Concomitant disease in diabetic cats

Concomitant disease is common in diabetic cats at the time of diagnosis [27]. This is partly attributable to the advanced age of most diabetic cats. It is also because some diseases predispose to diabetes, (eg, pancreatic neoplasia, hyperadrenocorticism) and diabetes predisposes to other diseases (eg, infection, bacterial cystitis). Diseases found concurrently at the time of diagnosis include hyperthyroidism, inflammatory bowel disease, eosinophilic granuloma complex, anemia, neoplasia, and renal failure [27].

Treatment

Therapy for diabetes should be instituted as soon as possible after diagnosis. The aims of therapy are to treat any underlying disease and to achieve good glycemic control. Administration of insulin and dietary modification are the principal therapies used for the management of diabetic cats. A recent study has shown that if good glycemic control is achieved early in newly diagnosed diabetic cats, high remission rates occur within 4 weeks of treatment [37]. Good glycemic control reverses the glucose toxicity suppressing β cells, and maximizes the chance of preserving β-cell function and achieving diabetic remission. Because clinical hypoglycemia can be life threatening, avoid aiming for perfect glycemic control, especially if using lente insulin, because the risk for hypoglycemia is increased. The use of longer acting insulin and low-carbohydrate diets may facilitate achieving better glycemic control while minimizing the chance of hypoglycemia. Cats that are not substantially dehydrated and are still eating can be treated with subcutaneous insulin or oral hypoglycemic drugs. Cats initially presented with diabetic ketoacidosis can be treated with subcutaneous insulin after stabilization.

Oral hypoglycemic drugs

The use of oral hypoglycemic drugs to treat feline diabetes has been limited for a number of reasons. Many owners find administering tablets more difficult than injecting the cat with insulin. Drugs that stimulate insulin secretion (eg, sulphonylureas) require adequate β-cell function to be effective, and if there is an inadequate glucose-lowering effect, persistent hyperglycemia can lead to continued β-cell loss through glucose and lipid toxicity. These drugs may also stimulate accelerated islet amyloid deposition, exacerbating β-cell loss.

The α-glucosidase inhibitors (eg, acarbose) reduce intestinal glucose absorption [38] and are generally not effective in the treatment of feline diabetes alone but can be used in conjunction with insulin or other oral agents to gain better glycemic control. Cats given acarbose and fed a low-carbohydrate diet had a reduced insulin requirement and improved glycemic control, but similar results were achieved feeding the low-carbohydrate diet alone [39].

Chromium and vanadium are transitional metals that potentiate insulin action. Chromium has been shown to produce small but significant decreases in blood glucose in healthy cats [40], but there are no reports of its efficacy in diabetic cats. Vanadium is reported to reduce the insulin requirement of diabetic cats [41]. There is renewed interest in both metals in human medicine, but further investigation into their use in veterinary medicine is required before definite conclusions and recommendations are made.

Insulin-sensitizing drugs (thiazolidinediones and biguanides) increase the response of muscle, liver, and fat cells to insulin [42,43]. Their main effect is to decrease peripheral insulin resistance and, in muscle, to increase glucose uptake stimulated by insulin. They also reduce hepatic glucose production. In theory, these drugs should be invaluable in reversing insulin resistance, but there are currently no reports of their successful use in diabetic cats. Insulin sensitivity and lipid metabolism can be improved in obese cats using the insulin-sensitizing drug darglitazone [44].

Insulin therapy

Insulin therapy remains the preferred initial and long-term treatment of choice for diabetes mellitus in cats. Many types of insulin are available and have been used in cats [45–47]. Achieving good glycemic control with shorter acting potent insulins, such as neutral protamine Hagedorn (NPH), lente, and ultralente, is often difficult and increases the risk of clinical hypoglycemia. Recent data suggest that the longer acting insulins glargine and protamine zinc insulin (PZI) provide better glycemic control and reduced risk of clinical hypoglycemia when administered twice daily and combined with a low-carbohydrate diet (R.D. Marshall, BVSc and J.S. Rand, BVSc, DVSc, unpublished data, 2004).

Insulin glargine

Glargine, a new long-acting synthetic insulin analogue, has shown exciting results in healthy and diabetic cats. Glargine is marketed for human use as a "peakless" insulin, with regard to its glucose-lowering effect. By contrast, studies in healthy cats have shown that there is a peak action at approximately 16 hours, with significant suppression of blood glucose concentrations up to 24 hours in most cats [37]. Initial results in diabetic cats suggest that glargine is a better choice than lente insulin in diabetic cats, because glycemic control is better and diabetic remission rates are higher [48]. Studies in healthy cats indicate that twice-daily dosing provides optimal glycemic control, and preliminary studies in diabetic cats also support twice-daily use [37,48]. Although many cats may potentially be able to be maintained or controlled on once-daily dosing with glargine, the limited data available suggest that optimal glycemic control with minimal risk of clinical hypoglycemia occurs with twice-daily dosing.

Insulin glargine cannot be mixed or diluted because its slow absorption is dependent on its low pH and the interaction with subcutaneous fat. Glargine should be refrigerated because it has a shelf life of 4 weeks once opened and kept at room temperature. We have found that opened vials kept refrigerated can be used for more than 6 months. If using an insulin pen, the manufacturer recommends that once a vial of insulin is used, the pen be kept at room temperature because temperature changes associated with refrigeration alter the volume administered by the pen.

Insulin glargine should be dosed according to initial blood glucose concentration and calculated for ideal body weight. If the blood glucose concentration is equal or greater than 360 mg/dL (20 mmol/L), start with 0.5 U/kg twice daily, and if the blood glucose concentration is less than 360 mg/dL (20 mmol/L), start with 0.25 U/kg twice daily. A 12-hour serial blood glucose curve should be obtained with samples taken every 4 hours. Because of the long duration of action and likely overlap of insulin action, the dose should not be increased for the first week. The dose should be decreased if the blood glucose concentration decreases below normal, however. Cats should stay in the hospital for 3 days, or home glucose curves can be obtained for the first 3 days to check the initial response. Repeat serial curves should be obtained at weeks 1, 2, and 4 and then as required. It is important to be aware that many cats have little decrease in blood glucose concentration during the first 3 days of treatment with glargine, even if remission is achieved within 4 weeks. Therefore, glargine should not be used as the initial insulin therapy in sick ketoacidotic diabetic cats until studies show that it reverses ketoacidosis despite its minimal initial glucose-lowering effect.

Monitoring therapeutic efficacy

Response to treatment can be evaluated in a number of ways, and no individual modality should be used as the sole parameter for adjusting therapy. A combination of owner assessment, clinical signs, and changes in body weight and water intake is often the best indicator of glycemic control. Dosage changes can be made based on a number of different blood glucose parameters and should optimally include more than one parameter. The preinsulin glucose concentration is important when using glargine and PZI, because there is often a persisting effect from the previous injection (Table 1).

Table 1
Parameters for changing insulin dosage when using glargine or protamine zinc insulin in diabetic cats

Parameter used for dosage adjustment	Change in dose
If preinsulin blood glucose concentration is >360 mg/dL (>20 mmol/L) and/or nadir blood glucose concentration is >180 mg/dL (>10 mmol/L)	Increase by 0.5–1 U
If preinsulin blood glucose concentration is 270 to <360 mg/dL (15 to <20 mmol/L) and/or nadir blood glucose concentration is 90–180 mg/dL (5–10 mmol/L)	Same dose
If preinsulin blood glucose concentration is 190–270 mg/dL(11–14 mmol/L) and/or nadir glucose concentration is 54–72 mg/dL (3–4 mmol/L)	Use nadir, water drunk, urine glucose concentration, and next preinsulin glucose concentration to determine if insulin dose is decreased or maintained
If preinsulin blood glucose concentration is <180 mg/dL (10 mmol/L) and/or nadir blood glucose concentration is <54 mg/dL (<3 mmol/L)	Reduce by 0.5–1 U or if total dose is 0.5–1 U, stop insulin and check for diabetic remission
If clinical signs of hypoglycemia are observed	Reduce by 50%
If water intake is <20 mL/kg on wet food or <70 mL/kg on dry food	Same dose
If water intake is >40 mL/kg on wet food or >100 mL/kg on dry food	Increase dose by 0.5–1 U
If urine glucose score is >3+ (scale of 0–4+)	Increase dose by 0.5–1 U
If urine glucose concentration is negative	Reduce dose by 1 U and check for diabetic remission if on a minimal insulin dose

Nadir (lowest) glucose concentration can be used for dosage adjustment in a way similar to that used with other insulin types. Water drunk and urine glucose concentrations are probably more useful for adjusting dose when using glargine and PZI than for other types of insulin, but for all insulins should receive consideration.

When using other insulins (eg, lente or NPH), dosage changes are usually based on nadir blood glucose concentration. Preinsulin glucose concentration, time to nadir, and time to return to baseline are also used when appropriate, and recommendations for their use are listed in Table 2.

Determining if diabetic remission has occurred

Insulin dose should be decreased sequentially if indicated based on Table 1. After a minimum of 2 weeks of insulin therapy, if the preinsulin blood glucose concentration is less than 200 mg/dL (12 mmol/L), and insulin dose is only 0.5–1 U/cat once or twice per day, insulin should be withheld and a 12-hour glucose curve performed. If the blood glucose concentration is

Table 2
Parameters for changing insulin dosage and frequency based on blood glucose measurements when using lente, neutral protamine Hagedorn, or ultralente in diabetic cats

Blood glucose parameter	Recommendation
If preinsulin blood glucose concentration is <210 mg/dL (<12 mmol/L)	Withhold insulin and check for diabetic remission
If preinsulin blood glucose concentration is 234–288 mg/dL (13–16 mmol/L)	Total dose should be no more than 1 U per cat twice daily
If nadir blood glucose concentration is <54 mg/dL (<3 mmol/L)	Dose should be reduced by 50%
If nadir blood glucose concentration is 54–90 mg/dL (3–5 mmol/L)	Dose should be reduced by 1 U
If nadir blood glucose concentration is 91–162 mg/dL (6–9 mmol/L)	Dose should remain the same
If nadir blood glucose concentration is >180 mg/dL (>10 mmol/L)	Dose should be increased by 1 U
If nadir blood glucose concentration occurs within 3 hours of insulin administration or blood glucose returns to baseline within 8 hours	Change to longer acting insulin (ie, glargine or protamine zinc insulin)
If the nadir blood glucose concentration occurs at 8 hours or later	Once-daily administration may be used, although twice-daily administration at a reduced dose is preferred

greater than 200 mg/dL (12 mmol/L) at the next scheduled dosing time, insulin can be administered at the rate of 1 U twice daily, and if the blood glucose level is less than or equal to 200 mg/dL, continue to withhold insulin and discharge with a follow-up visit in 1 week.

Some cats may have a preinsulin glucose concentration less than 12 mmol/L within 2 weeks, but it is suggested that insulin therapy be maintained for a minimum of 2 weeks to give the β cells more time to recover fully from glucose toxicity. The dose can be reduced to 0.5 to 1 U once or twice daily.

Feeding

Although the ideal combination of macronutrients (protein, fat, and carbohydrate) to feed diabetic cats is not known, diets low in carbohydrates and high in protein reduce postprandial hyperglycemia and insulin concentrations in healthy cats [22]. Initial data from diabetic cats also suggest that low-carbohydrate–high-protein diets result in better clinical control, reduced insulin requirements, and increased rates of diabetic remission [39,48,49]. Thus, a commercial low- carbohydrate food should be used in diabetic cats unless contraindicated by other disease. During the first few weeks of treatment, diabetic cats may have a reduced appetite, and if they refuse these commercial low-carbohydrate diets, they should be offered any palatable food with a preference for a high protein, meat-based diet. Once appetite has returned, the cat can be transitioned to a balanced, low carbohydrate diet.

Care should be taken with cats diagnosed with renal disease, because diets high in protein may have a deleterious effect. For these cats, dietary management of renal disease using a restricted protein diet should take precedence over dietary management of diabetes.

Obesity in cats markedly reduces insulin sensitivity; hence, calories should be restricted so that obese cats achieve a 1% to 2% loss of body weight per week. Because of the decreased postprandial hyperglycemia and improved satiety with a low-carbohydrate diet, it is suggested that diets with less than 20% of calories from carbohydrate (eg, Hill's m/d [Topeka, KS], Purina DM [St. Louis, MO], Royal Canin diabetic [France]) should be used for obese diabetic cats. Currently, most feline weight loss diets are low-fat–high-carbohydrate diets. Weight loss improves insulin sensitivity and may reduce insulin requirements. In some cats, diabetic remission is obtained after weight loss and short-term insulin or oral hypoglycemic therapy.

Water intake

Daily water drunk is often overlooked but is an important tool for evaluating diabetic cats. Blood glucose concentrations higher than the renal threshold (14–16 mmol/L in cats) result in glycosuria, osmotic diuresis, and compensatory polydipsia. Measurement of water consumption at home is simpler, less expensive, and less stressful to measure for the owner, cat, and practitioner and correlates better with mean daily glucose concentration than does fructosamine concentration.

Water drunk should be measured over consecutive days, because there is considerable daily variation. Ideally, it should be measured for at least 48 hours before a serial blood glucose curve. In general, water intake of less than 40 mL/kg/d correlates with good glycemic control, and the insulin dose should not be changed. Water intake in excess of 100 mL/kg/d indicates poor glycemic control, and adjustment of the insulin dose is required.

Wet (canned) foods contain significant water; hence, the type of diet also needs to be taken into account. A healthy nondiabetic cat drinks, on average, less than 10 mL/kg every 24 hours if fed canned food and less than 60 mL/kg every 24 hours if fed dry food. Diabetic cats with excellent glycemic control drink, on average, less than 20 mL/kg every 24 hours when eating canned food and less than 70 mL/kg every 24 hours if eating dry food. Care also needs to be taken to identify cats with renal disease that lack the ability to concentrate urine and are overtly polydipsic even with good glycemic control.

Urine glucose measurements when using glargine

With shorter acting insulins, urine glucose concentration is usually only useful for recognition of poor control or exemplary control and remission, but when using glargine, urine glucose concentration may be used as a parameter on which to base dosage adjustments. Because of the long duration of action of glargine, the blood glucose concentration should remain below the renal threshold almost all day when good glycemic control has been achieved. A urine glucose score of 2+ or more (scale of 0–4+) likely indicates the need for a dose increase. A negative urine glucose concentration occurs with exemplary glycemic control and also in diabetic remission.

Treating and evaluating fractious cats using glargine

Traditionally, failure to obtain sufficient blood glucose curves for monitoring the response to treatment makes achieving good glycemic control more difficult. The most common cause is a fractious cat, in which multiple venipunctures are impossible. Glargine offers new hope for cats in which blood samples cannot be collected, because dosage changes can be made relatively safely based on water intake, urine glucose concentration, and clinical assessment. Fractious cats can be successfully treated and monitored as outpatients using water intake. Start with an insulin dose of 2 U per cat per injection twice daily, and record daily water intake. Increase the dose by 1 U per injection 1 week later if indicated based on water intake and then every 2 to 4 weeks until water intake is below 70 mL/kg/d (dry food) or 20 mL/kg/d (canned food), and then maintain at this dose. If water intake falls below 20 mL/kg/d, the insulin dose should be reduced by 1 U per injection at each recheck. Change in water intake over time in an individual cat is more valuable than comparing absolute values between cats. Urine glucose concentration may help to identify cats that are overdosed with insulin or are going into remission.

Summary

Feline diabetes is a multifactorial disease with genetic and environmental factors, including diet, excess body weight, and physical inactivity, involved in its pathogenesis. Although type 2 diabetes is most common in cats, most cats are insulin-dependent at the time of diagnosis. If good glycemic control can be achieved early after diagnosis, a substantial proportion of diabetic cats go into clinical remission. Diabetic remission may be facilitated by using a low-carbohydrate–high-protein diet combined with a long-acting insulin, such as glargine, administered twice daily. Rather than just controlling clinical signs, these new treatment modalities make curing feline diabetes a realistic goal for practitioners.

References

[1] Rand JS, Bobbermein LM, Hendrikz JK. Over-representation of Burmese in cats with diabetes mellitus in Queensland. Aust Vet J 1997;75(6):402–5.

[2] Baral R, Rand J, Catt M, Farrow H. Prevalence of feline diabetes mellitus in a feline private practice [abstract]. J Vet Intern Med 2003;17(3):433–4.

[3] Panciera DL, Thomas C, Eiker S, et al. Epizootiologic patterns of diabetes mellitus in cats: 333 cases (1980–1986). J Am Vet Med Assoc 1990;197(11):1504–8.

[4] Wade C, Gething M, Rand JS. Evidence of a genetic basis for diabetes mellitus in Burmese cats [abstract]. J Vet Intern Med 1999;13:269.

[5] Prahl A, Glickman L, Guptil L, et al. Time trends and risk factors for diabetes mellitus in cats. J Vet Intern Med 2003;17(3):434.

[6] Lederer R, Rand J, Hughes I, et al. Chronic or recurring medical problems, dental disease, repeated corticosteroid treatment, and lower physical activity are associated with diabetes in Burmese cats. J Vet Intern Med 2003;17(3):433.

[7] Rand JS. Current understanding of feline diabetes mellitus: Part 1, pathogenesis. J Feline Med Surg 1999;1:143–53.

[8] O'Brien TD, Hayden DW, Johnson KH. High dose intravenous tolerance test and serum insulin and glucagon levels in diabetic and non-diabetic cats: relationships to insular amyloidosis. Vet Pathol 1985;22:250–61.

[9] Feldman EC, Nelson RW. Feline diabetes mellitus. In: Canine and feline endocrinology and reproduction. St. Louis (MO): WB Saunders; 2004. p. 539–79.

[10] Feldhahn J, Rand JS, Martin GM. Insulin sensitivity in normal and diabetic cats. J Feline Med Surg 1999;1:107–15.

[11] Porte DJ. Beta-cells in type 2 diabetes mellitus. Diabetes 1991;40:166–80.

[12] Brand Miller JC, Colagiuri S. The carnivore connection: dietary carbohydrate in the evolution of NIDDM. Diabetologia 1994;37:1280–6.

[13] Appleton DJ, Rand J, Sunvold G, et al. Determination of reference values for glucose tolerance, insulin tolerance and insulin sensitivity tests in clinically normal cats. Am J Vet Res 2001;62(4):630–6.

[14] Van Baak M, Borghouts L. Relationships with physical activity. Nutr Rev 2000;58(3 Suppl): S16–8.

[15] Hoenig M, Wilkins C, Holson JC, et al. Effects of obesity on lipid profiles in neutered male and female cats. Am J Vet Res 2003;64(3):299–303.

[16] Johnson KH, O'Brien T, Betsholtz C, et al. Islet amyloid, islet-amyloid polypeptide and diabetes mellitus. N Engl J Med 1989;321:513–8.

[17] Lederer R, Rand JS, Hughes IP, et al. Pancreatic histopathology of diabetic Burmese and non-Burmese cats. J Vet Intern Med 2004;18(3):443.

[18] Lorenzo ARB, Weir GC, Yanker BA. Pancreatic islet cell toxicity of amylin associated with Type 2 diabetes mellitus. Nature 1994;368:756–60.

[19] Goossens MMC, Nelson RW, Feldman EC, et al. Response to treatment and survival in 104 cats with diabetes mellitus (1985–1995). J Vet Intern Med 1998;12:1–6.

[20] Unger RH, Grundy S. Hyperglycaemia as an inducer as well as a consequence of impaired islet cell function and insulin resistance: implications for the management of diabetes. Diabetologia 1995;28:119–21.

[21] Link KRJ. Feline diabetes: diagnostics and experimental modelling [doctoral thesis]. Queensland: The University of Queensland; 2001. p. 58–159.

[22] Farrow HA, Rand JS, Sunvold GD. The effect of high protein, high fat or high carbohydrate diets on postprandial glucose and insulin concentrations in normal cats. J Vet Intern Med 2002;16(3):360.

[23] Leidinger K, Nolte I, Eigenbrodt E. Klinische und labordiagnostiche Untersuchungen zum Phaenomen der Hyperglykaemie der Katze. Klienterpraxis 1989;34:457–64.

[24] Link KR, Rand JS. Reference values for glucose tolerance and glucose tolerance status in cats. J Am Vet Med Assoc 1998;213:492–6.

[25] Rand JS, Kinnaird ER, Baglioni A, et al. Acute stress hyperglycaemia in cats is associated with struggling and increased concentrations of lactate and norepinephrine. J Vet Intern Med 2002;16:123–32.

[26] Krauth SA, Cowgill LD. Renal glucose transport in the cat. In: Proceedings of the American College of Veterinary Internal Medicine Forum. Blacksburg (VA): American College of Veterinary Internal Medicine; 1982. p. 78.

[27] Crenshaw KL, Peterson ME. Pretreatment clinical and laboratory evaluation of cats with diabetes mellitus: 104 cases (1992–1994). J Am Vet Med Assoc 1996;209:943–9.

[28] Lutz TA, Rand JS, Ryan E. Fructosamine concentrations in hyperglycemic cats. Can Vet J 1995;36:155–9.

[29] Elliott DA, Nelson RW, Feldman EC, et al. Glycosylated hemoglobin concentration for assessment of glycemic control in diabetic cats. J Vet Intern Med 1997;11:161–5.

[30] Hasegawa S, Sako T, Takemura N, et al. Glycated hemoglobin fractions in normal and diabetic cats measured by high performance liquid chromatography. J Vet Med Sci 1992;54:789–90.

[31] Akol KG, Waddle JR, Wilding P. Glycated hemoglobin and fructosamine in diabetic and non-diabetic cats. J Am Anim Hosp Assoc 1992;28:227–31.

[32] Christopher MM, Broussard JD, Peterson ME. Heinz body formation associated with ketoacidosis in diabetic cats. J Vet Intern Med 1995;9:24–31.

[33] Hoyer-Otto MA, Reusch C, Minkus G. Glykosylierte Hamoglobine (GHb) bei der Katze: Affinitatschromatographische Bestimmung bei gesunden, permanent (Diabetes mellitus) und passager hyperglykamischen Katzen [Affinity chromatography of glycated hemoglobin in the blood of cats with permanent hyperglycemia (diabetes mellitus) or transient hyperglycemia]. Tierarztl Prax 1995;23:155–61.

[34] Donaghue S, Kronfeld DS. Feeding the hospitalised cat. In: Wills J, Wolf A, editors. Handbook of feline medicine. Oxford: Pergamon Press; 1993. p. 42–4.

[35] Martin G. Clinical management of feline diabetes mellitus [doctoral thesis]. Queensland: The University of Queensland; 2001. p. 126–43.

[36] Feldman EC, Nelson RW. Diabetic ketoacidosis. In: Canine and feline endocrinology and reproduction. Philadelphia: WB Saunders; 2004. p. 580–615.

[37] Marshall R, Rand J. Comparison of the pharmacokinetics and pharmacodynamics of glargine, protamine zinc and porcine lente insulins in normal cats [abstract]. J Vet Intern Med 2002;16(3):358.

[38] Greco DS. Oral hypoglycemic therapy in cats. In: Sellon DC, Paradis MR, editors. Proceedings of the 17th American College of Veterinary Internal Medicine Forum, Lakewood (CO): American College of Veterinary Internal Medicine; 1999. p. 647–9.

[39] Mazzaferro EM, Greco DS, Turner AS, et al. Treatment of feline diabetes mellitus using an α-glucosidase inhibitor and a low-carbohydrate diet. J Feline Med Surg 2003;5(3):183–9.

[40] Appleton DJ, Rand JS, Sunvold GD. Dietary chromium tripicolinate supplementation reduces glucose concentrations and improves glucose tolerance in normal-weight cats. J Feline Med Surg 2002;4:13–25.

[41] Greco D. Treatment of non-insulin dependent diabetes mellitus with oral hypoglycemic agents. In: Proceedings of the 15th Annual Veterinary Medical Forum, Lakewood (CO): American College of Veterinary Internal Medicine; 1997. p. 252–4.

[42] Saltiel A, Olefsky J. Thiazolidinediones in the treatment of insulin resistance and type II diabetes. Diabetes 1996;45(12):1661–9.

[43] Kahn C, Meyerovitch J, Shechter Y. A family of polypeptide substrates and inhibitors of insulin receptor kinase. Biochemistry 1990;29(15):3654–60.

[44] Hoenig M, Ferguson DC. Effects of darglitazone on glucose clearance and lipid metabolism in obese cats. Am J Vet Res 2003;64(11):1409–13.

[45] Broussard JD, Wallace MS. Insulin treatment of diabetes mellitus in the dog and cat. In: Bonagura J, editor. Kirk's current veterinary therapy XII. Philadelphia: WB Saunders; 1995. p. 393–8.

[46] Moise NS, Riemers TJ. Insulin therapy in cats with diabetes mellitus. J Am Vet Med Assoc 1983;182:158–64.

[47] Nelson RW, Feldman EC, Devries SE. Use of ultralente insulin in cats with diabetes mellitus. J Am Vet Med Assoc 1992;200(12):1828–9.

[48] Marshall R, Rand J. Insulin glargine and a high protein–low carbohydrate diet are associated with high remission rates in newly diagnosed diabetic cats [abstract]. J Vet Intern Med 2004;18:401.

[49] Frank G, Anderson W, Pazak H, et al. Use of a high-protein diet in the management of feline diabetes mellitus. Vet Ther 2002;2(3):238–46.

ELSEVIER
SAUNDERS

Vet Clin Small Anim
35 (2005) 225–269

VETERINARY
CLINICS
Small Animal Practice

Feline Hepatic Lipidosis

Sharon A. Center, DVM

College of Veterinary Medicine, Cornell University, PO Box 33, Ithaca, NY 14853, USA

Feline hepatic lipidosis (FHL) is a common and potentially fatal cholestatic syndrome afflicting domestic cats; overconditioned animals have an increased risk. Although FHL was initially described as an idiopathic condition, it is now clear that most cats (>95%) have an illness or circumstance directly causing a catabolic state. Inappetence, malassimilation, or maldigestion imposed by a variety of disease processes usually precedes syndrome development. Although predisposing factors remain incompletely understood, it is clear that there is an imbalance between peripheral fat stores mobilized to the liver, hepatic use of fatty acids (FAs) for energy, and hepatic dispersal of triglycerides (TGs). Successful treatment involves provision of balanced nutritional support, correction of acquired metabolic dysregulations, and treatment of any underlying primary disease. Most cats can recover with early diagnosis followed by aggressive supportive care, particularly when the syndrome is recognized in its earliest phase.

Pathomechanisms

A number of nutritional studies suggest metabolic associations with FHL. Of primary importance are feline nutritional idiosyncrasies associated with the evolution of cats as pure carnivores [1,2]. These influence hepatic FA metabolism and requirements for essential FAs and protein. Adult cats require two to three times more dietary protein than omnivorous species, maintain a greater basal nitrogen (protein) requirement than dogs, and have a high requirement for essential amino acids and essential FAs. The importance of high protein intake in feline metabolism has been demonstrated in several studies of rapid weight reduction in obese cats as well as in experimentally modeled FHL [2–5]. Unable to adapt their urea cycle enzymes or aminotransferases to reduced protein intake, cats possess limited ability to

---

E-mail address: sac6@cornell.edu

adjust protein metabolic pathways for conserving nitrogen. This peculiarity explains the rapid onset of protein malnutrition in anorectic cats and is an important feature of the FHL syndrome. The subnormal serum albumin concentrations demonstrated by 60% or more of cats with FHL, even in the presence of dehydration, likely reflect this process. In most cats with FHL, a sequential decline in albumin concentration occurs during the first week of therapy, reflecting rehydration and a gradual restoration of positive nitrogen balance.

Hastened use coupled with an inability to conserve certain amino acids, including taurine, arginine, methionine, and cysteine, necessitates a higher dietary intake for cats compared with most other species. In experimentally produced and spontaneous FHL, plasma concentrations of alanine, arginine, citrulline, taurine, and methionine become markedly reduced ($\geq 50\%$ reduction) [6,7]. Cats are unable to synthesize taurine adequately, yet they obligatorily use this amino acid for bile acid conjugation. Plasma bile acid concentrations in cats with FHL are remarkably increased, whereas their plasma taurine concentrations are profoundly low [7]. Arginine, essential for normal urea cycle function, cannot be synthesized in quantities sufficient to mediate ammonia detoxification in the face of an arginine-deficient high-protein load. Because feline arginine requirements are not significantly blunted during starvation, hyperammonemia may be provoked by feeding an arginine-deficient yet high-protein ration, a situation that may be encountered when human enteral nutrition modules or other custom-designed rations are used. Methionine is essential for methylation reactions and substrate entrance into the transsulfuration and aminopropylation pathways through its catabolic generation of s-adenosylmethionine (SAMe). Methionine (SAMe, synthesized from methionine) and cysteine function as essential thiol donors necessary for hepatocellular glutathione (GSH) and sulfate synthesis (Fig. 1). GSH and sulfates play important roles in conjugation and detoxification functions in the liver and elsewhere in the body. Cats with FHL may develop remarkably low hepatic GSH concentrations [8]. Carnitine (CN) is required for transport of long-chain FAs into the mitochondria, where they undergo β-oxidation. CN also is important as a shuttling mechanism for transport of FA esters from mitochondria into the hepatocyte cytosol and from the hepatic cytosol into plasma. Although CN can be synthesized in the kidneys as well as the liver of the cat, this process requires several B-vitamins, iron, lysine, and SAMe, which may be deficient in the FHL syndrome. In the circumstance of hepatic dysfunction and a coexistent high rate of FA oxidation imposed by catabolic mechanisms, available free CN may not be sufficient for optimal FA use (β-oxidation), for the systemic dispersal of acyl-CN as energy to other tissues, or for acyl-CN urinary excretion (assisting in the hepatic egress and systemic disposal of excess FAs).

Cats seemingly require higher amounts of several B-vitamins compared with other species and are predisposed to depletion during prolonged

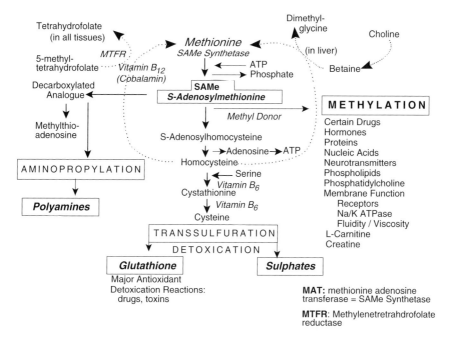

Fig. 1. Metabolic derivation of s-adenosylmethionine (SAMe) from methionine and the important metabolic pathways involving SAMe (transsulfuration, transmethylation, and aminopropulation); derivation of glutathione and L-carnitine; and the important interactions involving cobalamin, folate, and pyridoxine. ATP, adenosine triphosphate; ATPase, adenosine triphosphatase; MAT, methionine adenosine transferase (SAMe synthetase); MTFR; methylenetetrahydrofolate reductase.

inappetence, maldigestion, or malassimilation. The low hepatic GSH concentrations in cats with FHL is likely hastened or worsened by vitamin B_{12} (cobalamin) deficiency [8]. Cobalamin is necessary for the synthesis of methionine from homocysteine, an essential reaction when methionine intake is diminished by starvation as occurs in FHL; thus, cobalamin deficiency possibly augments the metabolic changes that promote syndrome onset. Limited methionine has an impact on the availability of SAMe and thereby secondarily limits the functioning of the transmethylation and transsulfuration pathways (see Fig. 1). Each of these pathways is important in the cat, in which there is high protein use and amino acid flux along degradative pathways, which require transmethylation reactions and a high turnover of cysteine.

SAMe is an essential precursor of L-CN, a conditionally essential nutrient necessary for β-oxidation of long-chain FAs and for the generation of hepatic GSH. Liver production of GSH is important for hepatocellular protection from oxidant injury as well as for a myriad of biochemical and molecular interactions influenced by reduction or oxidation (redox) status. The impact of compromised hepatic GSH synthesis is polysystemic, because most of the hepatic synthesized GSH is exported via bile and to the systemic circulation to provide systemic antioxidant protection and is catabolized to substrates for GSH synthesis in other tissues. In addition to these effects, several amino acids are degraded through a cobalamin-dependent pathway from propionyl–coenzyme A (CoA) to succinyl CoA, with the latter being an important intermediary of the Krebs cycle. Blockade of this pathway generates methylmalonic acid, a universally recognized marker of cobalamin insufficiency.

Obese cats accumulate a significantly greater hepatic TG content than do lean cats [4]. In lean cats, obese cats, obese cats after rapid weight loss, and cats with FHL, approximately 2.5%, 5%, 10%, and from 34% to 49% of liver weight, respectively, is comprised of fat [3,4]. Cats with FHL are known to develop significantly increased serum concentrations of nonesterified FA and β-hydroxybutyric acid consistent with enhanced peripheral fat mobilization and ketogenesis [7,9,10]. These phenomena are coupled with an apparent inability to counterbalance hepatic fat accretion. Multiple factors compromise appropriate regulation and function of FA β-oxidation, ketogenesis, and hepatic FA dispersal. Although high circulating and hepatic tissue CN concentrations and increased urinary elimination of acyl-CN occur in cats with FHL, it remains unclear whether shifts in CN dispersal, synthesis, or availability are appropriate in magnitude for the metabolic circumstances [7,10,11]. Because lipoprotein particle composition in FHL and adipose fat composition are not unusual, it is unlikely that an absolute protein phospholipid deficiency impairs lipoprotein egress from the liver [9,12]. A recent study investigating the influence of n3 polyunsaturated fatty acid (n3-PUFA) on FHL concluded that a dietary deficiency may promote syndrome development [1]. This study corroborates prior nutritional work with experimentally modeled FHL in suggesting that the quantity and quality of dietary protein during weight loss importantly influence liver and adipose tissue FA profiles and also suggests that modulation of FA desaturase enzyme activity may be involved.

Distention of hepatocytes with TG in FHL is associated with a significant reduction in the number of organelles involved with the formation, packaging, and egress of lipoproteins and with the conduction of FA oxidation and synthetic functions [13]. In addition, cell expansion compresses canaliculi and restricts bile flow. Some of these changes also have been observed in hepatocyte mitochondria from obese cats, in cats undergoing rapid weight loss, in obese healthy cats after food deprivation, and in cats during weight gain when a diet restricted in n3-PUFA was fed [1,4]. These morphologic changes may reflect impaired organelle function and membrane integrity or may represent a response to membrane injury. The impact on specific organelle functions has not been determined.

The inherent feline susceptibility to oxidant injury may augment the pathophysiologic mechanisms at play in FHL. Cats with spontaneous FHL often demonstrate increased numbers of circulating Heinz bodies and frequently are intolerant of xenobiotics that impose oxidant challenge (eg, phenol derivatives and drugs containing a propylene glycol carrier). Low hepatic GSH concentrations are consistent with the mitochondrial oxidative injury documented in many models of liver disease [14]. In FHL, it is possible that impaired synthesis of adenosine triphosphate (ATP) is exacerbated by starvation and is also promoted by development of a refeeding phenomenon (discussed elsewhere in this article). Although unproven in cats, in other species, food deprivation enhances mitochondrial oxidative stress when tissues are challenged by imposing circumstances, such as ischemia or reperfusion injury. In fact, oxidative damage is heightened by chronic food deprivation [15]. Coupling this information with evidence derived from a rodent model of hepatic lipidosis, it is likely that starvation and hepatic steatosis independently impair hepatic antioxidant defense [16]. Synergistic mechanisms may deplete essential antioxidants in FHL, predisposing inappetent cats to oxidative systemic injury imposed by their primary or underlying illness. Considering the primary disease processes associated with FHL (Table 1), enhanced systemic oxidant challenge would be expected in many cats. The importance of oxidant injury as a confounding factor in FHL is supported by study of a rodent HL model that convincingly demonstrates antioxidant benefit from supplemental SAMe, N-acetylcysteine (NAC), or direct GSH administration; animals experienced reduced tissue injury and reduced expression of tumor necrosis factor (TNF) associated with cytokine-mediated tissue damage [16].

Clinical characteristics

Although cats of any age may be affected, most are middle-aged adults (median = 7 [range: 0.5–20] years). A history of overconditioning prevails, with body condition scores of 4 to 5 (5-point scale) or greater (median body weight = 4.5 [range: 0.9–8.7] kg), inappetence ranging from 2 to 7 days (>90%), loss of 25% of body weight (hydration and body condition, fat lost primarily from peripheral depots rather than from the abdominal cavity), and variable gastrointestinal signs (vomiting [38%], diarrhea, and constipation) Other historical features reflect the underlying or primary disease processes [17]. Overt jaundice is noted in approximately 70% of cases on initial presentation, and most cats have a nonpainful and smoothly contoured hepatomegaly. Cats with severe electrolyte derangements develop profound head or neck ventroflexion, and some display remarkable ptyalism without provocation when stressed or when stimulated with food (Fig. 2). Ptyalism may reflect nausea or hepatic encephalopathy. Severe weakness and recumbency may develop in cats symptomatic for electrolyte disturbances (eg, potassium, phosphate) or thiamine deficiency (Fig. 3). Cats with neck ventroflexion have limited stress tolerance and may become dyspneic as a result of ventilatory muscle weakness or may collapse during routine

Table 1
Conditions associated with the severe hepatic lipidosis syndrome in 157 cats, Cornell
University, 1990–2004 (some cats demonstrated more than a single underlying disease process
or condition)

Condition	*n*
Other hepatic disorders	31
Cholangitis/cholangiohepatitis syndrome	27
Extrahepatic bile duct occlusion	3
Portosystemic vascular anomaly	1
Pancreatitis	17
Gastrointestinal related	59
Inflammatory bowel disease	44
Peritonitis	5
Gastrointestinal foreign body	2
Esophageal necrosis/stricture	2
Stomatitis	1
Chronic diaphragmatic hernia	1
Jejunostomy site sepsis	1
Intestinal abscess	1
Chronic jejunal intussusception	1
Constipation/obstipation	1
Diabetes Mellitus	4
Respiratory Related	6
Asthma	2
Chylothorax	2
Pleural effusion	1
Laryngeal hemiplegia	1
Septicemia	4
Urologic/renal related	7
Glomerulosclerosis/glomerulonephritis	3
Nephritis, acute renal failure	2
Hydronephrosis	1
Feline lower urinary tract syndrome	1
Neoplasia	22
Lymphosarcoma	10
Lung carcinoma	3
Liver carcinoma	1
Adenocarcinoma	5
Pancreatic	2
Small intestine	1
Carcinomatosis	1
Osteochondroma	1
Metastatic transitional cell carcinoma	1
Cardiovascular	4
Hypertrophic cardiomyopathy	3
Restrictive cardiomyopathy	1
Hyperthyroid	3
Anemia	5
Neurologic disease	4
Social interactions in home: new pet or house, menacing pet or person	8
Miscellaneous	13
Trauma	2
Steatitis	1

Table 1 (*continued*)

Condition	n
Metronidazole toxicity	1
Hypothyroidism	1
Painful tooth	1
Declaw complications	1
Cat lost (1 week)	2
Antibiotics: vomiting/anorexia	2
Trichobezoar	1
Chronic feline infectious peritonitis	1
Idiopathic (no cause for anorexia identified)	2

diagnostic or therapeutic procedures, restraint, or in response to menacing or barking dogs.

Clinicopathologic features

Because FHL lacks necroinflammatory liver lesions, clinicopathologic features predominantly reflect cholestasis imposed by hepatocellular TG

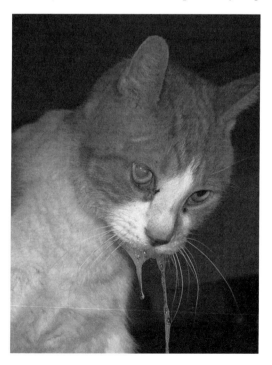

Fig. 2. Severe head and neck ventroflexion and ptyalism in a cat with hepatic lipidosis complicated by severe electrolyte depletions. (Courtesy of New York State College of Veterinary Medicine, Ithaca, NY, 2004.)

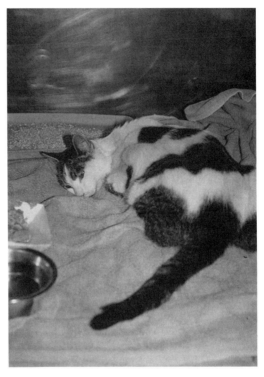

Fig. 3. Cat with hepatic lipidosis collapsed secondary to severe electrolyte depletions. In addition to general recumbency, this cat had impaired ventilatory capability as a result of marked muscle weakness. (Courtesy of New York State College of Veterinary Medicine, Cornell University, Ithaca, NY, 2004.)

accumulation, catabolism, fluid and electrolyte depletions, and the underlying or primary disease process causing anorexia.

Common hematologic abnormalities include poikilocytosis (reported on the initial complete blood cell count [CBC] in 63% of cats but developing during FHL treatment in most) and a predisposition to erythrocyte Heinz body formation. In fact, Heinz bodies can appear within hours and lead to symptomatic anemia and death after exposure to oxidant challenge imposed by drug or anesthetic agents. In addition, a number of common feline illnesses complicated by FHL are associated with Heinz body formation (eg, diabetes mellitus, hyperthyroidism, pancreatitis, other forms of liver disease) [18]. Anemia is present on initial evaluation in 22% of cats and develops in most during treatment as a result of phlebotomy for sequential testing, hemolysis associated with Heinz bodies or severe hypophosphatemia, or blood loss associated with feeding tube placement. Approximately 25% of cats in the author's hospital have required whole blood or packed red cells for severe acute anemia or bleeding during feeding tube placement. The leukogram reflects any underlying disease process.

Common biochemical features on presentation include increased liver enzyme activities (alkaline phosphatase [ALP] in ≥80% of cases, alanine aminotransferase [ALT] in ≥72% of cases, and aspartate aminotransferase [AST] in ≥89% of cases), subnormal blood urea nitrogen (58%) despite initial dehydration (impaired urea cycle function presumed), and high total bilirubin (variable magnitudes in ≥95% of cats) (Fig. 4). There is no diagnostic value in fractionating bilirubin into its unconjugated and conjugated forms (Fig. 5). Cats with underlying necroinflammatory liver disease (eg, cholangiohepatitis, major bile duct occlusion, bile duct carcinoma), pancreatitis, or pancreatic adenocarcinoma develop high gamma-glutamyltranspeptidase (GGT) activity, with 48% having a twofold or greater increase [19]. This feature is useful in identifying primary diseases. The concentration of globulins, cholesterol, and glucose reflects primary disease processes; few cats present with hypoglycemia (see Fig. 4). Some cats develop modest to marked increases in creatinine kinase (CK) activity reflecting tissue injury associated with intravenous catheter or feeding tube placement, catabolism (muscle mobilization), recumbency, or rhabdomyolysis secondary to severe electrolyte depletion (eg, severe hypophosphatemia).

Electrolyte abnormalities are an important cause of patient morbidity and mortality. Hypokalemia, hypophosphatemia, or hypomagnesemia may be identified initially (30%, 17%, and 28%, respectively) or may become apparent after initial volume expansion (crystalloid fluid therapy) or subsequent to a refeeding syndrome (discussed elsewhere in this article). Severe hypokalemia and hypophosphatemia increase the risk for red blood cell (RBC) hemolysis (hypophosphatemia), muscle weakness, enteric atony and vomiting, ventroflexion of the head or neck, and neurobehavioral changes that can be confused with hepatic encephalopathy. Although many disorders can provoke head and neck ventroflexion in the cat, low serum potassium, low phosphate concentrations, or thiamine deficiency is responsible in FHL. Prior studies in our hospital have proven that hypokalemia is significantly associated with failure to survive [17].

Urine sediment examination in cats with FHL often discloses lipiduria (refractile fat globules in urine). A buoyant lipid phase may be observed in urine after centrifugation.

Prolonged clotting time is detected more reliably with a coagulation test sensitive to vitamin K deficiency (PIVKA [proteins invoked by vitamin K antagonism or absence] clotting test; Thrombotest; Nycomed AS, Oslo, Norway). A comparison of standard laboratory bench coagulation assay and PIVKA testing in FHL patients is shown in Fig. 6A. Prolonged coagulation times respond to parenteral vitamin K_1 administration as demonstrated in Fig. 6B; posttreatment PIVKA values followed three doses of vitamin K_1 (1.0 mg/kg administered intramuscularly at 12-hour intervals). Within the first 48 hours after presentation, coagulation assessments have been replaced by routine administration of vitamin K_1 to facilitate uneventful catheter and feeding tube placement and hepatic aspiration sampling. Because of the high

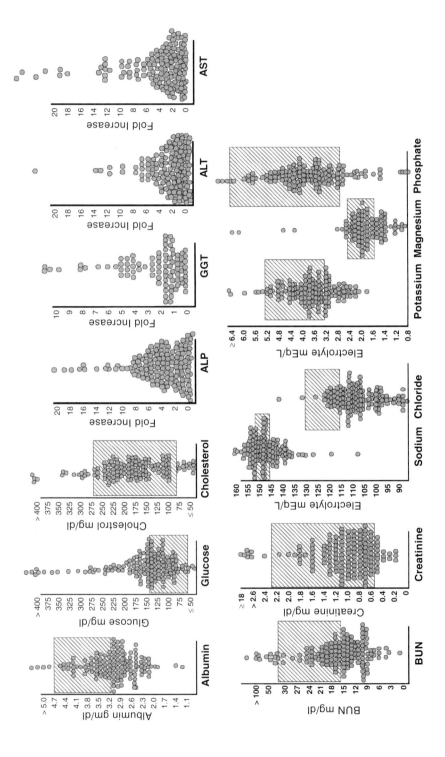

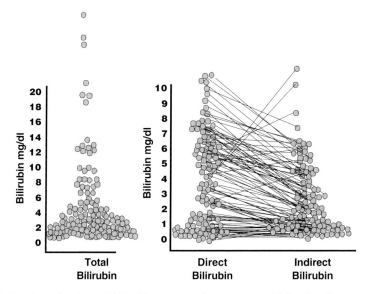

Fig. 5. Total and fractionated bilirubin concentrations (conjugated [direct] and unconjugated [indirect]). Bilirubin fractionation does not assist in differentiating feline liver disease from other causes of hyperbilirubinemia (*Data from* New York State College of Veterinary Medicine, Cornell University, Ithaca, NY, 2004).

frequency of coagulation test abnormalities, initial venipuncture should be performed only using peripheral veins that allow pressure wrap–assisted hemostasis. Cystocentesis, jugular catheter insertion, urethral catheterization, and feeding tube placement should be delayed for 12 to 36 hours after vitamin K_1 administration and until severe electrolyte perturbations are improved.

Secondary bile acids are formed by enteric bacterial dehydroxylation of primary bile acids in the alimentary canal. Fractionation of serum bile acids in cats with FHL demonstrated a marked reduction of secondary bile acids consistent with impaired enterohepatic bile acid circulation as occurs with major bile duct obstruction (Fig. 7) [21]. This concurs with the association between FHL and vitamin K–responsive coagulation abnormalities, suggesting an increased risk for malabsorption of fat-soluble vitamins. As a result, oral treatment with fat-soluble vitamins may be less effective than expected. Concern over impaired enterohepatic bile acid circulation underlies recommendations for administration of parenteral vitamin K_1 early in syndrome treatment as well as an oral water-soluble form of vitamin E.

Fig. 4. Clinicopathologic features in cats with hepatic lipidosis. Each circle represents a single clinical patient (data derived from the New York State College of Veterinary Medicine, Cornell University, Ithaca, NY, 2004). ALP, alkaline phosphatase; ALT, alanine aminotransferase; AST, aspartate aminotransferase; BUN, blood urea nitrogen; GGT, gamma-glutamyltranspeptidase.

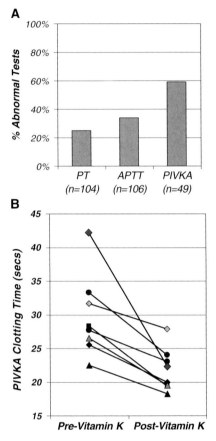

Fig. 6. (*A*) Percentage of tested cats with abnormal coagulation tests. APTT, activated partial thromboplastin time; PIVKA (proteins invoked by vitamin K antagonism or absence) Thrombotest (Nycomed AS) clotting time; PT, prothrombin time. The PIVKA test is more sensitive for detection of coagulation abnormalities in cats with liver disease [20]. Abnormal PIVKA clotting times usually correct in hepatic lipidosis after vitamin K administration (*Data from* New York State College of Veterinary Medicine, Cornell University, Ithaca, NY, 2004). (*B*) PIVKA clotting time in cats with hepatic lipidosis before and after parenteral administration of vitamin K_1. Marked improvement in the PIVKA clotting time is realized within 48 hours of vitamin administration (*Data from* New York State College of Veterinary Medicine, Cornell University, Ithaca, NY, 2004).

Special blood or urine tests

Serum or urine bile acids

Routine submission of serum or urine bile acids in severe FHL offers no diagnostic advantage, because these patients are hyperbilirubinemic, with most being overtly jaundiced.

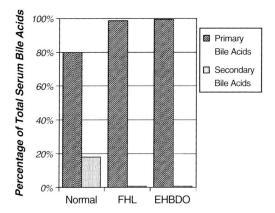

Fig. 7. Percentage of total serum bile acids comprising primary and secondary moieties in healthy cats and cats with feline hepatic lipidosis (FHD; *Data from* New York State College of Veterinary Medicine, Cornell University, Ithaca, NY, 2004) [21]. EHBDO, extrahepatic bile duct occlusion.

Ammonia testing

Cats with experimentally induced FHL developed hyperammonemia on challenge with ammonium chloride [6]. This was not unique, however, because fasted healthy cats also demonstrated similar ammonia intolerance. These findings relate to the necessity of arginine for adequate hepatic ammonia detoxification (urea cycle function) in the cat [6]. Determining the ammonia status or tolerance in clinical feline patients is not recommended as a test of hepatic insufficiency. The unreliability of enzymatically determined ammonia measurements and the lability of ammonia compromise test conduction and interpretation. Furthermore, the propensity for anorectic cats to become hyperammonemic strongly contraindicates ammonium chloride challenge and obfuscates the usefulness of hyperammonemia as an indication of liver dysfunction.

Vitamin B_{12} status

Cats malnourished secondary to inflammatory or infiltrative bowel disease are at risk for vitamin B_{12} (cobalamin) deficiency [22]. This easily diagnosed and rectified disorder has the potential to influence feline intermediary metabolism. Because cobalamin deficiency predisposes ill anorectic cats to metabolic aberrations associated with FHL and may itself promote anorexia, a blood cobalamin concentration should be evaluated when intestinal or pancreatic disease is suspected. Cobalamin concentrations in 35 cats with confirmed FHL are shown in Fig. 8; subnormal cobalamin in 57% of these cats derived from severe inflammatory bowel disease or enteric lymphoma. It is important to acquire a sample for cobalamin measurement before empirically treating the FHL cat with vitamin B_{12}, because the need

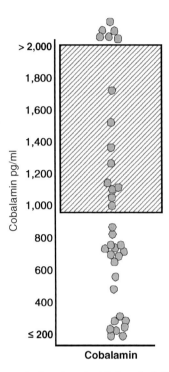

Fig. 8. Plasma cobalamin concentrations in cats with hepatic lipidosis; all cats with subnormal values had enteric disease causing the lipidosis syndrome (*Data from* New York State College of Veterinary Medicine, Cornell University, Ithaca, NY, 2004).

for long-term parenteral therapy can only be deduced from sequential plasma measurements. Although estimation of vitamin B_{12} status by measuring plasma cobalamin concentration is less sensitive and specific for detecting metabolic cobalamin sufficiency compared with measuring methylmalonic acid in blood or urine, prompt analyses are widely available for cobalamin only [23].

Because the liver contains most of the body's cobalamin, FHL may impose a high risk for symptomatic cobalamin deficiency. Confirmation of deficiency may be problematic, however, considering that human beings with severe liver disease have discordant blood and liver cobalamin concentrations (eg, high plasma levels, low tissue levels). Thus, interpretation of plasma cobalamin concentrations in the context of FHL may not be reliable; a normal plasma cobalamin concentration cannot exonerate the presence of a metabolic cobalamin-deficient state.

It remains unclear as to what form of cobalamin is best for therapeutic supplementation in metabolically compromised patients. The usual therapeutic form of cobalamin, cyanocobalamin, contains a cyanide molecule and a cobalt molecule. Before metabolic use, the cyanide molecule must be removed and eliminated. This detoxification process involves GSH conjugation and may be compromised by low hepatic GSH concentrations in patients with FHL. Thus, despite appropriate therapy, a functional co-balamin-deficient state may persist. The customarily used veterinary assay (chemiluminescence) for detecting cobalamin cannot differentiate between cyanocobalamin and the metabolically active adenosyl- and methylcobala-min forms of vitamin B_{12}. Thus, normal or even high vitamin values are found in supplemented animals that may be unable to derive an immediate metabolic benefit. To guard against this scenario, FHL patients receiving cobalamin should also be treated with a thiol donor and α-tocopherol. Experimental evidence suggests that α-tocopherol may augment the formation of active cobalamin from therapeutically administered synthetic cobalamin.

Trypsin-like immunoreactivity

Although a high concentration of feline trypsin-like-immunoreactivity (FTLI) helps to support a diagnosis of pancreatitis, this test cannot be endorsed for definitive confirmation or exclusion of feline pancreatitis as an underlying cause of FHL. The inability of FTLI to correlate histologically with confirmed pancreatitis, along with broad clinical experience demon-strating inconsistent correlation with biopsy-confirmed disease, dictates cautious test interpretation [24]. For best utility, FTLI should be used adjunctively with ultrasonographic abdominal imaging and other hemato-logic and biochemical indicators of pancreatic disease.

Diagnostic imaging

Abdominal radiography commonly discloses hepatomegaly and may indicate the presence of an underlying or primary disease. Rarely, an ab-dominal effusion may be detected. Of 157 cats reviewed for this article, only 6 developed an abdominal effusion. In 4 of these cats, onset of pure transudate followed crystalloid fluid therapy and likely reflected overhydration coupled with impaired sinusoidal perfusion. Otherwise, abdominal effusion reflected an underlying primary illness, such as neoplasia.

Abdominal ultrasonography usually discloses a hyperechoic hepatic parenchyma, comparing liver tissue echogenicity relative to falciform fat (Fig. 9). Renal tubule lipid accumulation compromises comparison of echogenicity between the liver and kidney. Careful evaluation of abdominal structures may disclose an underlying or primary disease. The exception is in cats with cholangitis or cholangiohepatitis, in which parenchymal hyper-echogenicity caused by hepatocyte TG storage can mask parenchymal, portal tract, or biliary tree irregularities that would otherwise be apparent. Cats with FHL unassociated with another hepatobiliary illness do not develop lesions associated with the gallbladder, common bile duct, or other biliary structures. Evaluation of the pancreas should always be undertaken, looking for

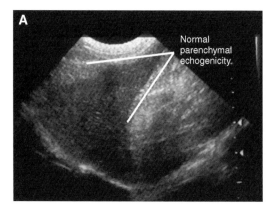

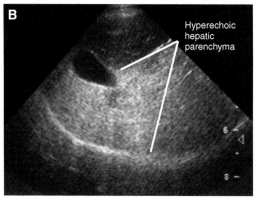

Fig. 9. Ultrasonographic appearance of liver tissue in a cat (*A*) and in a cat with hepatic lipidosis (*B*) demonstrating hyperechoic hepatic parenchyma commonly associated with diffuse lipid accumulation. Normal hepatic parenchyma is delineated between white lines. (Courtesy of New York State College of Veterinary Medicine, Cornell University, Ithaca, NY, 2004.)

evidence of pancreatitis or neoplasia. Pancreatic disease may be evidenced by altered echogenicity (hypoechoic or focal hyperechoic change), mass lesions, general gland enlargement, pancreatic duct prominence or dilation, hyperechoic peripancreatic fat, or hypoechoic peripancreatic effusion. Although these findings support a diagnosis of feline pancreatitis, they cannot confirm its presence, because many cats with clinically significant pancreatitis lack identifiable lesions on careful abdominal ultrasonography [25].

Should a liver aspirate or liver biopsy be collected to diagnose feline hepatic lipidosis?

Cats with severe FHL are in metabolic crisis and pose considerable risk for anesthetic and surgical complications; collection of a liver biopsy or other surgical samples is inappropriate until the patient is stabilized. The author rarely pursues a liver biopsy in the FHL syndrome and now relies on ultrasound-guided needle aspiration sampling to confirm the obvious diffuse hepatocellular TG vacuolation characteristic of this syndrome. Liver biopsy is pursued only in recalcitrant cases in which appropriate treatment does not resolve or improve clinicopathologic markers of liver disease after 10 days of treatment. It is important to remember that cytologic diagnosis of other hepatobiliary disorders can be remarkably discordant with biopsy specimens.

Liver aspirates should only be collected after vitamin K_1 therapy, after a response interval has been allowed. In the author's hospital, aspirates are not collected at the time of the initial ultrasonographic investigation performed during immediate patient evaluation. Hepatic aspirate collection is done without systemic analgesia or sedation in moribund patients but with local anesthesia. Systemic analgesia, sedation, or anesthesia is restricted to intractable cats or cats struggling in response to handling and restraint despite local analgesia. Simple hepatic aspirates are sprayed on glass slides; thin smears are then prepared, rapidly air dried, and stained with DIFF Quik (Dade Behring, Newark, DE). At least 80% of hepatocytes must have cytosolic vacuolation with empty fat vacuoles (TG does not take up water-soluble stain) to warrant a diagnosis of FHL syndrome (Fig. 10). Because ill cats have a propensity to accumulate TG vacuoles in their hepatocytes, it is important to estimate the number of affected cells. Several aspirates from different sites should be collected. It is essential that hepatocytes be identified, because aspiration of falciform or subcutaneous fat may erroneously be interpreted as a "fatty" sample representing FHL. In some cats with a primary necroinflammatory liver disease or lymphoma, a reactive inflammatory or abnormal cell population may also be identified. Definitive diagnosis of these hepatic disorders requires liver biopsy, however. If pancreatitis is an associated concern, a pancreatic aspirate is collected from an abnormal area identified by ultrasonographic imaging. Cytology from cats with symptomatic pancreatitis often discloses inflammatory cells (neutrophils and macrophages) containing engulfed fat (refractile "empty" fat vacuoles) and acinar cells containing granules (zymogens).

Liver biopsies collected with core needle devices are not necessary for the diagnosis of FHL if an adequate ultrasound examination has been completed; a representative cytologic specimen has been secured; and the signalment, history, and clinicopathologic features are consistent with FHL. Core biopsy procedures carry a high risk for iatrogenic injury in cats (inadvertent sampling of major vessels, gallbladder, and enteric structures) because of their small body size and liver mass. Furthermore, high discordance between core needle and larger tissue samples in cats with cholangitis or cholangiohepatitis has been clearly demonstrated [26]. Surgical biopsies collected during the early stages of FHL management are undesirable, because these cats have a high risk of death as a result of their debilitated state, inability to metabolize anesthetic agents, electrolyte

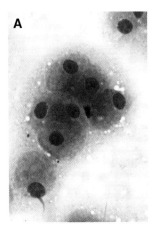

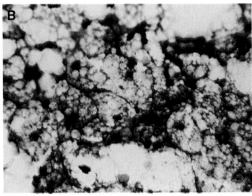

Fig. 10. Photomicrographs showing cytologic preparations stained with Diff Quik (Dade Behring) displaying hepatocytes from a healthy cat (*A*) and from a cat with hepatic lipidosis (*B*) (original magnification ×100). Note the large number of "empty" vacuoles in the hepatocytes from the cat with hepatic lipidosis, where triglyceride does not take up the stain. (Courtesy of New York State College of Veterinary Medicine, Cornell University, Ithaca, NY, 2004.)

derangements, bleeding tendencies, and catabolism resulting in poor tissue healing. Liver biopsy is reserved for cats making a partial but not full recovery from FHL and is used to detect an underlying hepatobiliary disease process. Tissue biopsy using laparoscopic technique is preferred to laparotomy if attempting to rule out concurrent cholangitis or cholangio-hepatitis syndrome or chronic pancreatitis; endoscopic intestinal biopsies should also be collected.

Fluid and electrolyte therapy

Polyionic crystalloid fluids are used to correct dehydration and provide for maintenance and contemporary losses associated with vomiting.

Impaired lactate metabolism is suspected in severe FHL based on high measured lactate concentrations in a few cats. Consequently, avoiding lactate-containing fluids seems prudent. Fluid supplementation with dextrose is contraindicated because this deregulates adaptation to FA oxidation, augments hepatic TG accumulation, aggravates preexisting glucose intolerance, and may induce an osmotic diuresis worsening preexistent electrolyte depletions, especially potassium.

Supplemental potassium chloride is added to fluids using the conventional sliding scale. Unfortunately, there is no accurate formula that can exactly calculate the amount of potassium necessary to replete an individual's status because of differences in urinary and enteric losses or influence of administered insulin in diabetics. The rate of potassium administration is critical and must not exceed 0.5 mEq/kg/h. Judicious titration of administered potassium chloride is individually tailored using twice-daily assessments of the potassium status during the first week. It is essential to correct hypokalemia because this is significantly associated with failure to survive [17]. Hypokalemia usually imparts overt neuromuscular signs (ie, skeletal muscle weakness, cardiac arrhythmias) when K^+ is 2.5 mEq/L or less because of impaired electrical conduction (membrane hyperpolarization). Additional effects include lethargy, anorexia, vomiting (associated with gastric, intestinal, or esophageal stasis), "silent" gut atony that thwarts feeding attempts, inability to concentrate urine, carbohydrate intolerance, hypoventilation as a result of impaired strength of ventilatory muscles, neck ventroflexion, and a demeanor easily confused with that of hepatic encephalopathy. Because severe hypokalemia can promote proximal renal tubular HCO_3^- reabsorption, it can augment the persistence of metabolic alkalosis that may be associated with vomiting. Metabolic alkalosis must be avoided because this partitions potassium intracellularly, may increase renal ammonia production and reabsorption, and enhances ammonia diffusion into the central nervous system (CNS). Continued administration of an alkalinizing fluid in a patient with a metabolic alkalosis perpetuates the potassium imbalance by promoting renal potassium wasting.

Hypophosphatemia may exist at initial presentation or develop secondary to a refeeding phenomenon [27]. Phosphorus is integral to cellular metabolism as a component of cell membranes, nucleic acids, and nucleoproteins. It is also involved in glycolysis and is a key component of vital enzyme systems involving ATP, 2,3-diphosphoglycerate (2,3-DPG), and CK. Therefore, its deficiency can provoke widespread organ dysfunction reflecting impaired cell energy pathways and diminished oxygen availability. Reduced RBC ATP may lead to cell membrane fragility, dysfunction, and hemolysis. Impaired skeletal muscle function manifesting as weakness, myopathy, and rhabdomyolysis has been observed in FHL. Hypophosphatemia can also induce weakness, vomiting, gastric atony, hemolysis, bleeding tendencies as a result of platelet dysfunction, and abnormal neurobehavioral signs. A starting dose of potassium phosphate ranging from 0.01 to

0.03 mmol/kg/h is given at the time of initial feeding in cats with severe FHL, because induced hypophosphatemia is quite common. Care must be given to avoid supplementation with too much potassium (reducing the amount of potassium chloride supplemented).

Hypomagnesemia also may be encountered and may be linked to a number of associated disorders, such as cholangiohepatitis, sepsis, inflammatory bowel disease, enteric or multicentric lymphoma, and acute pancreatitis. Low magnesium is important because of magnesium's status as an enzyme cofactor. Although the mechanisms responsible for hypomagnesemia remain unclarified, they are likely multifactorial and involve transcellular shifts of magnesium into cells with glucose. Hypomagnesemia can provoke many clinical manifestations, including muscle weakness, impaired diaphragm contractility, worsening of preexistent cardiomyopathy (muscle weakness coupled with an increased susceptibility to cardiac arrhythmias), and impaired mental acuity feigning hepatic encephalopathy. All these effects can be mistakenly attributed to disorders of potassium or phosphate. Additionally, severe hypomagnesemia can impair response to potassium supplementation because it perpetuates renal potassium wasting. Acute management of hypomagnesemia requires intravenous magnesium using magnesium sulfate (8.13 mEq/g) and magnesium chloride (9.25 mEq/g) salts, both of which are available as 50% solutions. These are administered as 20% solutions (or lower) in 5% dextrose and water. A recommended dose is 0.75 to 1.0 mEq/kg/d administered by constant rate infusion for the first day. Because of slow restitution of magnesium stores (several days in a patient that is truly deficient), a lower dose of 0.3 to 0.5 mEq/kg/d is given for an additional 2 to 5 days. Higher doses advocated for life-threatening ventricular arrhythmias (0.15–0.3 mEq/kg [100 mg/kg] given over 5–15 minutes) have not been necessary in cats with FHL. Daily monitoring of serum magnesium is essential during supplementation, because overdosing may precipitate hypocalcemia, hypotension, atrioventricular and bundle branch blocks, and respiratory muscle weakness. Overdoses are treated with calcium gluconate given intravenously as a 50-mg/kg slow bolus, followed by a 10-mg/kg/h constant rate infusion.

Rarely, cats with FHL secondary to acute pancreatitis may become hypocalcemic. Because calcium is an important cofactor in zymogen and protease activation, however, treatment is ill advised unless hypocalcemia is symptomatic.

General nutritional recommendations

Nutrition is the cornerstone of treatment as well as prevention of FHL. Feeding 25% of maintenance energy as high-quality protein attenuates FHL but does not ameliorate it [3]. Studies with obese cats undergoing weight loss and diabetic cats support that providing 33% to 45% of calories as protein is preferable [5,28,29]. Fortunately, this level of protein intake can be provided with several commercial cat food products (eg, CliniCare, Abbott Laboratories, Animal Health, Abbott Park, IL; Maximum Calorie, The Iams Co., Dayton, OH; Prescription diet a/d, Hills Pet Nutrition, Topeka, KS; Diabetes Management, DM diet, Nestlé Purina PetCare Company, Checkerboard Square, St. Louis, MO; Prescription diet M/d, Hills Pet Nutrition, Topeka, KS). The response of diabetic cats to high-protein low-carbohydrates diets also should be kept in mind, because cats with diabetes are recognized as a disease group at risk for FHL. Feeding energy-dense diets in which 44% to 66% of the calories derive from fat also is successful and does not promote increased hepatic lipid accumulation if the protein content is sufficient. Carbohydrates should not be used to increase the energy density of the diet for a cat with FHL. Trickle feeding (ie, feeding by slow constant rate infusion) of a liquid diet (CliniCare) containing 34% protein and 45% fat calories also has proven effective. This approach is routinely used by the author during the initial few days of therapy via nasogastric tube.

The quantity of food ingested must provide adequate energy and protein to avoid catabolism. Although the exact energy requirements of cats with liver disease have not been determined, using metabolizable energy at a rate of 60 to 80 kcal/kg of ideal body weight provides a successful target. It is important to adopt the concept of feeding the highest or "optimal" amount of protein that the individual cat can tolerate. Protein restriction is only used when hepatic encephalopathy is overtly encountered or in the rare circumstance of ammonium urate crystalluria. Feeding a balanced and complete feline ration as opposed to a "designer" diet is recommended, because the latter may be unexpectedly restricted in an essential nutrient. Most liquid enteral formulas for people lack adequate taurine for cats and may contain arginine or citrulline in quantities insufficient to sustain feline urea cycle function. If such products are used, taurine at a rate of 250 mg/d and arginine at a rate of 1 g per 8–fl oz can (250 mg per 100 kcal) of diet is recommended. If designer diets are preferred, such as for cats with known inflammatory bowel disease, basic ingredients can be formulated using a nutritional tool provided as a free service on the Internet (Nutritional Analysis Tool 2, available at: http://nat.crgq.com/). Care should be taken to consult a reputable feline nutritional reference to ensure provision of appropriate feline vitamins and other essential nutrients.

Nutritional support

Oral "forced" alimentation

Some cats, albeit only a few, can be rescued from FHL using oral alimentation. Although this has been successful for some owners able to coax their cat into accepting syringe feeding, it may precipitate the onset of a food aversion syndrome. This learned avoidance response to oral food intake may result in rejection of a particular type or brand of food and may delay the return to self-alimentation. Consequently, routes for more efficient enteral feeding are usually necessary.

Nasogastric tubes

Because of patient status and the risk of bleeding during the first few days of treatment, a nasogastric feeding tube is used for feeding during the first few days of hospitalization. The small tube lumen (5–8 French scale for cats) limits feeding to a liquefied diet. These tubes are placed after administration of a local anesthetic to the nasal passage (eg, 0.5% proparacaine [Ophthaine]) and lubrication with a small amount of topical lidocaine gel. Long-term feeding using this route is discouraged because of the associated discomfort from nasal and pharyngeal irritation, potential for tube displacement (retroflexion during emesis), and necessity for an Elizabethan collar to guard against self-removal of the tube. Nevertheless, some cats have been recovered using only this method of feeding.

Sedation/anesthesia for esophagostomy/endoscopic gastrostomy tube placement

After hydration, electrolyte, and coagulation problems are improved, short-term anesthesia permits placement of a feeding tube with a larger lumen. Avoiding injectable agents that require hepatic metabolism or impose an oxidant challenge is paramount in patients with FHL; prolonged anesthetic recovery has been observed with oxymorphone, propofol, diazepam, etomidate, and ketamine. Life-endangering hemolytic anemia may follow injection of diazepam and etomidate preparations that contain 40% to 35% vol/vol propylene glycol, respectively, as well as after injection of propofol, a phenol derivative. Hemolytic crisis typically is identified from 4 to 12 hours after drug administration. Persistent hypotension, recumbency, and weakness may occur after use of injectable anesthetic regimens.

A preferred anesthesia protocol involves administering a small dose of butorphanol (0.05 mg/kg) only if necessary in frightened or stressed cats, followed by mask induction and maintenance of short-term anesthesia with isoflurane. Administration of anticholinergics, such as glycopyrrolate and atropine, should be avoided because they promote gastric atony that may last for several days, thwarting nutritional support.

Esophagostomy tube

The tube size ranges between 10 and 12 French scale. Care should be given to avoid the use of highly pliable silicone tubes that are easily retroflexed. Esophagostomy tubes (E-tubes) can be placed and secured within 10 to 15 minutes, are relatively pain-free, are easy to care for and use, and are rarely complicated by infection or retroflexion. A thoracic radiograph is mandatory after tube placement to verify appropriate positioning of the tube tip cranial to the gastroesophageal junction (Fig. 11). Tube insertion into the stomach must be avoided because this increases the risk of reflux esophagitis. Careful cervical placement is necessary to avoid laceration of large vessels; transillumination may assist careful placement.

Gastrostomy tube

Gastrostomy tubes (G-tubes) are preferred by some clinicians because their larger tube lumen (≥20 French scale) permits easier feeding and greater food variety and they are more amenable to the trickle feeding approach necessary for some cats. G-tubes are best placed percutaneously using endoscopic guidance in cats with FHL. During endoscopic placement, biopsies of the stomach and duodenum may be collected if enteric disease is considered to be an underlying primary disease. G-tubes placed surgically impose excessive risk because of prolonged anesthesia and tissue injury and may be placed too ventrally in the stomach, distorting its normal position

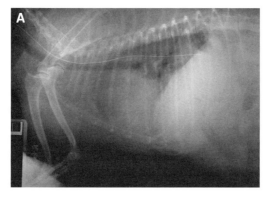

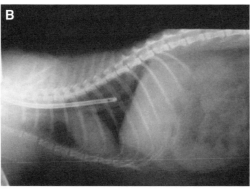

Fig. 11. Thoracic radiograph showing a malpositioned esophagostomy tube (E-tube) placed through the gastroesophageal junction (*A*); a well-placed E-tube is also shown (*B*). (Courtesy of New York State College of Veterinary Medicine, Cornell University, Ithaca, NY, 2004.)

and causing discomfort. Surgically placed tubes also may not achieve rapid body wall adhesion as compared with those placed endoscopically. Premature tube removal (within 2–3 weeks) may lead to septic peritonitis. Surgical placement of gastrostomy tubes in cats with FHL has been associated with the highest mortality in the author's hospital, seemingly because of the tenuous metabolic status of affected cats and their heightened risk and slow recovery from anesthetic and surgical procedures.

General maintenance for esophagostomy and gastrostomy tubes

E-tubes and G-tubes must be securely anchored to their puncture sites, and the surrounding area must be kept clean and protected during the first 2 weeks. The puncture site should be inspected daily for infection or retrograde food infiltration, a small amount of triple antibiotic ointment applied to the puncture site and suture areas, and an aseptic supporting bandage applied. Any discharge should be cytologically examined to detect infection. Owners must be taught appropriate appliance care and bandaging procedures. Tubes must be cleansed after use by flushing with a small amount of lukewarm water, and the insertion site and tube must be protected from patient mutilation. Simple provision of an infant's tee-shirt is not an effective deterrent; bandage stabilization is preferred. Despite protective bandaging, some patients require an Elizabethan collar to prohibit tube mutilation or self-removal. The supportive bandage covering a G-tube should have the tube silhouette drawn on it to avoid inadvertent damage during bandage change.

Feeding regimen

Initial feeding of lukewarm water at a rate of 15 mL at 2-hour intervals two to three times discloses the likelihood of emesis and presence of gastric atony. When using a G-tube, it is useful to aspirate gastric contents before each water feeding to appraise gastric emptying. Food is progressively introduced over a 2- to 4-day interval to achieve intake of between 250 and 400 kcal/d for the average-sized cat. Initial feeding is delayed for 24 hours after G-tube insertion to allow return of gastric motility and to permit formation of an initial wound seal around the insertion site. Feeding through an E-tube may be initiated after full recovery from the anesthetic restraint.

Daily food intake should be divided into four or more small meals; however, some cats do not tolerate meal feeding but accept trickle or continuous feeding. This may be accomplished using nasogastric E-tube or G-tube routes. During trickle feeding via a G-tube, gastric atony may be monitored by aspirating gastric contents every 8 to 12 hours to determine residual gastric volume. If a volume more than the hourly delivery rate is encountered, feeding is temporarily discontinued for several hours, electrolytes are evaluated to determine a cause for enteric atony, and the hourly feeding rate is reduced by 20%. A continued trend of high residual gastric volume warrants evaluation of tube position by ultrasound or radiographic contrast (a sterile water-soluble contrast material, such as Hypague-76 [66% diatrizoate meglumine and 10% diatrizoate sodium sterile solution; Amersham Health, Princeton, NJ]) to investigate for tube-induced pyloric outflow obstruction.

Management of vomiting

Repeated vomiting after commencement of feeding should initiate investigation of electrolyte disturbances (eg, hypokalemia, hypophosphatemia), feeding tube complications (eg, kinking, retroflexion, painful positioning), or an underlying disease, such as inflammatory bowel disease or pancreatitis. If a causal factor is not found, metoclopramide is administered at a rate of 0.01 to 0.02 mg/kg/h by constant rate infusion (0.2–0.5 mg/kg/d). Alternatively, metoclopramide can be administered by subcutaneous injection (0.2–0.5 mg/kg up to three times daily) 30 minutes before feeding to meal-fed cats. Metoclopramide accelerates the emptying of liquid material into the duodenum, centrally inhibits emesis via dopaminergic receptors in the chemoreceptive trigger zone, and may diminish the severity of vomiting by preventing the retrograde peristalsis that precedes vomiting. Side effects caused by overdosing include muscle fasciculations (first noted in the whiskers, ears, and face), body tremors, facial expression of "trismus," and seizures.

Alternative antiemetics include ondansetron (Zofran; GlaxoSmithKline, Research Triangle Park, NC) and butorphanol. Ondansetron, a serotonin (5-HT$_3$) receptor antagonist, mediates nausea and vomiting through its influence on the chemoreceptive trigger zone and is associated with fewer side effects than metoclopramide. A dose of 0.1 to 0.2 mg/kg administered every 6 to 12 hours has been used. Butorphanol provides an antiemetic effect when combined with other antiemetics; a low dose of 0.1 mg/kg administered every 12 hours has been used. Careful observation is warranted to avoid patient sedation.

Exercise may stimulate enteric motility in cats with FHL and is easily included in the treatment regimen. Fifteen to 30 minutes of free-walking exercise in a nonstressful environment (eg, no barking dogs) during owner visitation and before feeding in meal-fed cats should suffice.

Appetite stimulants

Appetite stimulants (eg, diazepam, clonazepam, cyproheptadine) are unreliable for ensuring adequate energy intake in cats. Diazepam requires hepatic biotransformation, specifically hepatic glucuronidation. Hepatic glucuronidation of some other drugs is known to be slower in cats compared with other species and likely is compromised in FHL. Use of diazepam also imposes a risk (albeit low) of idiopathic fulminant hepatic failure in cats, and the injectable form delivers an oxidant challenge (propylene glycol carrier) [30]. Idiopathic hepatotoxicity associated with fulminant hepatic failure also has been observed in a cat given clonazepam and in a cat given cyproheptadine as appetite stimulants (unpublished data, S.A. Center, DVM). Propofol has been suggested to provide an antianorexic effect in inappetent cats, but such use is strongly contraindicated in FHL because of the pro-oxidant effects of propofol in these patients, heightened risk of aspiration pneumonia in sedated cats secondary to choking or emesis, delayed hepatic metabolism of the drug, and propensity to cause Heinz body anemia. Furthermore, adverse effects of propofol on mitochondrial function may also be relevant [31].

Water-soluble vitamin supplementation

Considering the importance of the liver for storage and activation of many of water-soluble vitamins and the apparent susceptibility of cats to thiamine and cobalamin depletion, a doubled daily maintenance dose of water-soluble vitamins is recommended in FHL. Water-soluble vitamins are usually administered with intravenous crystalloid fluids each day; typically, a fortified B-complex solution (2 mL) is mixed with each liter of fluids. Fluids containing B-vitamins should be protected from direct light. Ingredients in a typical fortified B-complex vitamin solution appropriate for addition to intravenous fluids are summarized in Table 2.

Thiamine (vitamin B_1)

Thiamine deficiency is recognized based on response to treatment. Converted intracellularly to its active form, thiamine pyrophosphate, thiamine acts as an essential coenzyme mediating carbohydrate metabolism. Thiamine depletion compromises cerebral and cerebellar energy metabolism and impairs synaptic nerve impulse transmission and DNA synthesis.

Table 2
Contents of a fortified B-vitamin complex used for supplementation of crystalloid fluids in cats with feline hepatic lipidosis

Thiamine hydrochloride (vitamin B_1)	50 mg
Riboflavin 5' phosphate sodium (vitamin B_2)	2.0–2.5 mg
Niacinamide (vitamin B_3)	50–100 mg
D-panthenol (vitamin B_5)	5–10 mg
Pyridoxine sodium chloride (vitamin B_6)	2–5 mg
Cyanocobalamin (vitamin B_{12})	variable, 0.4–50 μg
(Low vitamin B_{12} values necessitate additional supplementation in deficient cats administered intramuscularly)	
Benzyl alcohol (preservative)	1.5%
(no adverse consequences noted in cats with FHL)	

Depletion of thiamine can derive from chronic anorexia, protein-energy malnutrition (eg, inappropriate diet, enteric disease-causing malabsorption), protracted vomiting, chronic polyuria causing accelerated renal losses, and carbohydrate loading in the presence of marginal thiamine stores (eg, refeeding after starvation as occurs in FHL). Symptomatic cats are weak or lethargic, may appear apathetic with signs confused with those of hepatic encephalopathy, or may be moribund. Neurologic manifestations include central vestibular signs, abnormal oculocephalic responses, dilated poorly responsive pupils, head or neck ventroflexion, abnormal postural reactions, and hypothermia (involvement of central temperature regulation nuclei; Fig. 12). Severe hypotension reflects abnormal sympathetic responses and reduced peripheral vascular resistance.

Unfortunately, a rare vasovagal anaphylactic response to intramuscular thiamine administration has been observed in a small number of cats when thiamine hydrochloride was administered subcutaneously, similar to a rare reaction described in human beings [33]. This potentially fatal reaction is characterized by cardiac arrest or severe bradycardia, cardiac arrhythmias, apnea, hypotension, collapse, seizure, and protracted neuromuscular weakness. Thiamine (50 mg/mL of B2-soluble vitamin solution) is provided using 1–2 mL of B-soluble vitamins per liter of crystalloid fluids.

Vitamin B_{12}

Chronically malnourished cats with primary enteric disease may have impaired cobalamin availability. The availability of cobalamin is influenced by enteric microbial flora [34]; high numbers of enteric microorganisms that bind intrinsic factor or metabolically consume vitamin B_{12} can reduce cobalamin availability. Healthy cats given oral metronidazole increase circulating B_{12} concentration by twofold as a result of altered colonic microflora [35]. Cobalamin supplementation is recommended for all cats with FHL that are suspected of having an underlying primary enteric disease; all suspected individuals should be tested by securing a diagnostic sample before cobalamin administration (see Fig. 8). A dose between 0.5 and 1.0 mg per cat is given on the first day of hospitalization. Based on plasma vitamin B_{12} concentrations, this dose is repeated at weekly or biweekly intervals until measured cobalamin concentrations document values within the normal range. Long-term supplementation is predicated on the basis of the underlying disease and the clinical ability to correct or ameliorate it.

Consideration of the concurrent status of GSH and α-tocopherol has importance in the cat with cobalamin deficiency as this may restrict thiol availability and impair methylation reactions essential for metabolic recovery [36]. Of special concern in FHL is that impaired proprionate metabolism derived from cobalamin deficiency (decreased L-methylmalonyl-CoA activity) may reduce availability of free-CN necessary for transport of long chain FA into mitochondria where they undergo β-oxidation. The

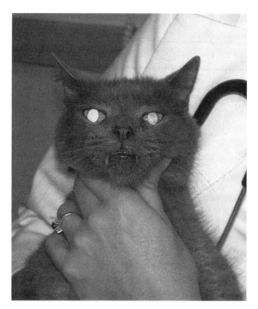

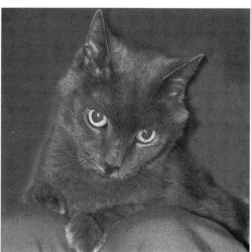

Fig. 12. Photographs of a cat with hepatic lipidosis demonstrating clinical signs consistent with thiamine deficiency. This cat had anisocoria, dilated unresponsive pupils, vestibular signs, neck ventroflexion, postural reaction deficits, and seizures that resolved with thiamine therapy. Underlying disorders were hyperthyroidism and severe inflammatory bowel disease. (Courtesy of New York State College of Veterinary Medicine, Cornell University, Ithaca, NY, 2004.)

resulting accumulation of FA products may impose an inhibitory influence on ammonia detoxification (inhibition of carbamyl phosphate synthetase, aspartate availability) [37–40]. The relationship between cobalamin sufficiency, CN, and hepatic lipidosis has been explored using a rat model of cobalamin deficiency where CN supplementation only partially reversed the metabolic blockade of FA oxidation and hepatic lipid accumulation without restitution of cobalamin [40].

Fat-soluble vitamin supplementation

Vitamin K₁

Vitamin K_1 is given to all cats with FHL during the first 12 hours of hospitalization. The intramuscular or subcutaneous route is recommended, because an apparent reduced enterohepatic circulation of bile acids likely compromises uptake of enterically administered fat-soluble vitamins and because intravascular injection may provoke anaphylaxis. A dose ranging between 0.5 and 1.5 mg/kg repeated three times at 12- hour intervals has been clinically proven to ameliorate coagulation abnormalities based on PIVKA testing (see Fig. 6B). It is important to calculate the dose of vitamin K carefully, because too much can induce oxidant injury to the liver, other organs, and erythrocytes.

Vitamin E

Hepatic and potentially systemic depletion of vitamin E (α-tocopherol) is suspected to complicate FHL based on circumstantial information, including (1) experimentally modeled hepatic lipidosis, (2) vitamin E status in human beings affected with a similar disorder, (3) reduced liver tissue GSH concentrations in FHL (representing essential antioxidant depletion), (4) the presence of vitamin K depletion (also a fat-soluble vitamin), and (5) serum bile acid fractionation profiles consistent with impaired assimilation of fat-soluble vitamins. Treatment with vitamin E is recommended because it has the ability to protect lipid-soluble and water-soluble cell constituents against oxidative damage and experimentally provides antioxidant protection in a number of different forms of liver injury, including those associated with cholestasis [41–43]. As an antioxidant, the amount of vitamin E needed to protect membrane PUFAs against oxidative damage ranges from 0.4 to 0.8 mg/g of PUFA fed [44]. Diets rich in long-chain PUFAs may require vitamin E at a rate greater than 1.5 mg per gram of PUFA. Because it is well established that diets supplemented with fish oils can lower hepatic and plasma α-tocopherol concentrations, use of fish oil supplements in cats with FHL may increase the vitamin E requirements, although this has not specifically been investigated [45]. The complex relation between vitamin E status and dietary (n3) PUFA intake (specific fish oils differentially influence vitamin E requirements) complicates definitive recommendations [46]. Furthermore, cholestasis associated with FHL may impose a heightened requirement for vitamin E similar to the situation in people with impaired enterohepatic bile acid circulation (documented in biliary tree occlusion or biliary atresia) [47]. A water-soluble form of α-tocopherol is desirable for enteric dosing, and a dose of α-tocopherol at a rate of at least 10 IU/kg/d of vitamin E is recommended but has not been critically evaluated for efficacy.

L-carnitine supplementation

CN supplementation is recommended for cats with FHL for several reasons. Hepatic CN synthesis may be limited in these catabolic cats because of hepatic dysfunction and impaired availability of one or more of its synthetic substrates: lysine, SAMe, Fe^{2+}, vitamin C, succinate, and pyridoxal phosphate. The ability of cats with FHL to provide CN appropriately for FA oxidation and FA dispersal to facilitate a net negative FA flux remains undetermined. Study of CN supplementation in obese cats undergoing weight loss demonstrated increased concentrations of acetyl-CN, the end product of FA oxidation, and led to a higher acyl-CN/total CN ratio consistent with an enhanced rate of FA oxidation (Fig. 13) [48]. Further work substantiates the finding that supplemental CN facilitates FA oxidation and fat mobilization, conserves lean body mass in obese cats undergoing weight reduction, and can attenuate the degree of hepatic lipid accumulation in modeled FHL [4,10,49,50]. Improved survival in cats with severe FHL has been achieved in the author's hospital by administering CN at a dose of 250 to 500 mg per cat per day. Medical grade CN should be used whenever possible, because there is a wide diversity in the bioavailability of different commercial products [51].

Amino acid supplementation

Short-term taurine supplementation is used by the author for cats with FHL, because these patients have low plasma taurine concentrations, obligatorily use taurine for bile acid conjugation as do all cats, and have high bile acid concentrations and a high flux of conjugated bile acids into their urine [52]. Taurine conjugates the membranocytolytic bile acids, mitigating their toxic effects on cells, and influences a number of other physiologic and metabolic processes important in FHL (eg, its influence on membrane calcium ion flux, membrane stabilization, detoxification reactions, and anti-oxidant protection).

The feline dietary requirement for taurine depends not only on the enteric dietary protein intake but also on the quality of protein ingested. It also is proven that the extent of protein digestion during food processing influences an individual cat's quantitative need for extra taurine [53,54]. Because taurine synthesis from sulfur-containing amino acids proceeds slowly in cats, protein supplementation alone cannot sufficiently meet their needs. Additionally, undigested proteins in the alimentary canal may increase the taurine requirements by physically binding bile acids or by enhancing the microbial catabolic use of taurine. Although the latter effect may occur in FHL

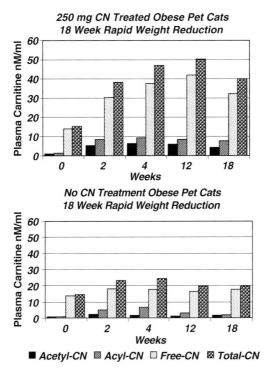

Fig. 13. Plasma carnitine (CN) moieties in obese pet cats undergoing weight loss; one group received supplemental L-CN (250 mg/d), and the other received an identical appearing placebo [48]. Higher plasma CN concentrations and percentage of acetyl-CN were achieved with supplementation. The increased acetyl-CN concentrations correspond with enhanced or preferential use of fat for energy.

secondary to enteric atony, it may be attenuated by the oral antibiotic treatment that is often empirically prescribed during the early phase of treatment. Based on the concern for taurine adequacy, supplementation with taurine at a rate of 250 mg/d day is provided during the first 7 to 10 days of FHL treatment.

Thiol antioxidant supplementation

Thiol-containing compounds (compounds containing S-H bonds or HS-SH disulfide bonds) have central importance in many biochemical and pharmacologic reactions. The disulfide bond, usually by incorporation of a cysteine moiety, is important in determining the tertiary structure of proteins (eg, molecule configuration, folding) and in influencing the pharmacologic effects of certain drugs. A significant number of proteins involved in cell signaling contain critical thiol sites; each of these can have its function dramatically altered by oxidation and the formation of mixed disulfides.

The most important nonprotein thiol source in most cells is GSH. Maintaining GSH homeostasis is essential for normal health and reparative responses to tissue injury. Conservation of reduced GSH as well as provision of substrates for GSH synthesis (cysteine, glutamic acid, and glycine) is important to ensure normal biologic functions. Although there is constant turnover of GSH in the body, the liver sits at the center of its dynamic flux. The liver has one of the highest organ contents of GSH and is unique in two ways: (1) it has the exclusive ability to convert methionine to cysteine (the direct substrate for GSH synthesis) via the transsulfuration pathway, and (2) it exports GSH into plasma and bile at a rate that accounts for nearly all its GSH biosynthesis [55,56]. Hepatic exportation of GSH accounts for 90% of the plasma GSH concentration [57]. Numerous experimental and clinical situations characterized by low GSH concentrations in liver tissue substantiate increased risk of liver injury from spontaneous disease and toxicity derived from therapeutic agents. It is clear that low hepatic GSH synthesis has polysystemic ramifications in cats with FHL.

Inappetence is known to deplete circulating and liver tissue GSH and SAMe concentrations as a result of diminished availability of cysteine and other precursor amino acids required for GSH synthesis. Starvation also enhances hepatic mitochondrial susceptibility to oxidant injury, with greater damage being incurred the longer food is deprived [15,58]. Kwashiorkor (protein calorie starvation in humans), which shares many similarities with FHL, is associated with impaired redox status and enhanced lipid peroxidation [59–61]. Experimental models of hepatic lipidosis demonstrate increased risk for mitochondrial oxidative injury because of enhanced production of reactive oxygen species (ROS) [16]. Experimental data substantiate that starvation also worsens mitochondrial function in animals with a fatty liver. Because mitochondrial oxidative metabolism represents the major source of cell energy, impaired organelle function compromises energy management and ATP availability. Oxidant injury is promoted by concurrent cobalamin deficiency because this compromises the ability to sustain adequate cell GSH concentrations [62].

Low hepatic GSH concentrations (Fig. 14) and high susceptibility to Heinz body hemolysis are the basis for thiol donor supplementation in FHL. Intravenous NAC is used as a crisis cysteine donor in FHL during the first few days of treatment. NAC may be a direct source of cysteine after hydrolysis or may reduce plasma cystine (the oxidized form of cysteine) through thiol-disulfide exchange, liberating endogenous cysteine [57]. Initially, NAC at a rate of 140 mg/kg (20% solution diluted at least 1:4 with saline or 5% dextrose) is given intravenously through a 0.2-μm non-pyrogenic filter over a 20-minute interval. Experimental work with NAC and SAMe in a steatotic liver model have each demonstrated benefit [63,64]. A longer infusion interval is contraindicated based on a recognized complication in human beings caused by impaired urea cycle ammonia detoxification [65]. Overdosing NAC may result in excessive cysteine catabolism in the liver,

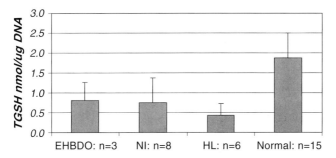

Fig. 14. Liver total GSH concentrations, spontaneous liver disease vs healthy cats. Total glutathione (TGSH) concentrations (mean, standard deviation) in liver tissue (per tissue DNA concentration) from healthy cats and clinical patients with various liver disorders, including extrahepatic bile duct occlusion (EHBDO), necroinflammatory liver disease (NI), and hepatic lipidosis (HL) as well as from healthy cats (normal). The remarkably low TGSH concentration in hepatic lipidosis is consistent with a substantial reduction in tissue antioxidant availability (*Data from* New York State College of Veterinary Medicine, Cornell University, Ithaca, NY, 2004) [14].

with the potential to produce an overabundance of protons favoring glutamine synthesis instead of ammonia detoxification in the urea cycle (Fig. 15). For this reason, giving bolus doses of NAC is thought to be safer than using a constant rate infusion in patients with liver disease [65]. Subsequent administration at 8- to 12-hour intervals is provided using a dose of 70 mg/kg; dosing frequency is highly variable depending on clinical signs.

Once enteric alimentation is established, enteric coated SAMe tablets replace NAC treatment. A 180-mg dose per cat (approximately 35–60 mg/kg)

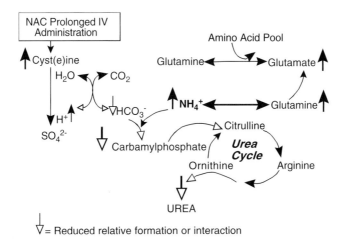

Fig. 15. Theoretic complication induced by slow constant rate infusion of N-acetylcysteine (NAC). Excessive cysteine catabolism yields an overabundance of protons blocking urea formation (reduced carbamyl phosphate necessary for ammonia condensation) and favoring glutamine synthesis.

is given orally one or two times daily. This dose of SAMe significantly increases hepatic GSH concentrations and influences the redox status of RBCs and liver tissue in healthy cats dosed after an overnight fast [66]. The tablets have an enteric coating, because food compromises the bioavailability of SAMe; crushing the tablets and administering them in the presence of gastric food reduces efficacy. Unfortunately, the specifics of dosing have not been evaluated in this scenario.

Ursodeoxycholic acid supplementation

Hydrophobic bile acids that accumulate in cats with FHL may impair formation of very low density lipoproteins (VLDLs) essential for TG egress from the liver. This is a concern in FHL, because suppression of hepatic TG secretion has been shown in human and rat hepatocytes exposed to increased but physiologically relevant bile acid concentrations [67–69]. Ursodeoxycholic acid (UDCA), a synthetic hydrophilic bile acid, is used therapeutically for gallstone dissolution in human patients and for attenuation of hepatotoxicity imposed by membranocytolytic bile acids accumulating in cholestatic disorders. A plethora of basic research has delineated cytoprotective, anti-inflammatory, antioxidant, antifibrotic, and antiapoptic benefits from UDCA [14]. Administration of UDCA to obese children with hepatic steatosis has not provided clinical benefit, however [70]. Furthermore, UDCA did not facilitate regression of hepatic steatosis in a standard rat model, although incorporation of UDCA in the diet initiating steatosis ameliorated the syndrome [71]. Clinical trials in adult human subjects with nonalcoholic steatohepatitis (NASH, a form of metabolic fatty liver) describe variable results with UDCA, including clinicopathologic and histologic benefits but no change in hepatic fat content after months of therapy [72,73]. The most recent multi-institutional prospective trial showed that UDCA had no benefit as a single-agent treatment after 2 years of administration in this disorder [74].

All bile acids have the potential to disrupt normal cellular processes. Cats with FHL have remarkably increased total serum bile acid concentrations similar in quantity and quality to those associated with major bile duct occlusion [21]. Treatment with UDCA is not recommended by the author for cats jaundiced as a result of FHL, because there is no evidence supporting its short-term efficacy or that it is innocuous in this syndrome.

Other concerns

Refeeding phenomenon

The refeeding phenomenon describes a potentially lethal condition characterized by severe electrolyte and fluid shifts invoked by sudden metabolic adaptations in malnourished patients undergoing initial refeeding (oral, enteral, or parenteral) [75]. Cats with FHL seem to have a heightened risk. The underlying pathomechanism involves conversion from a purely catabolic state invoked by prolonged anorexia to rapid-onset carbohydrate use. Shifted metabolism promotes insulin release and cell uptake of glucose, phosphate, potassium, magnesium, and water as well as enhanced protein synthesis. Nutritional provision magnifies cell requirements for phosphate, potassium, glucose, and water and increases the demand for ATP, 2,3-DPG, and CK.

Hypokalemia, by far the most common electrolyte abnormality in FHL, is magnified in severity because of refeeding. Although less common on initial presentation than hypokalemia, severe hypophosphatemia also can produce a plethora of clinical signs as previously defined. Hypophosphatemia induced by the refeeding phenomenon typically appears within the first 48 hours of initial feeding; effects are clinically overt when phosphate is 1.5 mg/dL or less. Least commonly associated with refeeding is symptomatic hypomagnesemia, although its effects can be profound and easily confused with those of hypokalemia and hypophosphatemia.

Hyperglycemia induced by carbohydrate intake, gluconeogenesis, diabetes mellitus, or fluids supplemented with glucose aggravates electrolyte depletion through osmotic diuresis. During the initial stages of feeding, this also may provoke symptomatic hypothiaminosis in cats with marginal thiamine reserves. Because thiamine functions as a cofactor for a number of enzymatic reactions necessary in glucose metabolism, thiamine supplementation is mandatory during initial refeeding and is provided using a B-soluble vitamin source. For reasons noted previously, glucose supplementation is strongly contraindicated in FHL.

Importance of body condition assessment

Body condition scores and estimation of the percentage of ideal body weight are useful in guiding appropriate fluid and drug dosing. This effort should guard against inappropriate drug and fluid dosing for the over-conditioned cat with FHL. Sequential body weight and hydration assessment is essential in tailoring fluid provision during initial hospitalization.

Drugs to avoid

Stanozolol (a 17-α–alkylated steroid), sometimes prescribed as an anabolic agent, seems to increase the risk of FHL and should be avoided [76]. Because several steroid hormones impose a dose-dependent inhibition of bile flow, careful consideration should be given before instituting such treatments [77].

In some cats, glucocorticoids given for a primary disease process have seemingly precipitated the onset of FHL. It is speculated that this reflects the inhibitory influence of glucocorticoids on mitochondrial matrix acyl-CoA dehydrogenases and β-oxidation (medium- and short-chain FAs) as demonstrated in vitro [78]. In addition to inhibiting initial β-oxidation of some FAs, dexamethasone has been shown to reduce hepatic egress of TG, inducing microvesicular steatosis and ultrastructural mitochondrial lesions in other species. Although glucocorticoids should warrant concern for their potentiating influence on FHL, patients with an underlying disease requiring glucocorticoid intervention usually improve as the primary disease process is brought under control and nutritional and metabolic support is provided.

Tetracyclines should be avoided in cats with FHL because of their steatogenic influence on hepatocytes in many mammals [79]. A concentration-dependent inhibition of mitochondrial β-oxidation has been proven in vitro using canine hepatocytes [78]. Accumulated nonesterified FAs converge into hepatocellular microvesicular TG stores.

Appetite stimulants, such as diazepam, clonazepam, and cyproheptadine, encourage a false sense of nutritional success in cats with FHL, and several impose the potential for hepatotoxicity. Sedation in response to benzodiazepines increases the risk for aspiration of vomited material. In addition to the acknowledged low feline ability to glucuronidate the metabolites of some drugs, FHL-induced hepatic dysfunction may increase the risk for drug toxicity. Diazepam, oxazepam, and cyproheptadine have each been associated with fulminant hepatic failure in individual patients.

Drugs imposing oxidant challenge include injectable diazepam or etomidate (propylene glycol carriers), propofol, benzene derivatives (eg, cetocaine, benzocaine), onion powder food flavoring, and foods and treats containing propylene glycol as well as others. These products increase RBC oxidant challenge and must be assiduously avoided. Propylene glycol carriers injected intravenously typically induce a hemolytic response within 4 to 12 hours of administration and may provoke acute anemia severe enough to cause death.

Caution is warranted in use of propofol in cats with FHL, because slow recovery (hours to days) and death have been observed in these patients when conservative doses have been used. It remains undetermined whether toxicity relates to the phenol derivative status of propofol (cats generally do not metabolize phenol derivatives well) or to impaired FA oxidation associated with a "propofol infusion syndrome" described in critically ill pediatric human patients [31,32]. In the latter syndrome, propofol impairs mitochondrial electron transport, oxidation of short-chain FAs, and mitochondrial transport of long-chain FAs. Affected human patients demonstrate metabolic acidosis, FA blockade, and fatal myocardial failure associated with lethal hypotension.

Careful dosing of vitamin K_1 is essential in FHL because of its oxidant capacity, considering that some cats present with low RBC GSH concentrations. Quinones are well-acknowledged oxidants having heightened toxicity in GSH-depleted cell systems [80,81]. Hemolytic reactions associated with Heinz body formation have developed in cats with FHL receiving

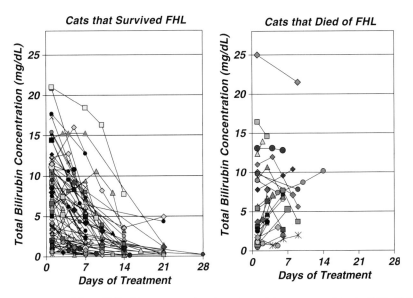

Fig. 16. Sequential total bilirubin concentrations in cats surviving or succumbing to FHL. Cats that survive demonstrate a 50% reduction in their total bilirubin concentration within 7 to 10 days. (*Data from* New York State College of Veterinary Medicine, Cornell University, Ithaca, NY, 2004.)

appropriate doses too frequently (eg, daily basis) or excessive individual doses (eg, >1.5 mg/kg per treatment beyond three doses at 12-hour intervals).

What to monitor

Recovery from FHL is best predicted by sequential measurement of the serum total bilirubin concentration (Fig. 16), along with the patient's vital

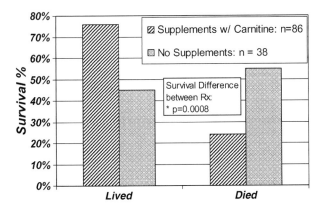

Fig. 17. Cats (n = 124) receiving treatments (33 of 157 cats died or were euthanized within 1 day). Survival percentage in cats receiving nutritional support with a premium cat food with or without metabolic supplements described in this article. Consult text for detailed discussion. (*Data from* New York State College of Veterinary Medicine, Cornell University, Ithaca, NY, 2004.)

Box 1. Treatment guidelines

Dos and Don'ts
1. Don't rush to sedate or anesthetize, place a central jugular line, apply an E- or G-tube for feeding, do cystocentesis, or aspirate liver until vitamin K has been given and a reasonable response interval permitted (12–24 hours).
2. Avoid using general anesthetics until electrolyte and hydration deficits are addressed and abnormalities are attenuated.
3. Consider that FHL is most often a secondary disorder. Look for an underlying cause.
4. A liver biopsy is not necessary initially to diagnose and treat FHL, although some cats have cholangitis/cholangiohepatitis or another hepatic disease that eventually requires biopsy. Liver aspiration cytology combined with signalment, history, typical clinicopathologic features, and ultrasound imaging provides enough information for a provisional diagnosis and aggressive treatment.
5. Avoid lactate containing fluids initially.
6. Do not supplement fluids with dextrose; this may promote further hepatic TG accumulation.
7. Correct electrolyte abnormalities early.
8. Anticipate electrolyte shifts associated with the refeeding syndrome (especially severe acute hypophosphatemia), and make efforts to thwart their occurrence.
9. Do feed a protein replete balanced feline diet. Avoid feeding a protein-restricted diet unless overt hepatic encephalopathy is recognized.
10. Ensure adequate B-soluble vitamins. Consider vitamin B_{12} deficiency and treat based on suspicion of such. Always collect a baseline blood sample for vitamin B_{12} determination for retrospective guidance regarding the need for chronic parenteral vitamin supplementation.
11. Anticipate antioxidant depletion, especially in cats showing Heinz body hemolysis. Provide a thiol donor substrate, such as NAC for crisis, followed more chronically with enteric SAMe dosing.

If neck ventroflexion is present, consider electrolyte or thiamine insufficiency
   Check electrolytes: potassium, phosphate, and magnesium; provide supplements as appropriate.

Administer thiamine: 100 mg in fluids (B-soluble vitamins
given slowly with crystalloid fluids). Parenteral
administration by the intramuscular route may result in
collapse, although this is rare.

B-soluble vitamins in fluid: consult Table 2 (2 mL B-soluble
vitamins/L crystalloid fluids).

Consider the possibility of other underlying disorders and
submit appropriate tests early in Illness: cervical weakness
(neurologic disease, vertebral injury), muscle weakness
(myopathy, myasthenia gravis [extremely rare]),
hyperthyroidism, organophosphate toxicosis, and even
hepatic encephalopathy.

signs. Total bilirubin concentrations usually decline by 50% during the first 7 to 10 days of treatment in cats destined to survive. Sequential monitoring of liver enzymes is unreliable as a predictor of survival. Cats with a poor prognosis usually decline or succumb within 7 days.

Does treatment with supplements make a difference?

There are no placebo-controlled studies of cats with severe hepatic lipidosis that compare feeding of premium protein-replete diets with similar feeding with the metabolic supplements suggested in this article. In the author's hospital, nutritional support using a premium cat food (eg, Maximum Calorie, Prescription diet a/d) has been combined with the discussed metabolic supplements in many affected cats over the past 15 years. A summary of patient survival with and without metabolic supplements (including L-CN) is presented in Fig. 17.

There was no difference in survival when this population was stratified according to method of alimentation; however, significantly greater survival is realized when metabolic supplements are prescribed, including L-CN. Review of these patients disclosed no significant determinants suggesting more severe disease in cats given supplement treatment. This finding contradicts the outcome in a retrospective study of 43 cats with hepatic lipidosis from a large referral hospital [82]. In that study, an 88% survival rate was achieved using only alimentation with a premium cat food. Differences in patient population (14% of cats had a normal total bilirubin concentration, only 30% had an identified concurrent illness, and 28% lacked an identifiable underlying problem causing anorexia [they were considered to have idiopathic FHL]). In the present referenced population, only 1.4% of 157 cats had a normal bilirubin concentration, 91% had an identified underlying illness, and only 1.3% were considered idiopathic. It is

Box 2. Supplements routinely used

Vitamin K: administer 0.5–1.5 mg/kg at 12-hour intervals
   parenterally (not intravenously and not orally) for two to three
   doses.
Vitamin E: administer 10 IU/ kg orally each day until convinced of
   recovery.
Water-soluble vitamins: 1–2 mL B-soluble vitamins/L crystalloid
   fluids; keep supplemented fluids covered from light exposure.
Thiamine: administer 100 mg orally and via B-soluble vitamins
   (see Table 2) in crystalloid fluids. Avoid subcutaneous or
   intramuscular injection, which may cause collapse (rare).
Vitamin B_{12}–cobalamin: administer 500–1000 µg (0.5–1.0 mg)
   total dose parenterally (intramuscularly or subcutaneously) in
   cats with suspected enteric disease as the underlying problem
   causing FHL catabolism (eg, severe inflammatory bowel
   disease or malabsorption because of infiltrative bowel disease,
   such as lymphoma). Affected cats often require chronic weekly
   or biweekly parenteral treatment (intramuscularly or
   subcutaneously). The frequency of dose administration is
   determined based on sequential plasma vitamin B_{12}
   concentrations. Consider that injectable vitamin B_{12} may not be
   activated without adequate GSH and vitamin E.
L-CN: administer 250 mg/d orally to promote fatty acid oxidation,
   urinary excretion of CN-FA esters in urine, and retention of lean
   body mass as well as for several other theoretic concerns.
Anticipate GSH insufficiency: consider use of a thiol donor to
   improve GSH substrate availability.
      Acute "crisis" thiol substrate: administer intravenously.
      NAC: administer 140 mg/kg intravenously and then 70 mg/kg
         intravenously at 8- to 12-hour intervals; give over 20
         minutes (not as a slow constant rate infusion) to guard
         against glutamine toxicity (see text). Dilute 10% NAC 1:4,
         and administer through a 0.2-µm nonpyrogenic filter.
      Chronic thiol substrate: administer orally.
      SAMe (Denosyl-SD4; Nutramax Laboratories, Edgewood,
         MD): administer 30–60 mg/kg orally once to twice daily
         when given with food using product pharmacologically
         proven to provide bioavailable SAMe. A high dose is
         recommended because of impaired bioavailability when
         given in the presence of food. SAMe replaces NAC therapy
         once an enteric route for dosing and feeding is established.

likely that the population scrutinized in the author's hospital and serving as the basis for current treatment recommendations had more severe hepatic TG accumulation and liver dysfunction typical of severe FHL. For important considerations, see Box 1, and for general treatment recommendations, see Box 2.

Summary

We have come a long way in understanding and managing the FHL syndrome since it was first described nearly 30 years ago. Increased sensitivity of clinicians for recognizing the syndrome has improved case outcome by arresting this metabolic syndrome in its earliest stages. Simply ensuring adequate intake of a complete and balanced feline diet can rescue cats just developing clinical signs; however, full metabolic support as described herein provides the best chance for recovery of cats demonstrating the most severe clinicopathologic features. It remains possible that adjustments in recommended micronutrient and vitamin intake for healthy cats may pivotally change feline susceptibility to FHL over the coming years.

References

[1] Szabo J, Ibrahim WH, Sunvold GD, et al. Effect of dietary protein quality and essential fatty acids on fatty acid composition in the liver and adipose tissue after rapid weight loss in overweight cats. Am J Vet Res 2003;64:310–5.

[2] Zoran DL. The carnivore connection to nutrition in cats. J Am Vet Med Assoc 2002;221: 1559–67.

[3] Biourge VC, Massat B, Groff JM, et al. Effects of protein, lipid, or carbohydrate supplementation on hepatic lipid accumulation during rapid weight loss in obese cats. Am J Vet Res 1994;55:1406–15.

[4] Ibrahim WH, Bailey N, Sunvold GD, et al. Effects of carnitine and taurine on fatty acid metabolism and lipid accumulation in the liver of cats during weight gain and weight loss. Am J Vet Res 2003;64:1265–77.

[5] Butterwick RF, Markwell PJ. Changes in the body composition of cats during weight reduction by controlled dietary energy restriction. Vet Rec 1996;138:354–7.

[6] Biourge V, Groff JM, Fisher C, et al. Nitrogen balance, plasma free amino acid concentrations and urinary orotic acid excretion during long-term fasting in cats. J Nutr 1994;124: 1094–103.

[7] Center SA, Thompson M, Wood P, et al. Hepatic ultrastructural and metabolic derangements in cats with severe hepatic lipidosis. In: Proceedings of the Ninth American College of Veterinary Internal Medicine Forum. New Orleans: American College of Veterinary Internal Medicine; 1991. p. 193–6.

[8] Center SA, Warner KL, Erb HN. Liver glutathione concentrations in dogs and cats with naturally occurring liver disease. Am J Vet Res 2002;63:1187–97.

[9] Pazak HE, Bartges JW, Cornelius LC, et al. Characterization of serum lipoprotein profiles of healthy, adult cats and idiopathic feline hepatic lipidosis patients. J Nutr 1998;128(Suppl): 2747S–50S.

[10] Blanchard G, Paragon BM, Milliat F, et al. Dietary L-carnitine supplementation in obese cats alters carnitine metabolism and decreases ketosis during fasting and induced hepatic lipidosis. J Nutr 2002;132:204–10.

[11] Jacobs G, Cornelius L, Keene B, et al. Comparison of plasma, liver, and skeletal muscle carnitine concentrations in cats with idiopathic hepatic lipidosis and in healthy cats. Am J Vet Res 1990;51:1349–51.

[12] Hall JA, Barstad LA, Connor WE. Lipid composition of hepatic and adipose tissues from normal cats and from cats with idiopathic hepatic lipidosis. J Vet Intern Med 1997;11: 238–42.

[13] Center SA, Guida L, Zanelli MJ, et al. Ultrastructural hepatocellular features associated with severe hepatic lipidosis in cats. Am J Vet Res 1993;54:724–31.

[14] Center SA. Metabolic, antioxidant, nutraceutical, probiotic, and herbal therapies relating to the management of hepatobiliary disorders. Vet Clin N Am Small Anim Pract 2004;34: 67–172.

[15] Domenicali M, Caraceni P, Vendemiale G, et al. Food deprivation exacerbates mito-chondrial oxidative stress in rat liver exposed to ischemia-reperfusion injury. J Nutr 2001; 131:105–10.

[16] Vendemiale G, Grattagliano I, Caraceni P, et al. Mitochondrial oxidative injury and energy metabolism alteration in rat fatty liver: effect of the nutritional status. Hepatology 2001;33: 808–15.

[17] Center SA, Crawford MA, Guida L, et al. A retrospective study of 77 cats with severe hepatic lipidosis. 1975–1990. J Vet Intern Med 1993;7:349–59.

[18] Christopher MM. Relation of endogenous Heinz bodies to disease and anemia in cats: 120 cases (1978–1987). J Am Vet Med Assoc 1989;194:1089–95.

[19] Center SA, Baldwin BH, Dillingham S, et al. Diagnostic value of serum gamma-glutamyl transferase and alkaline phosphatase activities in hepatobiliary disease in the cat. J Am Vet Med Assoc 1986;188:507–10.

[20] Center SA, Warner K, Corbett J, et al. Proteins invoked by vitamin K absence and clotting times in clinically ill cats. J Vet Intern Med 2000;14:292–7.

[21] Center SA, Thompson M, Guida L. 3 alpha-hydroxylated bile acid profiles in clinically normal cats, cats with severe hepatic lipidosis, and cats with complete extrahepatic bile duct occlusion. Am J Vet Res 1993;54:681–8.

[22] Simpson KW, Fyfe J, Cornetta A, et al. Subnormal concentrations of serum cobalamin (vitamin B_{12}) in cats with gastrointestinal disease. J Vet Intern Med 2001;15:26–32.

[23] Elin RJ, Winter WE. Methylmalonic acid: a test whose time has come? Arch Pathol Lab Med 2001;125:824–7.

[24] Swift NC, Marks SL, MacLachlan NJ, et al. Evaluation of serum feline trypsin-like immunoreactivity for the diagnosis of pancreatitis in cats. J Am Vet Med Assoc 2000;217: 37–42.

[25] Saunders HM, Van Winkle TJ, Drobatz K, et al. Ultrasonographic findings in cats with clinical, gross pathologic, and histologic evidence of acute pancreatic necrosis: 20 cases (1994–2001). J Am Vet Med Assoc 2002;221:1724–30.

[26] Cole TL, Center SA, Flood SN, et al. Diagnostic comparison of needle and wedge biopsy specimens of the liver in dogs and cats. J Am Vet Med Assoc 2002;220(10):1483–90.

[27] Adams LG, Hardy RM, Weiss DJ, et al. Hypophosphatemia and hemolytic anemia associated with diabetes mellitus and hepatic lipidosis in cats. J Vet Intern Med 1993;7: 266–71.

[28] Frank G, Anderson W, Pazak H, et al. Use of a high-protein diet in the management of feline diabetes mellitus. Vet Ther 2001;2:238–46.

[29] Mazzaferro EM, Greco DS, Turner AS, et al. Treatment of feline diabetes mellitus using an alpha-glucosidase inhibitor and a low-carbohydrate diet. J Feline Med Surg 2003;5: 183–9.

[30] Center SA, Elston TH, Rowland PH, et al. Fulminant hepatic failure associated with oral administration of diazepam in 11 cats. J Am Vet Med Assoc 1996;209:618–25.

[31] Wolf A, Weir P, Segar P, et al. Impaired fatty acid oxidation in propofol infusion syndrome. Lancet 2001;357:606–7.

[32] Kang TM. Propofol infusion syndrome in critically ill patients. Ann Pharmacother 2002;36: 1453–6.

[33] Hoffman RS. Thiamine hydrochloride. In: Goldfrank L, editor. Goldfrank's toxicologic emergencies. 5th edition. New York: Prentice Hall; 1997. p. 825–6.

[34] Kapadia CR, Donaldon RM. Disorders of cobalamin (vitamin B_{12}) absorption and transport. Annu Rev Med 1985;36:93–110.

[35] Johnson KL, Lamport AI, Ballevre OP, et al. Effects of oral administration of metronidazole on small intestinal bacteria and nutrients of cats. Am J Vet Res 2000;61:1106–12.

[36] Doi T, Kawata T, Tandano N, et al. Effect of vitamin B_{12} deficiency on S-adenosylmethionine metabolism in rats. J Nutr Sci Vitaminol 1989;35:1–9.

[37] Glasgow AM, Chase HP. Effect of propionic acid on fatty acid oxidation and ureagenesis. Pediatr Res 1976;10:683–6.

[38] Walajtys-Rode, Coll KE, Williamson JR. Effects of branched chain α-ketoacids on the metabolism of isolated rat liver cells. Interactions with gluconeogenesis and urea synthesis. J Biol Chem 1979;254:11521–9.

[39] Martin-Requero A, Corkey BE, Cerdan S, et al. Interactions between alpha-ketoisovalerate metabolism and the pathways of gluconeogenesis and urea synthesis in isolated hepatocytes. J Biol Chem 1983;258:3673–8.

[40] Brass EP, Allen RH, Ruff LJ, et al. Effect of hydroxocobalamin [c-lactam] on propionate and carnitine metabolism in the rat. Biochem J 1990;266:809–15.

[41] Lavine JE. Vitamin E treatment of nonalcoholic steatohepatitis in children: a pilot study. J Pediatr 2000;136:734–8.

[42] Sokol RJ, Devereaux M, Khandwala RA. Effect of dietary lipid and vitamin E on mitochondrial lipid peroxidation and hepatic injury in the bile duct-ligated rat. J Lipid Res 1991;32:1349–57.

[43] Sokol RJ, McKim JM, Goff MC, et al. Vitamin E reduces oxidant injury to mitochondria and the hepatotoxicity of taurochenodeoxycholic acid in the rat. Gastroenterology 1998;114: 164–74.

[44] Weber P, Bendich A, Machlin LJ. Vitamin E and human health: rationale for determining recommended intake levels. Nutrition 1997;13:450–60.

[45] Alexander DW, McGuire SO, Cassity NA, et al. Fish oils lower rat plasma and hepatic, but not immune cell alpha-tocopherol concentration. J Nutr 1995;125:2640–9.

[46] McGuire SO, Alexander DW, Fritsche KL. Fish oil source differentially affects rat immune cell alpha-tocopherol concentration. J Nutr 1997;127:1388–94.

[47] Davit-Spraul A, Cosson C, Couturier CM, et al. Standard treatment of alpha-tocopherol in Alagille patients with severe cholestasis is insufficient. Pediatr Res 2001;49:232–6.

[48] Center SA, Harte J, Watrous D, et al. The clinical and metabolic effects of rapid weight loss in obese pet cats and the influence of supplemental oral L-carnitine. J Vet Intern Med 2000; 14:598–608.

[49] Center SA, Sunvold GD. Investigations of the effect of l-carnitine on weight reduction, body condition and metabolism in obese dogs and cats. In: Reinhart GA, Carey DP, editors. Recent advances in canine and feline nutritional research, vol. III. 2000 Iams Nutritional Symposium Proceedings. Wilmington, OH: Orange Frazier Press; 2000. p. 113–22.

[50] Center SA, Warner KL, Randolph JF, et al. Influence of l-carnitine on metabolic rate, fatty acid oxidation, body condition, and weight loss in obese cats [poster]. Presented at the World Small Animal Veterinary Congress. Vancouver, August 8–11, 2001.

[51] Millington DS, Dubay G. Dietary supplement l–carnitine: analysis of different brands to determine bioavailability and content. Clinical Research and Regulatory Affairs 1993;10: 71–80.

[52] Trainor D, Center SA, Randolph JF, et al. Urine sulfated and nonsulfated bile acids as a diagnostic test for liver disease in cats. J Vet Intern Med 2003;17:145–53.

[53] Kim SW, Rogers QR, Morris JG. Maillard reaction products in purified diets induce taurine depletion in cats which is reversed by antibiotics. J Nutr 1996;126:195–201.

[54] Backus RC, Morris JG, Kim SW, et al. Dietary taurine needs of cats vary with dietary protein quality and concentration. Vet Clin Nutr 1998;5:18–22.

[55] Meister A. On the biochemistry of glutathione. In: Taniguchi N, Higashi R, Sakamoto Y, et al, editors. Glutathione centennial. San Diego: Academic Press; 1989. p. 3–21.

[56] Fernandez-Checa J, Lu SC, Ookhtens M, et al. The regulation of hepatic glutathione. In: Tavoloni N, Berk PD, editors. Hepatic anion transport and bile secretion: physiology and pathophysiology. New York: Marcel Dekker; 1992. p. 363–95.

[57] Deleve LD, Kaplowitz N. Glutathione metabolism and its role in hepatotoxicity. Pharmacol Ther 1991;52:287–305.

[58] Grattagliano I, Vendemiale G, Caraceni P, et al. Starvation impairs antioxidant defense in fatty livers of rats fed a choline-deficient diet. J Nutr 2000;130:2131–6.

[59] Becker K, Leichsenring M, Gana L, et al. Glutathione and associated antioxidant systems in protein energy malnutrition: results of a study in Nigeria. Free Radic Biol Med 1995;18: 257–63.

[60] Lenhartz H, Ndasi R, Anninos A, et al. The clinical manifestations of the kwashiorkor syndrome are related to increased lipid peroxidation. J Pediatr 1998;132:879–81.

[61] Fechner A, Bohme CC, Gromer S, et al. Antioxidant status and nitric oxide in the malnutrition syndrome kwashiorkor. Pediatr Res 2001;49:237–73.

[62] Treacy E, Arbour L, Chessex P, et al. Glutathione deficiency as a complication of methylmalonic acidemia: response to high doses of ascorbate. J Pediatr 1996;129:445–8.

[63] Nakano H, Nagasaki K, Yoshida K, et al. N-acetylcysteine and anti-lCAM-1 monoclonal antibody reduce ischemia-reperfusion injury of the steatotic rat liver. Transplant Proc 1998; 30:3763.

[64] Nakano H, Yamaguchi M, Kaneshiro Y, et al. S-adenosyl-L-methionine attenuates ischemia-reperfusion injury of steatotic livers. Transplant Proc 1998;30:3735–6.

[65] Droge W, Holm E. Role of cysteine and glutathione in HIV infection and other diseases associated with muscle wasting and immunological dysfunction. FASEB J 1997;11:1077–89.

[66] Center SA, Warner K, Hoffman WE. Influence of SAMe on erythrocytes and liver tissue in healthy cats [abstract]. J Vet Intern Med 2000;14, in press.

[67] Fettmann MJ, Valerius KD, Ogilvie GK, et al. Effects of dietary cysteine on blood sulfur amino acid, glutathione, and malondialdehyde concentrations in cats. Am J Vet Res 1999;60: 328–33.

[68] Lin Y, Havinga R, Verkade HJ, et al. Bile acids suppress the secretion of very-low-density lipoprotein by human hepatocytes in primary culture. Hepatology 1996;23:218–28.

[69] Lin Y, Havinga R, Schippers IJ, et al. Characterization of the inhibitory effects of bile acids on very-low-density lipoprotein secretion by rat hepatocytes in primary culture. Biochem J 1996;316(Part 2):531–8.

[70] Vajro P, Franzese A, Valerio G, et al. Lack of efficacy of ursodeoxycholic acid for the treatment of liver abnormalities in obese children. J Pediatr 2000;136:739–43.

[71] Okan A, Astarciouglu H, Tankurt E, et al. Effect of ursodeoxycholic acid on hepatic steatosis in rats. Dig Dis Sci 2002;47:2389–97.

[72] Laurin J, Lindor KD, Crippin JS, et al. Ursodeoxycholic acid or clofibrate in the treatment of non-alcohol-induced steatohepatitis: a pilot study. Hepatology 1996;23:1464–7.

[73] Kiyici M, Gulten M, Gurel S, et al. Ursodeoxycholic acid and atorvastatin in the treatment of nonalcoholic steatohepatitis. Can J Gastroenterol 2003;17:713–8.

[74] Lindor KD, Kowdley KV, Heathcote EJ, et al. Ursodeoxycholic acid for treatment of nonalcoholic steatohepatitis: results of a randomized trial. Hepatology 2004;39:770–8.

[75] Marinella MA, et al. The refeeding syndrome and hypophosphatemia. Nutr Rev 2003;61: 320–3.

[76] Harkin KR, Cowan LA, Andrews GA, et al. Hepatotoxicity of stanozolol in cats. J Am Vet Med Assoc 2000;217:681–4.

[77] Vore M, Liu Y, Huang L. Cholestatic properties and hepatic transport of steroid glucuronides. Drug Metab Rev 1997;29:183–203.

[78] Letteron P, Brahimi-Bourouina N, Robin MA, et al. Glucocorticoids inhibit mitochondrial matrix acyl-CoA dehydrogenases and fatty acid beta-oxidation. Am J Physiol 1997;272: G1141–50.

[79] Amacher DE, Martin BA. Tetracycline-induced steatosis in primary canine hepatocyte cultures. Fundam Appl Toxicol 1997;40:256–63.

[80] Cho Y-S, Kim M-J, Lee J-Y, et al. The role of thiols in protecting against simultaneous toxicity of menadione to platelet plasma and intracellular membranes. J Pharm Exp Ther 1997;280:1335–40.

[81] Chung S-M, Lee J-Y, Lee M-Y, et al. Adverse consequences of erythrocyte exposure to menadione: involvement of reactive oxygen species generation in plasma. J Toxicol Environ Health 2001;63:617–29.

[82] Kuehn NF. Nutritional management of feline hepatic lipidosis. In: Reinhart GA, Carey DP, editors. Recent advances in canine and feline nutrition, vol. III. 2000 Iams Nutrition Symposium Proceedings. Wilmington, OH: Orange Frazier Press; 2000. p. 333–8.

ELSEVIER
SAUNDERS

Vet Clin Small Anim
35 (2005) 271–279

VETERINARY
CLINICS
Small Animal Practice

Index

Note: Page numbers of article titles are in **boldface** type.

A

Abdomen
  feline infectious peritonitis effects on, 48–49

Acid(s)
  urine bile
    in feline hepatic lipidosis, 236

Acromegaly
  feline, 181–187
    clinical signs of, 181–185
    diagnosis of, 185–186
    pathogenesis of, 181
    prognosis of, 187
    treatment of, 186–187

α-Adrenoceptor agonists
  for pain in feline patients, 140

β-Adrenoceptor blocking agents
  for feline hyperthyroidism, 176

Amino acid(s)
  in feline hepatic lipidosis, 254–255

Amitriptyline
  for interstitial/idiopathic cystitis, 158–159

Ammonia testing
  in feline hepatic lipidosis, 237

Analgesic(s)
  for pain in feline patients, 131–137

Anesthesia/anesthetics
  for esophagostomy/endoscopic
    gastrostomy tube placement
    in feline hepatic lipidosis, 246
  local
    for pain in feline patients, 139–140

Antibody(ies)
  in blood
    in feline infectious peritonitis
      diagnosis, 56–57
  in CSF
    in feline infectious peritonitis
      diagnosis, 58

  in effusion
    in feline infectious peritonitis
      diagnosis, 57–58
  in feline infectious peritonitis
    diagnosis, 55–58

Antibody antigen complex detection
  in feline infectious peritonitis
    diagnosis, 59

Antidepressant(s)
  tricyclic
    for pain in feline patients, 141

Antigen(s)
  detection of
    in feline infectious peritonitis, 59–61
  in tissue
    in feline infectious peritonitis, 60–61

Anti-inflammatory drugs
  nonsteroidal (NSAIDs)
    for pain in feline patients, 137–139

Antithyroid therapy
  trial course of
    in feline hyperthyroidism, 175

Antiviral chemotherapy
  for feline infectious peritonitis, 63–65

Appetite stimulants
  for feline hepatic lipidosis, 249–250
    avoidance of, 260

B

Bacteria
  zoonoses due to
    control of, 12–14

Bile acids
  urine
    in feline hepatic lipidosis, 236

Blood
  antibodies in

Changing Your Address?

Make sure your subscription changes too! When you notify us of your new address, you can help make our job easier by including an exact copy of your Clinics label number with your old address (see illustration below.) This number identifies you to our computer system and will speed the processing of your address change. Please be sure this label number accompanies your old address and your corrected address—you can send an old Clinics label with your number on it or just copy it exactly and send it to the address listed below.

We appreciate your help in our attempt to give you continuous coverage. Thank you.

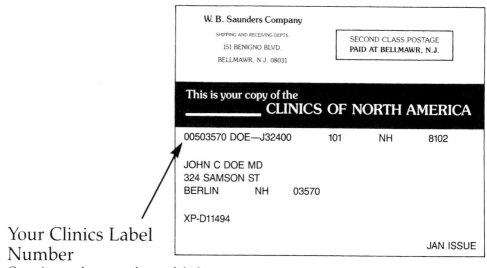

W. B. Saunders Company

SHIPPING AND RECEIVING DEPTS.

151 BENIGNO BLVD.

BELLMAWR, N.J. 08031

SECOND CLASS POSTAGE
PAID AT BELLMAWR, N.J.

This is your copy of the
CLINICS OF NORTH AMERICA

00503570 DOE—J32400   101   NH   8102

JOHN C DOE MD
324 SAMSON ST
BERLIN   NH   03570

XP-D11494

JAN ISSUE

Your Clinics Label Number

Copy it exactly or send your label
along with your address to:
W.B. Saunders Company, Customer Service
Orlando, FL 32887-4800
Call Toll Free 1-800-654-2452

Please allow four to six weeks for delivery of new subscriptions and for processing address changes.